CARDIAC AND RENAL FAILURE:
AN EXPANDING ROLE
FOR ACE INHIBITORS

MEDAC
Medical Advisory Council
1988

Series Editor: LOUIS M. SHERWOOD, M.D., F.A.C.P.

Senior Vice President
Medical & Scientific Affairs
Merck Sharp & Dohme International
Rahway, New Jersey, U.S.A.

ABOUT THE EDITORS

Prof. Sir Colin T. Dollery, M.B., Ch.B., F.R.C.P.

Dr. Dollery received his medical education at the Birmingham University Medical School, Birmingham, England. Knighted by the Queen in 1987, he is currently Professor of Medicine at the Royal Postgraduate Medical School and Chairman of the Department of Medicine at Hammersmith Hospital in London. His initial appointment as Professor of Clinical Pharmacology at the Royal Postgraduate Medical School was in 1969, and he ran the program until 1987 when he became Chairman of Medicine. Internationally known in cardiopulmonary disease and clinical pharmacology, he has also served as President of the European Society for Clinical Investigation. Dr. Dollery has been a MEDAC member since its inception in 1973.

Louis M. Sherwood, M.D., F.A.C.P.

Dr. Sherwood received his medical education at the Columbia College of Physicians and Surgeons in New York and is presently Executive Vice President, Worldwide Development, Merck Sharp & Dohme Research Laboratories. He was formerly Professor of Medicine at the University of Chicago and Chairman of the Department of Medicine at Michael Reese Medical Center (1972–80) and Baumritter Professor of Medicine and Biochemistry, and Chairman of the Department of Medicine at the Albert Einstein College of Medicine and Physician-in-Chief at Montefiore Medical Center (1980–87). Internationally known in endocrinology and calcium metabolism, he has also served as President of the American Society for Clinical Investigation.

Cardiac and Renal Failure: An Expanding Role for ACE Inhibitors

Merck Sharp & Dohme International
Medical Advisory Council
Kronberg im Taunus, Federal Republic of Germany

October 17 and 18, 1988

Editors

Colin T. Dollery, M.B., Ch.B.
Louis M. Sherwood, M.D., F.A.C.P.

Hanley & Belfus, Inc.   Philadelphia

Library of Congress Cataloging-in-Publication Data

Main entry under title:

Cardiac and renal failure: an expanding role for ACE inhibitors.

"Merck Sharp & Dohme International Medical Advisory Council, Kronberg im Taunus, FDR, October 17 and 18, 1988.
Includes bibliographies and index.
1. Angiotensin converting enzyme—Inhibitors—Therapeutic use—Congresses.   2. Heart failure—Chemotherapy—Congresses.
3. Kidneys—Diseases—Chemotherapy—Congresses.
I. Dollery, Colin T.   II. Sherwood, Louis M.   III. Medical Advisory Council (Merck, Sharp & Dohme International)   IV. Series: Medical Advisory Council (Series): 1988.

RC684.A53C37   1989   616.1'29061—dc20   89-15425

ISBN 0-932883-99-0

Published by Hanley & Belfus, Inc., 210 South 13th Street, Philadelphia, Pennsylvania 19107, USA

Contents

v

Contributors and Participants

DR. FRANCOIS ALHENC-GELAS
*Institut National de la Santé et de la Recherche Médicale,
Hôpital Lariboisière, Paris, France*

DR. JACQUELINE ALLEGRINI
*Institut National de la Santé et de la Recherche Médicale,
Hôpital Lariboisière, Paris, France*

PIERRO ANVERSA, M.D.
*Department of Pathology
New York Medical College
Valhalla, New York, U.S.A.*

DR. DIANE DE LA BASTIE
*Institut National de la Santé et de la Recherche Médicale,
Hôpital Lariboisière, Paris, France*

SIR RICHARD BAYLISS,
K.C.V.O., M.D., F.R.C.P.
*Honorary Consultant Physician and Endocrinologist
Westminster Hospital
London, England, U.K.*

ALEXANDER G. BEARN, M.D.,
F.R.C.P., F.A.C.P.
*Professor of Medicine
Cornell University Medical College
Professor (Adjunct Faculty)
The Rockefeller University
New York, New York, U.S.A.*

HANS R. BRUNNER, M.D.
*Associate Professor of Medicine
Head, Hypertension Division
Centre Hospitalier Universitaire
Lausanne, Switzerland*

DR. CRAMER K. CHRISTENSEN
*Medical Department M,
Second University Clinic of Internal Medicine,
Kommunehospitalet, Aarhus C, Denmark*

DR. JENS SANDAHL CHRISTIANSEN
*Medical Department M,
Second University Clinic of Internal Medicine,
Kommunehospitalet, Aarhus, Denmark*

JAY N. COHN, M.D.
*Head, Cardiovascular Division
Professor of Medicine
University of Minnesota Medical School
Minneapolis, Minnesota, U.S.A.*

PIERRE CORVOL, M.D.
*Director
Vascular Pathology and Renal Endocrinology Unit
Institut National de la Santé et de la Recherche Medicale
Paris, France*

PAUL E. DeJONG, M.D.
*Associate Professor in Nephrology
State University Hospital
Groningen, The Netherlands*

PROF. SIR COLIN T. DOLLERY,
M.B., Ch.B., F.R.C.P.
*Director
Department of Medicine
Royal Postgraduate Medical School
Hammersmith Hospital
London, England, U.K.*

CALVIN ENG, M.D.
Department of Medicine
Albert Einstein College of Medicine
Bronx, New York, U.S.A.

STEPHEN M. FACTOR, M.D.
Department of Medicine
Albert Einstein College of Medicine
Bronx, New York, U.S.A.

DETLEV GANTEN, M.D., Ph.D.
Professor, Department of
  Pharmacology
University of Heidelberg
Scientific Director, German Institute
  for High Blood Pressure Research
Heidelberg, Federal Republic of
  Germany

DR. KLAVS WÜRGLER HANSEN
Medical Department M,
Second University Clinic of Internal
  Medicine,
Kommunehospitalet, Aarhus C,
  Denmark

JAN E. HEEG, M.D.
Department of Medicine,
Division of Nephrology,
State University Hospital,
Groningen, The Netherlands

DR. CHRISTINE HUBERT
Institut National de la Santé et de la
  Recherche Médicale,
Hôpital Lariboisière, Paris, France

PAUL G. HUGENHOLTZ, M.D.,
  F.E.S.C., F.A.C.C.
Professor of Cardiology
President, Societe pour la Recherche
  Cardiologique
Nyon, Switzerland

HIROO IMURA, M.D.
Professor and Chairman
Second Division
Department of Medicine
Kyoto University
School of Medicine
Kyoto, Japan

JOHN D. IRVIN, M.D., Ph.D.
Group Director, Clinical Research—
  Cardiovascular, Renal,
  Endocrinology, and Metabolic
Merck Sharp & Dohme Research
  Laboratories
Blue Bell, Pennsylvania, U.S.A.

COLIN I. JOHNSTON, M.B., B.S.,
  F.R.A.C.P.
Professor of Medicine
University of Melbourne
Chairman, Division of Medicine
Austin Hospital
Heidelberg, Victoria, Australia

BERTRAM L. KASISKE, M.D.
Division of Nephrology
Department of Medicine
Hennepin County Medical Center
University of Minnesota Medical
  School
Minneapolis, Minnesota, U.S.A.

WILLIAM F. KEANE, M.D.
Professor of Medicine and Pharmacy
Department of Medicine
Division of Nephrology
Hennepin County Medical Center
University of Minnesota Medical
  School
Minneapolis, Minnesota, U.S.A.

JOHN KJEKSHUS, M.D.
Senior Consultant of Cardiology
Department of Medicine
Baerum Hospital
Oslo, Norway

MICHAEL J. S. LANGMAN, M.D.,
F.R.C.P.
Professor of Internal Medicine
University of Birmingham
Queen Elizabeth Medical Centre
Birmingham, England, U.K.

JOHN G. G. LEDINGHAM, M.D.,
F.R.C.P.
May Reader in Medicine
University of Oxford
Honorary Consultant Physician
Oxford Area Health Authority
Oxford, England, U.K.

THIERRY LE JEMTEL, M.D.
Departments of Medicine and
Pathology
Albert Einstein College of Medicine
Bronx, New York, U.S.A.

JOHN LENNANE, M.B.,
F.R.A.C.P., M.D.
Managing Director,
SOCAR S.A.,
Nyon, Switzerland

KLAUS LINDPAINTNER, M.D.
German Institute for High Blood
Pressure Research and Department
of Pharmacology,
University of Heidelberg,
Heidelberg, Federal Republic of
Germany

ANNE-MARIE LOMPRE, Ph.D.
Institut National de la Santé et de la
Recherche Médicale,
Hôpital Lariboisière,
Paris, France

JACOBUS LUBSEN, M.P.H., M.D.
Professor of the Theory of Clinical
Practice,
Erasmus University,
Rotterdam, The Netherlands

RUEDI P. LÜTHY, M.D.
Professor of Medicine
Chief, Division of Infectious Diseases
Department of Medicine
University Hospital
Zurich, Switzerland

ERROL S. McKINNEY
Executive Director
Marketing Planning
Merck Sharp & Dohme International
Rahway, New Jersey, U.S.A.

JEAN-JACQUES MERCADIER,
Ph.D., M.D.
Institut National de la Santé et de la
Recherche Médicale,
Hôpital Lariboisière,
Paris, France

KALMAN C. MEZEY, M.D.
Clinical Professor of Medicine
University of Medicine & Dentistry
of New Jersey
Newark, New Jersey, U.S.A.

ALBERT MIMRAN, M.D., Ph.D.
Professor of Internal Medicine
University Hospital Lapeyronie
Montpellier, France

CARL ERIK MOGENSEN, M.D.
Professor of Medicine
Second University Clinic of Internal
Medicine
Department M
Aarhus Kommunehospital
Aarhus, Denmark

TREFOR O. MORGAN, M.D.
Professor, Department of Physiology
Faculty of Medicine
University of Melbourne
Parkville, Victoria, Australia

GEORGES MOURAD, M.D.
Department of Medicine,
Centre Hospitalier Universitaire,
Hopital Lapeyronie,
Montpellier, France

DR. JOHN MULLINS
German Institute for High Blood
* Pressure Research and Department*
* of Pharmacology,*
University of Heidelberg,
Heidelberg, Federal Republic of
* Germany*

KAZUWA NAKAO, M.D.
Second Division, Department of
* Medicine,*
Kyoto University Faculty of Medicine,
Kyoto, Japan

GERJAN NAVIS, M.D.
Department of Medicine,
Division of Nephrology,
State University Hospital,
Groningen, The Netherlands

S. RAGNAR NORRBY, M.D., Ph.D.
Professor and Chairman
Department of Infectious Diseases
University of Umea
Umea University Hospital
Umea, Sweden

J. DEREK K. NORTH, M.D., D.Phil.
Dean and Professor of Medicine
School of Medicine
University of Auckland
Auckland, New Zealand

DR. J. NUSSBERGER
Cardiovascular Research Group and
* Hypertension Division,*
University Hospital,
Sausanne, Switzerland

MICHAEL P. O'DONNELL, M.D.
Division of Nephrology
Department of Medicine
Hennepin County Medical Center
University of Minnesota Medical
* School*
Minneapolis, Minnesota, U.S.A.

CARLO PATRONO, M.D.
Professor of Molecular Pharmacology
Catholic University School of
* Medicine*
Rome, Italy

DR. MARGRETHE MAU
  PEDERSEN
Medical Department M,
Second University Clinic of Internal
* Medicine,*
Kommunehospitalet, DK-8000
* Aarhus C, Denmark*

DAVID KEITH PETERS, M.B.,
  F.R.C.P.
Regius Professor of Physic
University of Cambridge School of
* Clinical Medicine*
Addenbrooke's Hospital
Cambridge, England, U.K.

ALESSANDRO PIERUCCI, M.D.
Catholic University School of
* Medicine*
Rome, Italy

PHILIP A. POOLE-WILSON, M.D.,
  F.R.C.P.
Professor of Cardiology
Cardiothoracic Institute and National
* Heart Hospital*
London, England, U.K.

JEAN RIBSTEIN, M.D.
Department of Medicine,
Centre Hospitalier Universitaire,
Hopital Lapeyronie,
Montpellier, France

HEONIR ROCHA, M.D.
Dean and Professor of Medicine
Faculty of Medicine
Medical School of the Federal
  University of Bahia
Bahia, Brazil

JANET E. RUSH, M.D.
Director,
Clinical Research-Cardiovascular,
Merck Sharp & Dohme Research,
West Point, Pennsylvania, U.S.A.

DR. ANITA SCHMITZ
Medical Department M,
Second University Clinic of Internal
  Medicine,
Kommunehospitalet, Aarhus C,
Denmark

KETTY SCHWARTZ, Ph.D.
Director of Research CNRS
Institut National de la Santé et de la
  Recherche Medicale
Unit 127
Hôpital Lariboisiere
Paris, France

EDWARD M. SCOLNICK, M.D.
President
Merck Sharp & Dohme Research
  Laboratories
Rahway, New Jersey, U.S.A.

LOUIS M. SHERWOOD, M.D.,
  F.A.C.P.
Senior Vice President
Medical & Scientific Affairs
Merck Sharp & Dohme International
Rahway, New Jersey, U.S.A.

YUICHI SHIOKAWA, M.D.
President, Japan Rheumatism
  Foundation
Chairman of the Board of Directors,
  Japan Inflammation Society
Professor Emeritus, Juntendo
  University
Tokyo, Japan

RONALD D. SMITH, M.D.,
  F.A.C.P.
Director, Clinical Research—Renal
Merck Sharp and Dohme Research
  Laboratories
Blue Bell, Pennsylvania, U.S.A.
Clinical Associate Professor of
  Medicine
Temple University Medical School
Philadelphia, Pennsylvania, U.S.A.

THOMAS W. SMITH, M.D.
Professor of Medicine
Harvard Medical School
Chief, Cardiovascular Division
Brigham and Women's Hospital
Boston, Massachusetts, U.S.A.

EDMOND SONNENBLICK, M.D.
Olson Professor of Medicine
Chief, Division of Cardiology
Albert Einstein College of Medicine
Bronx, New York, U.S.A.

DR. FLORENT SOUBRIER
Institut National de la Santé et de la
  Recherche Médicale,
Hôpital Lariboisière, Paris, France

KARL SWEDBERG, M.D.
Ostra Sjukhuset
Goteborg, Sweden

CHARLES S. SWEET, Ph.D.
Senior Scientist
Department of Pharmacology
Merck Sharp & Dohme Research
  Laboratories
West Point, Pennsylvania, U.S.A.

DR. LEIF THUESEN
Medical Department M,
Second University Clinic of Internal
  Medicine,
Kommunehospitalet, Aarhus C,
Denmark

KLAUS THURAU, M.D.
Professor of Physiology and Chairman
Department of Physiology
August Lenz Foundation
University of Munich
Munich, Federal Republic of Germany

JAN G.P. TIJSSEN, Ph.D.
Centre for Clinical Decision Analysis
 and Department of Cardiology
 (Thoraxcentrum),
Erasmus University and Academic
 Hospital,
Rotterdam, The Netherlands

DR. TH. UNGER
German Institute for High Blood
 Pressure Research and Department
 of Pharmacology,
University of Heidelberg,
Heidelberg, Federal Republic of
 Germany

DR. B. WAEBER
Cardiovascular Research Group and
 Hypertension Division
University Hospital, Lausanne,
 Switzerland

PETER-CLAUS WEBER, M.D.
Professor and Director
Institute for Prophylaxis and
 Epidemiology of Coronary Heart
 Disease
Head, August Lenz Foundation
University of Munich
Munich, Federal Republic of Germany

DICK DE ZEEUW, M.D.
Department of Medicine,
Division of Nephrology,
State University Hospital,
Groningen, The Netherlands

Foreword

This volume on the expanding role of ACE inhibitors focuses primarily on two important clinical applications of these anti-renin system drugs. It is particularly timely to take stock of these applications and related issues ten years after the introduction of this class of drugs into clinical practice. The experience to date involves largely captopril and enalapril, with many other analogs to follow. To date, it appears that all ACE inhibitors act similarly; however, important differences are related to bioavailability, distribution, pharmacokinetics, and side effects.

Captopril and enalapril have important differences that could become significant as more data accumulate. Captopril acts more rapidly orally and has a sulfhydryl grouping which, among other things, may produce penicillamine-like side effects. On the other hand, enalapril is sulfhydryl-free, has a much greater affinity for the converting enzyme, and has a longer half-life.

The explosive growth in the use of these drugs to treat patients has probably never been matched. As I write, both captopril and enalapril have passed one billion dollars in annual sales and look to be headed much higher. They are the first billion dollar cardiovascular drugs. This is a far cry from the consensus view of the potential for this type of therapy in 1975. At that time I presented results to Squibb on the striking anti-renin–related antihypertensive actions of teprotide, the first converting enzyme inhibitor, which had to be given intravenously. Most scientists did not share our views on either the central importance of the renin system for blood pressure control, on the pathogenesis of hypertension, or on the efficacy of teprotide. There was little support for further pursuit, and other major pharmaceutical companies rejected an opportunity to share in the project. However, two scientists who shared our view proceeded without sanction to design captopril, the first orally active analog of teprotide.

Because of their dramatic actions to dilate arterioles and lower blood pressure, and thereby to relieve the failing heart as well, this class of drugs has generated a huge volume of clinical and basic research, resulting in exciting new knowledge about the drugs themselves. New questions have been raised about the mechanisms of hypertensive disorders and congestive heart failure. This, in turn, has raised new issues, many of which are probingly discussed in these pages.

From the beginning, a most important research question has been whether any important component of ACE inhibitor action can be ascribed to mechanisms unrelated to inhibition of the circulating renal renin system. When some groups reported high bradykinin levels in patients treated with ACE inhibitors, some of their depressor action was attributed to the persistence of bradykinin through inhibition of converting enzyme. Such claims have not been retracted even though numerous studies, using proper methods, have shown no bradykinemia in ACE inhibitor treated patients. More important, bradykinin skin wheals are only rarely and transiently observed after the first dose, and there is no tachycardia, an almost universal effect of bradykinin infusion. Furthermore, after billions of doses worldwide, no treated patient has reported a bradykinin-type reaction to a bee sting or to other trauma including major surgery. Accordingly, bradykinin accumulation is unimportant for the antihypertensive action, except perhaps in very special, as yet undefined, circumstances.

Another more persistent minority viewpoint on ACE inhibitor action questions whether blockade of the circulating renin system can account for the effect on blood pressure. This viewpoint postulates a functioning, intrinsic vascular tissue-renin system as an important factor in circulatory homeostasis. The fact that various components of the renin system (converting enzyme, renin substrate, angiotensin II) are found in many tissues, including vascular tissues, has been used to support this concept. However, the crucial evidence, i.e., the demonstration of significant amounts of renin and/or of renin mRNA in vascular tissues, is still lacking. This could, in fact, be studied readily with the modern techniques of molecular biology. It has not been difficult to demonstrate renin gene expression and large amounts of prorenin or renin in other tissues such as the ovaries, adrenals, placenta, and uterus.

Actually, if the circulating renin system functions like other endocrines, circulating renal renin is very likely taken up by vascular tissues, as the Skeggs and Swales groups have demonstrated, just as insulin is taken up by muscles. This most likely explains many of the observations made by proponents of vascular renin and obviates the need to postulate a separate vascular tissue system operating in concert, in opposition, or independently of the circulating endocrine mechanism. I believe that studies which claim local tissue formation of active renin require its demonstration 48 hours after bilateral nephrectomy. This has not been done.

Beyond the lack of direct evidence, other physiologic studies provide us with no evidence, or teleologic need for a separate vascular wall-renin system. Thus, in bilaterally nephrectomized humans or animals, plasma renin is always zero, and converting enzyme inhibitors and renin inhibitors are totally inactive against blood pressure. Moreover, salt loading (with a falling plasma renin) wipes out the antihypertensive action of ACE inhibitors in normal subjects and in congestive heart failure. In primary aldosteronism, where plasma renin is zero, ACE inhibitors also fail to lower pressure.

All of this fits with the clinical experience in hypertension which establishes that hypertensive patients with high plasma renin respond dramatically, whereas those with low values respond significantly but less well, to ACE inhibitors. The main situation, where plasma renin values are not strongly predictive of ACE inhibitor effectiveness, is in hypertensive patients with so-called "normal" plasma renin levels. In these patients, ACE inhibitors often reduce blood pressure. Let us consider why this is so:

Evidence indicates that *any* secretion of renin by the kidneys is abnormal in the face of a raised arterial pressure. Thus, the contralateral normal kidney of patients or animals with unilateral renovascular Goldblatt hypertension reduces its renin secretion to zero as it should. This implies that the failure to turn off renin secretion is a special characteristic of the kidney of the patient with essential hypertension. In fact, this can be demonstrated by either giving a saline infusion or feeding extra dietary sodium to hypertensive patients; they do not suppress their renin nearly as well as normal subjects do. We have postulated that this inappropriate persistence of renin secretion in essential hypertension is related to nephron heterogeneity. Inappropriate renin secretion arising from a subpopulation of ischemic hypofiltering nephrons acts on the neighboring normal nephrons to promote sodium retention and impair their compensatory adaptive hypernatriuresis. Hypertension is then sustained by an inappropriately "normal" (unsuppressed) plasma renin level in relation to the abnormal sodium-volume retention. ACE inhibitors can be expected to be effective here by deleting the adverse effects of the normal renin level on the adapting nephrons. This ACE blockade relaxes the arterioles, and, by also removing ANG II's direct effect on tubular sodium reabsorption, enables a diuresis which, in turn, offsets further the pressor action of any residual renin activity.

There are still other new areas of knowledge about the renin system that have blossomed in the past ten years that may help the reader to analyze, understand, and enjoy the material in this volume. One that attracts me is the demonstration of a potent action of ANG II on the proximal tubules to promote sodium bicarbonate reabsorption. This local sodium retaining action, added to that occurring via aldosterone, very likely causes subtle but significant sodium retention in those hypertensive patients who exhibit inappropriately "normal" plasma renin levels. (Remember, in hypertension renal renin secretion should be zero.) Very likely there may prove to be an intrarenal renin system also, coordinating intrarenal phenomena with the goals of the simultaneously operating circulating renin system. Here, too, prorenin might be a key player, as it seems to be in the other separated and protected tissue renin systems, such as that in the ovary.

Another intriguing finding is the fact that angiotensin II receptors have been demonstrated in many nonvascular tissues. The possibilities for a range of nonvascular angiotensin actions have to be taken seriously. This could involve such diverse things as brain function (e.g., mentation, mood) and intestinal fluid absorption. Alternatively, many of these receptors could be processing or clearance receptors of the type recently described by Maack for the atrial natriuretic hormone.

I do not feel qualified to comment specifically on all of the papers in this symposium. Actually, an excellent job was done on this in the published question and answer periods and the panel discussions. However, I would perhaps make a few comments.

The fine work by Pierre Corvol and his colleagues suggesting two catalytic sites for angiotensin converting enzyme raises again the possibility of more than one catalytic function for converting enzyme — a finding in keeping with its broad distribution beyond the vascular system. I particularly enjoyed the paper by Hans Brunner and colleagues, because, using a sensitive assay for plasma angiotensin II, this study demonstrates that a reduction in *circulating* ANG II is a consistent and commensurate prerequisite for any blood pressure reduction observed after converting enzyme treatment. Once again this puts into focus the importance of the circulating renin system in cardiovascular homeostasis. I share Detlev Ganten's hopes for the potentials of transgenic mice transfected with the human renin gene. But, I do not share his enthusiasm for brain renin. It is very clear that there is angiotensin II in brain tissue. How it gets there and what it does is not clear, although some of it could be bloodborne. However, the evidence for renin gene expression in the brain is also controversial. There could possibly be another tissue protease that hydrolyzes renin substrate to form angiotensin.

A series of papers in this volume provide an excellent review of the pathophysiology of congestive heart failure and of the beneficial effects of ACE inhibitors. Here too, most if not all of the benefits of ACE inhibitors seem to be the result of reducing plasma ANG II levels. The Consensus study convincingly showed that enalapril can prolong the duration and enhance the quality of life in these patients. This is a most important contribution of these drugs to patient care.

The paper by Keane and associates is of interest because it raises the possibility that lipid lowering agents may have a beneficial effect on the progressive renal injury occurring in Dahl-S salt-fed hypertensive animals. Mogenson and his group present their impressive body of data in diabetic patients with nephropathy. ACE inhibitors certainly improve proteinuria, presumably by reducing glomerular pressure. However, in his hands, there is as yet no indication that any particular antihypertensive drug is superior for preserving renal function provided arterial pressure and glomerular pressure are similarly reduced.

It is apparent that we need to learn more definitively what ACE inhibitor therapy does to the heart, brain, and kidneys, especially in disease, and whether the effects are unique or merely the result of the reduced blood pressure and improved blood flow. The data in this book are provocative and will suggest some good new experiments. Lou Sherwood is to be complimented for his choices of participants and the agenda.

John H. Laragh, M.D.
New York

Opening Remarks

The last two decades have witnessed major changes in our approach to acute and chronic cardiovascular disease. Barely three decades old, the coronary care unit has become a standard feature of university and community hospital alike, and the care of patients with acute cardiovascular disorders, both diagnostic and therapeutic, has undergone dramatic change. Invasive and noninvasive diagnostic testing and monitoring as well as invasive and pharmacologic intervention have grown in complexity and potency, with substantial benefit to the patient. Likewise, the management of chronic cardiovascular diseases, particularly hypertension, coronary artery disease, and cardiac and renal failure has been much more aggressive and successful.

We are in a new era in which the results of large, randomized, placebo-controlled multicenter clinical trials have documented the efficacy of new therapeutic approaches. We have had an opportunity to demonstrate improvement, not only in the quality of life for patients with cardiovascular disease, but also in number of years of survival. The major risk factors for coronary heart disease have been firmly identified and emphasized in long-range epidemiologic studies such as the Framingham study and others, and assiduous attention to these risk factors has made a significant difference in morbidity and mortality. The impact of such recommendations has been appreciated to varying degrees around the world, depending on the responses of physicians and patients to the new "data" generated and the medical and cultural values and environment in which they practice or live.

In focusing, therefore, on cardiovascular disease as a major area of emphasis, we have chosen to look in depth at approaches to the renin-angiotensin system, particularly at inhibitors of angiotensin converting enzyme (ACE). The development of these new agents in the last decade has resulted in significant therapeutic advances, and the application of their therapeutic effects continues to expand. While it has been appreciated for some years that inhibitors of the renin-angiotensin system are useful in dealing with hypertension as a major cardiovascular risk factor, only more recently have they been shown to be of benefit in the management of congestive heart failure and in circulatory disorders involving the kidney, particularly its microcirculation and function. This year's meeting is focused on two major organs—the heart and the kidney. These are obviously closely linked, as Homer Smith mused in his classic comment that "the function of the heart is to drive blood to the kidney."

We have assembled for this discussion a truly distinguished group of international investigators whose knowledge spans a broad range of areas pertinent to the topic. These include the biochemistry and molecular biology of the renin-angiotensin system and its critical enzymes, the molecular and cellular biology of the heart and kidney, the physiology and interrelationships of the micro- and macrocirculatory systems, the effects of constrictors and dilators

1

of these systems, the clinical pharmacology and action of ACE inhibitors in animals and man, and, finally, the pathogenesis, clinical assessment, and therapy of cardiac and renal failure. After an exhaustive discussion of these issues, we hope to expand the horizons even further by looking for new therapeutic areas in which to use these potent pharmacologic agents.

There were a number of critical questions that we set out to address at this meeting. They included:

1. What new information useful in regulating ACE will come from studies of its molecular biology?

2. How do ACE inhibitors control hypertension, particularly in patients with low circulating renin?

3. What is the physiologic significance of the renin-angiotensin system in various extravascular tissues?

4. Are we all agreed that ACE inhibitors are first-line therapy in hypertension in 1988?

5. What are the molecular and biochemical changes that occur in the failing heart?

6. What is the role of ventricular remodeling and cardiac hypertrophy in the pathogenesis of cardiac failure?

7. How do animal models of heart failure help us with the therapy of human disease?

8. What are the best methods for detecting early heart failure and what modes of therapy should be used at various stages, particularly New York Heart Association Classes I to III.

9. Will earlier intervention with ACE inhibitors in patients with asymptomatic or early heart failure lead to long-term improvements in left ventricular function and survival? How early must these drugs be started? Could they be considered first-line therapy in congestive heart failure, and, if not, what additional data are needed?

10. Is the activation of the renin-angiotensin system in early heart failure due to disease or to diuretic treatment?

11. What are the mechanisms by which ACE inhibitors decrease ventricular arrhythmias?

12. Do ACE inhibitors reduce the incidence of sudden death?

13. What is the role of the glomerular microcirculation and its regulatory factors in the pathogenesis of renal failure?

14. What is the potential benefit of ACE inhibitors in varying types of renal disease? Will glomerular dysfunction in diabetes improve with ACE inhibitors?

15. What precautions need to be taken in the therapy of patients with cardiac and renal failure to prevent adverse results?

16. What benefit might there be in intervening at sites other than angiotensin-converting enzyme in the renin-angiotensin system?

17. What other areas of possible benefit may be found for ACE inhibitors, and what are the most critical areas of future research?

Louis M. SHERWOOD
October 1988

Cardiac and Renal Failure: An Expanding Role for ACE Inhibitors, edited by C. T. Dollery and L. M. Sherwood, Hanley & Belfus, Inc., Philadelphia.

Biotechnology in Pharmaceutical Research: Past, Present, and Future

Edward M. Scolnick

Generally, what scientists mean by biotechnology is the impact that two technologies have had on biomedicine: the discovery of monoclonal antibodies in 1976 by Milstein and Kohler and the gene splicing and transfer of an antibiotic resistance gene between two bacterial species performed by Cohen and Boyer in 1973. This paper focuses on the latter technology.

MAJOR APPLICATIONS OF RECOMBINANT DNA TECHNOLOGIES

There have been five significant protein products approved for human use by major sophisticated regulator agencies (Table I). The first is *human insulin,* approved in 1982 after being produced and developed by Genentech and Eli Lilly. The synthesis, development, and registration of insulin were accomplished in just nine years from the time the first gene splicing and joining experiment was carried out. In pharmaceutical discovery and development, this time frame would be admirable even for a conventional small organic chemical; for the practical application of a new technique, this accomplishment is certainly a tour de force. In the last four years, four other products have been developed and registered.

Human growth hormone (HGH) was developed by Genentech. During the development program for this product, medical students realized that the natural GH extracted from pituitary glands was contaminated with the agent(s) that cause Jacob-Creutzfeldt disease. This unexpected contamination threatened the supply of HGH for the treatment of the hormone deficiency in man. Thus the availability of HGH made by recombinant DNA was most propitious.

In 1986 the first vaccine developed for human use using recombinant DNA technology was licensed when Merck and Chiron developed their *hepatitis B*

3

TABLE I.   *Biotechnology products – approved*

Product	Year Approved	Company	Expression	Use
Insulin	1982	Lilly/Genentech	*E. coli*	Type 1 diabetes
Growth hormone	1985	Genentech	*E. coli*	Growth hormone deficiency
Hepatitis B vaccine	1986	Merck/Chiron	Yeast	Hepatitis B virus prophylaxis
α-Interferon	1986	Biogen/Genentech	*E. coli*	Hairy cell leukemia
Tissue plasminogen activator	1987	Genentech	Chinese hamster ovary	Myocardial infarctions

vaccine. The vaccine is highly immunogenic in man and has been shown to protect infants at risk of contracting hepatitis B infection. The availability of the vaccine obviated the need to rely on infected human plasma as the source of starting material for a vaccine against hepatitis B infection. The development of Recombivax moved recombinant DNA technology from *Escherichia coli* to a eukaryocytic yeast as the host. Recently the vaccine was licensed for use in Japan, marking the first licensure in Japan for a vaccine manufactured by a foreign company.

α-Interferon was licensed in 1986. α-Interferons are made in *E. coli* for the treatment of hairy cell leukemia.

The most recent addition to this list is *tissue plasminogen activator* (tPA), licensed in 1987 by Genentech for the treatment of the acute occlusion of coronary arteries, the cause of potentially life-threatening acute myocardial infarctions. The enzyme is made in a tumor-cell line, Chinese hamster ovary cells. From the point of view of industrial application of recombinant DNA technology, the licensure of a product made in this sort of cell line is also a significant benchmark. The licensure of tPA means that products made in bacteria, yeast, and mammalian cells have now been developed and approved. The impact of the technology is remarkable both in its rapid execution and in the speed with which the sociopolitical and regulatory questions were answered.

Some of the public health issues that were raised in the earliest days of recombinant DNA research are outlined in Table II. Shortly after the earliest gene-splicing experiments, a number of concerned scientists questioned the potential threat to public health of *some* of the contemplated experiments. After a conference at Asilomar in 1975, guidelines for use of recombinant DNA technology were formulated, and, for about two to three years, many potential applications could not be pursued practically. Significant scientific analyses took place during these two years to assure concerned individuals of the safety of the technology to public health before gene splicing could be

TABLE II. *Recombinant DNA safety*

1973	First public concern expressed regarding safety of DNA recombinant experiments
1974	Concerned scientists called for a worldwide moratorium on certain recombinant experiments
	• insertion of SV40 DNA into prokaryotic host (*E. coli*)
1975	Asilomar Conference held. Scientists requested that NIH develop guidelines for recombinant DNA research
	• Certification of safe host-vector systems
	• Definition of practices and containment
1976	NIH released first guidelines
1978	Major revision of guidelines by NIH
	• Relaxation of Containment Requirements

During all this time, recombinant DNA experiments never stopped; rather activity was curtailed on a voluntary basis. For example, the polyoma risk assessment studies of Malcolm Martin and Mark Israel proceeded at the NIH but were performed at a Biosafety Level 4.

applied widely outside Phase IV containment facilities. With the licensure of tPA, a major regulatory barrier to the use of mammalian tumor-cell lines to produce products for human use was also overcome.

With these contributions to human health behind us, what can we look forward to in the coming years from biotechnology? A few of the most interesting protein products to be developed (Table III) are discussed below.

FUTURE TRENDS

1. *Erythropoietin* (EPO). This naturally occurring hormone stimulates the growth and differentiation of red cell precursors. The hormone has been used in clinical trials and has shown efficacy in patients. The first indication for its use will probably be to ameliorate the anemia accompanying chronic renal failure. Clearly this will be a major contribution. Although diagnostic methods to detect infectious agents contaminating the blood supply for trans-

TABLE III. *Recombinant DNA products under development*

Product	Use
Erythropoietin (EPO)	Anemia
Colony stimulating factors (CSF)	Granulopoiesis
Granulocyte-macrophage (GMCSF)	
Granulocyte (GCSF)	
Interleukin 2	Cancer therapy
Factor VIII	Hemophilia
Epidermal growth factor (EGF)	Wound healing
Fibroblast growth factor (FGF)	Wound healing

fusions are very good, the detection methods are not perfect. The use of recombinant EPO will significantly increase safety for those patients requiring transfusions.

2. There are two major *white cell stimulatory growth factors*—granylocyte colony stimulating factor (G-CSF) and granulocyte macrophage colony stimulating factor (GM-CSF). These hormones are undergoing early clinical trials and have shown efficacy in humans; they stimulate the proliferation and differentiation of neutrophil precursors in human bone marrow. Their safety and exact clinical benefit remain to be defined. G-CSF and GM-CSF are being tried in clinical settings of bone marrow suppression caused by cancer chemotherapy or from other causes. There is an increased incidence of infections in patients with depressed bone marrows. Because these hormones stimulate proliferation of the leukocyte lineage, if they lessen the clinical consequences of the low white cell numbers, then G-CSF and GM-CSF will have a major clinical role.

3. *Factor VIII.* HIV contamination of the blood supply prior to the development of appropriate diagnostic tests led to the inadvertent contamination of replacement therapy for hemophiliacs. This contamination has been disastrous for hemophiliac patients. Fortunately, improved methods for preparation of factor VIII, along with HIV detection methods, have dramatically lessened the risks of replacement therapy for these patients. When the technological problems associated with factor VIII production by recombinant DNA have been fully solved, the product made by this route will contribute significantly to health.

4. Another white cell growth factor, *interleukin 2* (IL-2), also shows some promise as a therapeutic agent. IL-2 activates lymphocytes known as natural killer (NK) cells. These cells play a role in the processes by which the body rids itself of potential tumor cells. IL-2-activated autologous NK cells are being tried as a new approach to solid tumor therapy.

5. *Growth factors for wound healing.* Epidermal growth factor and fibroblast growth factor are two hormones that have been shown in animals to accelerate the process of wound healing. Each is in the early stage of development. There are many clinical settings such as burns, decubitus ulcers, or ulcers in diabetic patients in which such growth factors may be clinically useful.

It is clear that major proteins have been developed for use in man, and several others are presently being developed for potential use in man. Thus far, the technology has cloned and produced for clinical use proteins that have been known for some time. Recombinant DNA technology has allowed better definition of the protein and the production of usable amounts. One of the challenges that faces biotechnology is that most of the known proteins that can be cloned have been cloned. In the future, the challenge will be to use molecular cloning along with cell biology to discover new proteins that have potential directly as therapeutic or prophylactic agents.

AIDS AND THE ROLE OF BIOTECHNOLOGY

An even greater challenge and opportunity for the pharmaceutical industry are to use the tools of biotechnology to help decipher and solve major medical problems. In 1988, there is no greater problem than immunodeficiency disease caused by the human immunodeficiency virus (HIV). The virus is a member of the retrovirus family. It has approximately 10,000 nucleotides, and with the knowledge of science and the tools of biotechnology, one can hope to know the molecular details of the life cycle of the virus in great detail and with great precision. The following discussion briefly examines how genetics and biotechnology are helping to solve the problem of AIDS.

Detection of Contaminated Blood Units

In the area of diagnostic testing major strides are being made (Table IV). The first diagnostic tests to screen out contaminated units of blood and blood products for human use were carried out with antigens prepared from live HIV. Now a second generation of tests is being developed using these antigens and new antigens made by recombinant DNA technology. A third and even more powerful set of tests is on the horizon. Using a thermostable DNA polymerase, the DNA amplification method known as the polymerase chain reaction (PCR) is being developed. This reaction will allow the nucleic acid of the HIV virus to be detected with exquisite sensitivity in infected blood and should allow the detection of seronegative but infected units of blood. When the test is perfected and available for widespread use, the safety of blood supplies will be even greater.

Production of Vaccine Against HIV

Another important objective in the AIDS field is the attempt to discover and produce a vaccine against HIV. Clearly, significant basic research will be required before a true vaccine candidate emerges. However, the immunology of the gp 120/160 coat protein of the virus, the interaction of the gp 120 with its T_4 lymphocyte receptor molecule CD4, and the definition of the diversity

TABLE IV. *Diagnostic tests for HIV infection*

First generation immunological tests	Structural proteins purified from live virus
Second generation immunological tests	Proteins produced by recombinant DNA
	Structural proteins
	Regulatory Proteins (not in virions)
Third generation molecular hybridization tests	Polymerase chain reaction technology

among HIV strains could not be proceeding at its current rate without the techniques of biotechnology.

Chemotherapeutic Agents Against HIV

It is probably in this area that biotechnology may have its greatest impact. There are three enzymes identified as being coded for by HIV that could be targets for antiviral chemotherapy (Table V). One of them, the reverse transcriptase, is the target for the first useful drug in treating AIDS: azidothymidine (AZT).

The viral protease can serve to illustrate how biotechnology can help to lay the groundwork for a future chemotherapeutic agent against AIDS. The first question is whether the enzyme really is necessary to the life cycle of the virus. Until recently, strong circumstantial evidence existed which suggested that the HIV protease was required for viral replication: namely, HIVs have been isolated that are noninfectious and have defective protease, and genetic deletions in analogous murine retroviruses that remove protease knock out viral infectivity. Such evidence is very compelling that the HIV protease is essential for the replication of HIV. In order to achieve more conclusive evidence, we examined the primary amino acid (AA) sequences of several proteases, including the HIV protease (Table VI). It is clear that there is a similarity between the AA sequence in HIV protease and those of the known proteases pepsin and renin. Thus, although the HIV protease is roughly half the size, it appears to be a member of the family of aspartyl proteases. In order to study the HIV protease, the enzyme was made by recombinant DNA methods.

We have gone on to test the hypothesis that HIV protease is an aspartyl active site enzyme by site-directed mutagenesis. By changing the single aspartic acid at the putative active site to an asparagine residue, we have rendered the enzyme inactive in assays that measure, *in vitro*, the enzyme's catalytic activity. Furthermore, when such a mutation is incorporated into a full-length DNA clone of HIV, we have shown that the clone can give rise to virus particles by DNA transfections, but that such particles are completely noninfectious for virus spread. As expected, the viral protease in such particles is

TABLE V. *Critical events in the life cycle of HIV*

• Receptor binding (attachment of virus to surface of cells)	
• Entry of virus into cell	
• Replication of DNA	Reverse transcriptase
• Integration of DNA into chromosome (dormant)	Integrase
• Activation of virus	
• Viral proteins are made as fusions	
• Proteins are processed involving proteolysis	Protease
• Virus leaves cell and kills it	

TABLE VI. *HIV protease*

HIV aa 20–34†	KEALLDTGADDTVLE
H-Pepsinogen	CQAIVDIGTSLLTGP
B-Chymosin	CQAILDTGTSKLVGP
H-Cathepsin D	CEAIVDTGTSLMVGP
H-Renin	CLAIVDTGASYISGS

*Similar to pepsin and renin (aspartyl proteases) but half the size. Works as a dimer.
†Asp25

inactive. Thus, a small molecule that specifically inhibits the protease should also render HIV noninfectious.

Can an anti-protease inhibitor be a drug? Vasotec, Merck's angiotensin converting enzyme inhibitor, is an extraordinarily safe and effective protease inhibitor drug. Thus, we *assume* that a protease inhibitor can also be found for the HIV protease, and, that if we find it, it too will be a safe as well as effective drug.

In diagnostic techniques of enhanced sensitivity and specificity, in vaccine research, and in research for new chemotherapeutic agents, biotechnology is playing a vital role in efforts to ameliorate the AIDS public health problem. In fact, major new solutions to the AIDS problem would not be achievable without biotechnology.

BIOTECHNOLOGY IN PHARMACEUTICAL RESEARCH

Biotechnology has an important role to play in the wider field of drug research. The approaches and techniques that are being used in research against HIV are highly relevant to drug discovery in general. Two specific examples are outlined below:

Receptor Research

One of the major problems of our aging population is Alzheimer's disease, a devastating CNS degenerative disease that leads to severe memory loss and loss of other intellectual functions. The cause of the disease is not clear, but one of the functional accompaniments is the loss of neurons that produce the neurotransmittor acetycholine (ACH). Many pharmaceutical companies are attempting to design appropriate cholinomimetic molecules as chemical replacement therapy in this disease. By molecular cloning, the ACH receptor subtypes at which such cholinomimetics might work actually have been defined as molecular entities long before potent and selective drugs are available. Such molecular definition has been achieved prior to pharmacological definition with selective ligands of the different receptor subtypes. Such information is of great benefit in cholinomimetic design. In the future, molecular definitions will almost always precede pharmacological definitions, thus allowing faster insights into molecular receptor targets for drug design.

Enzyme Deficiency

Recombinant DNA technology will play an increasingly important role in defining the biological rationale for the choice of a target for drug development. Too often, at early stages of drug development projects, it is impossible to be certain of the importance of a given enzyme to a given biological process in mammalian cells or in man. The reason is clear. No mutant deficiency exists in animals or man that allows the consequences of blockade of a given pathway to be predicted. Sometimes, however, such evidence does exist (Table VII).

Years ago a syndrome of sexual dysfunction was recognized in man known as male pseudohermaphroditism. One form of this syndrome was found to be caused by the lack of a steroid metabolizing enzyme called steroid 5α reductase. The enzyme reduces testosterone to dihydrotestosterone (DHT). From the understanding of this naturally occurring mutation in man, it was realized that DHT is required for normal growth of the prostate gland. With this knowledge, Merck set out to develop a specific chemical inhibitor of the enzyme as a way to treat benign prostatic hypertrophy, a disease that today requires surgical intervention. Merck's potential drug, MK-906, recently has been shown to block 5α reductase in man and to shrink the prostate gland. In this case, because of the background of information about the genetic deficiency of the enzyme, the consequences in the prostate of the chemical blockade could be firmly predicted. In many other inhibitor discovery programs, no such prior genetic information exists.

Transgenic Research

However, in 1988 new technologies are on the horizon that can potentially provide such background genetic information. The creation of animals with newly inserted heritable genes is called transgenic research. Initial studies in creating transgenic animals have allowed the detection of physiological changes in the new animals carrying newly inserted and newly expressed

---

TABLE VII.   *Role of genetics in drug discovery*

- Recognition of male pseudohermaphroditism
  - Physically appearing males with abnormal development of external genitalia and small prostate glands
  - Deficiency of steroid 5α reductase leading to lack of dihydrotestosterone
- Testosterone $+ 5\alpha$ Reductase $\rightarrow$ dihydrotestosterone
- Synthesis of a specific inhibitor of 5α reductase — MK-906
- Proof in man that MK-906 inhibits 5α reductase and shrinks enlarged protaste glands

---

genes. More recently, methods are being developed for creation of genetic deficiencies and biochemical deficiencies in animals by gene insertion and cell transplantation methods. Such deficiencies will elucidate the biological role of *reduced* activity of specific enzymes and receptors long before drug molecules are available. The availability of such knowledge will greatly aid the choice of targets for pharmaceutical drug development efforts.

CONCLUSIONS

The practical application of biotechnology to diagnostic problems and to the development of prophylactic agents and therapeutic agents for human medicine is a reality in the 1980s. It is important to realize that the practical applications could not have been developed without government support for basic research for decades preceding the practical applications. No one could have foreseen the breadth of applications of studies in bacteriophage or in pneumococci that took place decades before the first therapeutic application in 1982. The taxpayers' dollars have been well spent—the results at hand speak for themselves. In the next decade the results for control of HIV may in fact be miraculous.

SUMMARY

The technology of gene splicing and transfer of an antibiotic resistance gene between two bacterial species are discussed. Some of the major applications of recombinant DNA technologies are reviewed, including a number of important protein products such as human insulin, growth hormone, and hepatitis B vaccine. The early days of recombinant DNA research are traced, and some of the recombinant DNA products currently under development, such as erythropoietin and white cell stimulatory growth factors, are described. Particular attention is focused on one of the greatest challenges to the pharmaceutical industry: immunodeficiency caused by HIV. A number of diagnostic tests are already available to detect contaminated blood supplies, and an infinitely more sensitive test using a method of DNA amplification, known as the polymerase chain reaction, is currently being perfected. The way in which biotechnology lays the groundwork for the development of future chemotherapeutic agents effective against AIDS is outlined. Enzymes in the virus's life cycle have been identified that potentially could be targets for antiviral chemotherapeutic agents. The progress that has been made in this area is presented. The value of biotechnology in the wider context of pharmaceutical research is addressed, particularly the fact that molecular cloning enables molecular definition to precede pharmaceutical definition and allows the role of reduced activity of specific enzymes and receptors to be detected long before drug molecules are available.

RÉSUMÉ

On traite ici de la recombinaison génétique et du transfert de gène de résistance antibiotique entre deux espèces bactériennes. On fait le point sur quelques-unes des principales applications des techniques de recombinaison de l'ADN, y compris un nombre importants de produits de protéines tels que l'insuline humaine, l'hormone de croissance, et le vaccin contre l'hépatite B. On retrace la recherche de la recombinaison génétique de l'ADN à ses débuts, et l'on décrit quelques produits de combinaison de l'ADN actuellement en voie de développement, tels que l'érythropoiétine et les facteurs de croissance de leucocytes. On s'attache particulièrement à l'un des plus grands défis de l'industrie pharmaceutique: l'immunodéficience causée par le virus de l'immunodéficience humaine VIH. Il existe déjà un certain nombre de tests de dépistage sérologique pour détecter la contamination sanguine, et actuellement, on est en train de perfectionner un test beaucoup plus précis utilisant une méthode d'amplification de l'ADN, connu sous le nom de réaction en chaîne de la polymérase. On décrit les voies ouvertes par la biotechnologie pour le développement de nouveaux traitements chimiothérapeutiques pour lutter contre le SIDA. On a identifié les enzymes du cycle de vie du virus qui pourraient conduire au développement d'agents chimiothérapeutiques contre le SIDA. On indique les progrès qui ont été faits dans ce domaine. On souligne l'importance de la biotechnologie dans ce domaine de la recherche pharmaceutique surtout du fait que le cloning moléculaire permet à la définition moléculaire de précéder la définition pharmaceutique et permet la détection du rôle de l'activité réduite d'enzymes spécifiques et de récepteurs bien avant le développement des molécules pharmaceutiques.

ZUSAMMENFASSUNG

Zur Diskussion stehen die Technologie der Genfusion und der Transfer eines Antibiotika-resistenten Gens zwischen zwei bakteriellen Spezies: Einige der wichtigsten Anwendungsgebiete rekombinanter DNA-Technologien werden besprochen; einschliesslich einiger wichtiger Proteinprodukte, wie menschliches Insulin, Wachstumshormon, und Impfstoff für Hepatitis B. Ein Bericht über die frühen Tage der rekombinanten DNA-Forschung wird gefolgt von einer Studie über einige der gegenwärtig in der Entwicklung befindlichen rekombinanten DNA-Produkte. Beschrieben werden unter anderem Erythropoietin und Wachstumsfaktoren, die weisse Zellen stimulieren. Besondere Aufmerksamkeit wird einer der grössten Herausforderungen der pharmazeutischen Industrie gewidmet: Immundefizienz, hervorgerufen durch HIV. Eine Reihe diagnostischer Tests für kontaminierte Blutkonserven sind bereits verfügbar; und zur Zeit ist ein sehr viel sensiblerer Test in der Perfektionsphase, bekannt unter dem Namen Polymerase-Kettenreaktion (PCR), der eine

Methode der DNA-Amplifikation verwendet. Eine Übersicht über die Art und Weise, in der die Biotechnologie eine Basis schafft für die Entwicklung zukünftiger chemotherapeutischer Mittel gegen AIDS wird gegeben. Identifiziert worden sind Enzyme im Lebenszyklus des Virus, die möglicherweise Ziel sein könnten für chemotherapeutische Anti-Virus-Wirkstoffe. Beschrieben wird der Fortschritt, der auf diesem Gebiet gemacht worden ist. Der Text bespricht die Bedeutung der Biotechnologie im weiteren Kontext der pharmazeutischen Forschung; insbesondere die Tatsache, dass Cloning die Möglichkeit eröffnet, dass molekulare Definition der pharmazeutischen Definition vorangeht, und damit die Rolle der reduzierten Aktivität spezifischer Enzyme und Rezeptoren festgestellt werden kann, lange bevor die Drogenmoleküle verfügbar sind.

RIASSUNTO

Verranno discussi la technologia della manipolazione genetica (gene splicing) ed il transferimento di un gene di resistenza antibiotica fra due specie batteriche. Verranno esaminate alcune delle principali applicazioni delle tecnologie DNA ricombinante, compreso un certo numero di importanti prodotti proteici quali l'insulina umana, l'ormone di crescita ed il vaccino dell'epatite B. Vengono ripercorsi i primi passi della ricerca sul DNA ricombinante e vengono descritti alcuni dei prodotti DNA ricombinante attualmente in corso di sviluppo, quali l'eritropoietina ed i fattori stimolatori della crescita dei globuli bianchi. Viene data particolare attenzione ad una delle grandi sfide che l'industria farmaceutica deve affrontare: l'immunodeficienza causata dall'HIV. E' già disponibile un certo numero di test diagnostici per rivelare scorte di sangue contaminato ed un test infinitamente più sensibile, facente uso di un metodo di amplificazione del DNA, noto come reazione a catena dei polimeri, è attualmente in corso di perfezionamento. Viene delineato il modo in cui la biotecnologia pone le basi per lo sviluppo di futuri agenti chemioterapeutici efficaci contro l'AIDS. Sono stati identificati degli enzimi nel ciclo vitale del virus che sono potenziali bersagli per agenti chemioterapeutici antivirali. Viene presentato il progresso compiuto in questo campo. Viene discusso il valore della biotecnologia nel più ampio contesto della ricerca farmaceutica, soprattutto il fatto che la clonazione molecolare consente alla definizione molecolare di precedere la definizione farmaceutica e permette di riconoscere il ruolo della ridotta attività di enzimi e recettori specifici molto prima che siano disponibili molecole per farmaci.

SUMÁRIO

Discute-se a tecnologia do entrançamento (splicing) de genes e da transferência de um gene de resistência antibiótica entre duas espécies de bactérias.

Revisam-se algumas das tecnologias mais importantes de DNA recombinante, inclusive uma série de produtos proteínicos importantes, tais como insulina humana, hormônio de crescimento e vacina contra a hepatite B. Traçam-se os primeiros dias da pesquisa do DNA recombinante e describemse alguns dos produtos de DNA recombinante que atualmente se encontram em desenvolvimento, tais como eritropoietina e fatores estimuladores do crescimento de leucócitos. Focaliza-se especial atenção a um dos desafios mais importantes à industria farmacêutica: a imunodeficiência ocasionada pelo HIV (vírus de immunodeficiência humana). Atualmente já dispõe-se de uma série de testes diagnósticos para detectar suprimentos de sangue contaminado, e vem-se aperfeiçoando um teste muito mais sensível que utiliza um método de amplificação de DNA, conhecido como a reação em cadeia da polimerasa. Esboça-se a maneira em que a biotecnologia estabelece as bases para o desenvolvimento de futuros agentes quimioterapêuticos eficazes contra AIDS. Têm-se identificado enzimas no ciclo de vida do vírus que potencialmente poderiam ser alvos para agentes quimioterapêuticos antivirais. Presenta-se o progresso que tem-se conseguido nesta área. Examina-se o valor da biotecnologia no contexto mais extenso da pesquisa farmacêutica, particularmente o fato que a duplicação (cloning) molecular permite que a definição molecular preceda a definição farmacêutica e permite a detecção do papel da atividade reduzida de enzimas e receptores específicos muito antes de que se dispõe de moléculas da droga.

RESUMEN

Se discute la tecnología de incorporación (splicing) de genes y transferencia del gen de resistencia antibiótica entre dos especies de bacterias. Se repasan algunas de las tecnologías más importantes de DNA recombinante, incluyendo un número importante de productos proteínicos tales como insulina humana, hormona de crecimiento y vacuna contra la hepatitis B. Se analizan los primeros días de la investigación de DNA recombinante y algunos de los productos de DNA recombinante que actualmente se hallan en desarrollo, tales como eritropoyetina y factores de estimulación del crecimiento de leucocitos. Se pone particular atención en uno de los retos más importantes que enfrenta la industria farmacéutica, la inmunodeficiencia causada por HIV (virus de inmunodeficiencia humana). Actualmente se cuenta con varios ensayos diagnósticos para detectar suministros de sangre contaminada, y se está perfeccionando un ensayo mucho más sensitivo que emplea un método de amplificación de DNA, conocido como reacción en cadena de la polimerasa. Se bosqueja la manera en que la biotecnología establece las bases para el desarrollo de futuros agentes quimioterapéuticos eficaces contra el SIDA. Se han identificado varias enzimas en el ciclo de vida del virus que podrían ser blancos potenciales para agentes quimioterapéuticos antivirales. Se presenta el progreso que se ha hecho en esta área. Se examina el valor de la biotecnología en el contexto más extenso de la investigación farmacéutica, particularmente el hecho de que la duplicación (cloning) molecular permite que la definición molecular preceda a la definición farmacéutica y permite la detección del papel de la reducción en la actividad de enzimas y receptores específicos mucho antes de que se disponga de las moléculas del fármaco.

要約

　ここでは，2種の細菌間での抗生剤耐性遺伝子の接合および転写技法について検討する。また，ヒトインスリンや成長ホルモン，B型肝炎ワクチンなどいくつかの重要なタンパク性物質など主要な組み換え DNA 技法の応用についても総説する。まず，初期の組み換え DNA 研究の歴史をふりかえり，さらに現在開発の進められている組み換え DNA 産物，たとえばエリスロポイエチンや白血球刺激成長因子などについても考察する。

　なかでもとくに，製薬業界への最大の挑戦であるヒト免疫不全ウイルス（HIV）による後天性免疫不全症候群（AIDS）の問題に焦点をあてる。すでに，いくつかの診断検査法により HIV 混入血液の検出が可能になっている。さらに現在，ポリメラーゼ鎖反応試験として知られる DNA 増幅法を用いた高感度の試験法によって完全な HIV 検査が可能になりつつある。また，将来 AIDS に対して有効な化学療法剤の開発に向けて，その基盤となる生体工学の果たす役割について概説する。

　まず，抗菌化学療法剤が標的とすべき，ウイルスの増殖・成長の生活環での必須酵素が明らかにされつつある。この分野での進歩について紹介する。

　今日，薬理研究の広範な分野における生体工学の意義が明確になってきた。とくに分子クローニングの技術は，薬理学的な分子同定を容易にし，薬剤分子の選定に先だって特定酵素の活性抑制および受容体の役割を明らかにすることを可能にした。

Cardiac and Renal Failure: An Expanding Role for ACE Inhibitors, edited by C. T. Dollery and L. M. Sherwood, Hanley & Belfus, Inc., Philadelphia.

History of Angiotensin-Converting Enzyme and Its Inhibition

Colin I. Johnston

Phylogenetically the renin angiotensin system is very old, having first appeared in bony fishes and teleosts and tetrapods.[1] Both renin and juxtaglomerular cells have been found in a variety of teleost fishes, but not in elasmobranchs or cyclostomes. It is probable that the original role of the renin-angiotensin system was that of vasoconstriction and maintaining pressure, and only later did it become important in steroidogenesis and sodium balance. Its history in medicine and science, however, is much shorter. Renin was discovered in 1898 by Tigerstedt and Bergman,[2] who showed that an extract of rabbit renal cortical tissue was pressor. Although Tigerstedt was a distinguished Scandinavian physiologist, little was made of this finding, and indeed it was described before enzymes were really understood. It is ironic that 83 years later, the most recently identified cardiovascular hormone, atrial natriuretic peptide (ANP) was discovered by the same technique of homogenizing tissues and performing a bioassay.[3]

Interest in the renin angiotensin system was not awakened until the classical experiments by Goldblatt in the 1930s, in which he produced a form of experimental renal hypertension by constricting the renal artery in a dog.[4,5] Although Goldblatt established that the hypertension was due to a humoral mechanism and associated with ischemia,[6] he did not associate the hypertension with increased renin secretion. This association was made by Pickering in 1938,[7] when he was repeating the experiments of Tigerstedt and Goldblatt and also by Braun-Menendez, *et al.*[8] About the same time, the Belgian morbid anatomist Goormaghtigh described the juxtaglomerular apparatus, suggesting that the juxtaglomerular cells in the afferent arteriole were secretory cells and noting their association with the lacis cells of the glomerulus and the macula densa in the kidney.[9] He rightly hypothesized that the juxtaglomerular cells were endocrine secretory cells and probably were also related to renal function, because of their close association with renal tubular cells.

Also during 1939 and 1940 the Braun-Menendez group[8,10] and Page's group[11] both recognized that renin was an enzyme and produced a vasoactive substance by acting on a substrate in plasma. Braun-Menendez named this substance hypertensin and the Page group called it angiotonin. It was not until much later in 1958 that the compromise name angiotensin was agreed to by these two distinguished scientists.[12] Despite recognition that renin was an enzyme acting on a plasma substrate, the active component was not purified until Skegg's work in the early 1950s. In 1954, Skeggs isolated hypertensin[13] from horse serum and showed by countercurrent electrophoresis that it contained two peptides. He also showed that the one of the peptides derived from the other due to a plasma contaminant that was a chloride dependent enzyme. In 1956, he described in addition the amino acid composition of hypertensin I and II and also partially purified the contaminant enzyme, which he named hypertensin converting enzyme.[14] Later in the same year, he published a paper on the preparation and function of hypertensin converting enzyme.[15] This probably was the first description of angiotensin-converting enzyme.

ANGIOTENSIN-CONVERTING ENZYME

From this humble beginning, angiotensin-converting enzyme (ACE) has now grown to be one of the most important enzymes in cardiovascular physiology. It is ubiquitously distributed, being found in all endothelial cells as well as a variety of epithelial cells, including the kidney, gastrointestinal and reproductive tracts, choroid plexus, and the placenta.[16,17] It has also been described in the testis[18] and spermatozoa, as well as in neuronal cells.[19] Angiotensin-converting enzyme (EC 3.4.15.1) is a zinc-containing dipeptidyl carboxypeptidase. In most sites it is an exopeptidase anchored to the plasma membrane. In this position on endothelial cells, it is strategically sited to act on peptides in the circulating blood. However, its role is now known to be much more extensive than this.

Although Skeggs had described the enzyme in 1956, it lay dormant until a decade later. At this time Vane in the Department of Pharmacology at the Royal College of Surgeons in London was conducting a series of experiments on vasoactive peptides in the circulation using his superfused blood bath technique. In 1968, Ng and Vane[20] showed that the rate of formation of angiotensin II (ANG II) by converting enzyme in the plasma was not rapid enough to account for the formation of ANG II in the circulation and demonstrated that it probably was due to the conversion of angiotensin I (ANG I) across the lung. Later in that year, Bakhle[21] showed that homogenates of lung were able to convert ANG I into ANG II. Vane also made the suggestion that the enzyme that converted ANG I to ANG II may be similar to or the same as an enzyme that had been described as breaking down bradykinin. This was because both enzymes appeared to cleave amino acids from the carboxy terminus of the peptide substrates, and to stop at a Pro-Phe sequence. Thus they were thought to be carboxypeptidases. Subsequently, however, it was shown that the enzyme cleaved dipeptides from the molecule.

Following the demonstration that the conversion of ANG I to ANG II probably occurred in the lung, many groups set about purifying the responsible enzyme. In the early 1970s several groups had purified the enzyme from lung and kidney and published that it cleaved dipeptides from ANG I and bradykinin.[22,23,24]

KININASE II

The discovery and history of the enzymes that destroy bradykinin followed a completely different path. In 1962, Erdos and Sloane[25] showed that bradykinin, the potent vasoactive nonapeptide isolated from snake venom by Roche de Silva, was inactivated by carboxypeptidases. Five years later, in 1967, Erdos and Yang[26] described a second bradykinin-degrading enzyme that they had isolated from the microsomal fraction of pig kidneys. They named this enzyme kininase II and later in the same year, Yang and Erdos[27] isolated the same enzyme from human blood plasma. However, it was not until the pharmacological studies initiated by Ferreira on bradykinin potentiating factor (BPF) that it became apparent that kininase II may be a similar or the same enzyme as the angiotensin-converting enzyme, first described by Skeggs. This was conclusively established enzymatically simultaneously by Yang et al.[28,29] and Elisseeva et al.[30] in 1970–71, when they published papers showing that in vitro kininase II, or carboxycathepsin, as the Russians had named their enzyme, and angiotensin-converting enzyme had identical catalytic activity on both ANG I and bradykinin.

BRADYKININ POTENTIATING FACTOR

At the same time, as this biochemical work was being performed in 1965, Ferreira, a young pharmacologist, commenced work in Roche de Silva's laboratory in Brazil. He started investigating some of the slowly reacting substances released by the venom of the South American pit viper *Bothrops jararaca*, which included bradykinin. He found that bradykinin was potentiated not only by metal-blinding agents such as dimercaprol (BAL) but also by the venom itself. He went on to show that the venom contained a factor that potentiated the pharmacological actions of bradykinin. He and Roche de Silva named this factor bradykinin-potentiating factor (BPF). He also demonstrated that it was probably a polypeptide, that it was specific for bradykinin, and that it did not affect the actions of histamine or acetylecholine.[31,32] Later, in 1967, while undertaking postdoctoral work in Vane's laboratory in London, Ferreira showed that bradykinin was destroyed in the blood,[33] particularly in the lung, but that it could be protected by bradykinin potentiating factor.[34]

It was the serendipity of Ferreira working on bradykinin and Ng on ANG I, both in Vane's laboratory, that the idea arose of the lung containing an enzyme that converts ANG I to ANG II and destroys bradykinin. However, Bakhle[21,35] in the same laboratory using lung homogenates was unable to unequivocally establish that the enzyme was indeed identical, because although BPF inhibited angiotensin-converting enzyme, he was unable to conclusively demonstrate that it prevented the destruction of bradykinin when incubated with pulmonary homogenates. Confirmation that it was the same enzyme had to be left to the biochemical enzymatic studies. When Ferreira returned to Brazil, he continued working on bradykinin-potentiating factor and in 1970[36] showed that the *Bothrops jararaca* venom consisted of a series of 9 peptides, from 5 to 13 amino acid residues per molecule. Later it was shown that the pentapeptide (BPP$_{5a}$) was the most potent inhibitor of bradykinin degradation and AI conversion.[37] However this peptide, although potent *in vitro*, had a very short life *in vivo* and had to be administered intravenously. BPP$_{9a}$, another peptide isolated from the venom, although not as potent, had a more prolonged action. Ferreira's group demonstrated the biological importance of inhibiting the enzyme by showing that it reduced blood pressure in a variety of animals with experimental hypertension,[38] and that the test had the possibility of being used as a diagnostic tool for the detection of renovascular hypertension in man.

Why the snake should have such inhibitory peptides in its venom is open to conjecture. However, one suggestion has been made that by natural selection those snakes whose venom contains both bradykinin and bradykinin-potentiating factor would have an evolutionary advantage because the bradykinin-potentiating factor would prevent the destruction of bradykinin, which would allow by its action on blood flow and vascular permeability more rapid access of poison into the circulation of the animal that is bitten.

ANGIOTENSIN-CONVERTING ENZYME INHIBITORS

Following the discovery of the importance of enzyme inhibition, Ondetti *et al.*[39] at the Squibb Institute of Medical Research in 1971 isolated six peptide inhibitors from the venom of the South American pit viper and proceeded to sequence and synthesise these inhibitory peptides. They showed that they all had potency *in vitro* and *in vivo* but that BPP$_{9a}$ (SQ20881) or teprotide, which was the second most potent, was resistent to peptidase activity and therefore had a prolonged action *in vivo*. Over the next few years unheralded and somewhat unencouraged, Ondetti, who had been joined by Cushman, pursued the synthesis and study of the peptides that would inhibit ACE. Their goal was to design a very potent, specific, orally-active compound to inhibit ACE.

At this state, however, support for the renin angiotensin system as a cause of hypertension had somewhat waned, except for the enthusiasm of John

Laragh.[40] The likelihood, therefore, of producing a useful and marketable product had diminished. Nevertheless by a superb piece of deductive reasoning, based on the known sequence of the snake venom peptide inhibitors, the similarity between carboxypeptidase A and ACE, Ondetti and Cushman were able to design a tailored drug to inhibit the enzyme. The active site of carboxypeptidase A had been well established and a dipeptide inhibitor had already been described for this enzyme.[41,42] By analogy and by using sequence data from the venom peptides, Ondetti et al.[43] designed a series of dipeptide analogues that were effective inhibitors of ACE. So in 1977 was borne captopril (SQ 14225), the first orally active, potent, and specific ACE inhibitor. This drug was rapidly shown to be effective in humans with hypertension[44,45] and in a variety of experimental animal hypertensive models.[46,47] Following captopril there has been a variety of second generation ACE inhibitors, which mainly differ from captopril in being pro-esterified drugs to assist their absorption and in lacking a sulphydryl group (such as enalapril). There are now third generation ACE inhibitors, some of which are nonpeptigenic.

CONCLUSION

It has become apparent that angiotensin-converting enzyme inhibitors have been a significant advance in the therapy of hypertension and congestive cardiac failure. The discovery of the ACE inhibitors is a perfect example of pursuing basic research and knowledge for its own sake. It is also a good example of university-based scientific research being further developed in a practical sense by industry. On the other hand, it illustrates the fallacy of naming an enzyme after a single substrate, and indicates why the idea that there is a rate-limiting step in an enzymatic cascade is probably too narrow and fixed. Renin has been for many years regarded as the rate-limiting step in the renin-angiotensin cascade. However, it is obvious that if one can sufficiently change or block some other enzyme in the cascade, this then becomes the rate-limiting process. Such is the example of ACE inhibition. Lastly, one should not conclude from the effectiveness of ACE inhibitors in lowering blood pressure in a variety of hypertensive states that the etiology of hypertension is due to over-activity of the renin-angiotensin system. What it does illustrate, however, is that the renin-angiotensin system is important in cardiovascular homeostasis in maintaining blood pressure, and if one effectively removes this system, as well as its interaction with the sympathetic nervous system, the blood pressure will fall.

WHAT OF THE FUTURE?

The angiotensin-converting enzyme inhibitors have rekindled interest in the enzyme. It is now possible by using radioinhibitor-binding techniques, combined with *in vitro* autoradiography, to accurately anatomically localize and map ACE. Some interesting results that may give leads to the future have emerged. The enzyme is found in high concentration in very highly localized areas of the brain and not in all cases is it related to the simultaneous occurrence of renin or angiotensin receptors. What function ACE is performing in the brain is still not known. Similarly, there are high concentrations of ACE in the reproductive tract, and in particular in the testis, and its role in this organ is also completely unknown. Whether or not the enzyme in the varying sites is merely an isoenzyme or whether it is a different enzyme has yet to be established. Indeed the very specificity of substrates for ACE is widening all the time.[17] ACE inhibitors may also have actions independent of their blocking effect on the enzyme. Lastly, the mode of action of the ACE inhibitors, although primarily due to inhibition of the enzyme, may involve many other systems because of the multiple physiological and biological affects of ANG II. Until effective renin inhibitors, ANG II-receptor antagonists, and kallikrein or bradykinin inhibitors are developed, it will not be possible to dissect out the exact mechanism of the hypotensive effect of ACE inhibitors.

REFERENCES

1. Nishimma H. Comparative endocrinology of renin and angiotensin. *Adv Exp Med Biol* 1980; **130**:29–74.
2. Tigerstedt R, Bergman PG, Niere und Kreislauf. *Scand Arch Physiol* 1898; **8**:223–271.
3. de Bold AJ, Borenstein BH, Veress AT, Sonnenberg H. A rapid and potent natriuretic response to intravenous injection of atrial myocardial extracts in rats. *Life Sci* 1981; **28**:89–94.
4. Goldblatt H, Lynch J, Hanzal RH, Summerville WW. Studies on experimental hypertension. I. The production of persistent elevation of systolic blood pressure by means of renal ischemia. *J Exp Med* 1934; **59**:347–380.
5. Goldblatt H. *The Renal Origin of Hypertension.* Springfield, Illinois: Charles C Thomas, 1948.
6. Goldblatt H. Studies on experimental hypertension. V. The pathogenesis of experimental hypertension due to renal ischemia. *Ann Intern Med* 1937; **11**:69–103.
7. Pickering GW, Prinzmetal M. Some observations on renin, a pressor substance contained in normal kidney, together with a method for its biological assay. *Clin Sci* 1938; **3**:211–227.
8. Munoz JM, Braun-Menendez E, Fasciolo JC, Leloir LF. Hypertensin: the substance causing renal hypertension. Nature 1939; **144**:980.
9. Goormaghtigh N. La fonction endocrine des arterioles renales. Son role dans la pathogenie de l'hypertension arterille. Louvain, kR. K Fonteyn and *Rev Belge Sci Med* 1944/1945; **16**:65–83.
10. Braun-Menendez E, Fasciolo JC, Leloir LF, Munoz JN. The substance causing renal hypertension. *J Physiol* 1940; **98**:283–289.
11. Page IH, Helmer OM. A crystalline pressor substance (angiotonin) resulting from the action between renin and renin-activator. *J Exp Med* 1940; **71**:29–42.
12. Braun-Menendez E, Page IH. Suggested revision of nomenclature—angiotensin. *Science* 1958; **127**:242.
13. Skeggs LT, Jr, Marsh WH, Kahn JR, Shumway NP. The purification of hypertension I. *J Exp Med* 1954; **100**:363–370.
14. Lentz, KE, Skeggs LT Jr, Woods KR, Kahn JR, Shumway NP. The amino acid composition of hypertensin II and its biochemical relationship to hypertensin I. *J Exp Med* 1956; **104**:183–191.
15. Skeggs LT Jr, Kahn JR, Shumway NP. The preparation and function of the hypertensin-converting enzyme. *J Exp Med* 1956; **103**:295–299.

16. Cushman DN, Cheung HJ. Concentration of angiotensin converting enzyme in tissues of the rat. *Biochim Biophys Acta* 1971; **250**:26–265.
17. Erdos EG, Skidgel RA. The angiotensin I converting enzyme. *Lab Invest* 1987; **56**:345–348.
18. Jackson B, Cubella RB, Sagakuchi K, Johnston CI. Characterization of angiotensin converting enzyme (ACE) in the testis and assessment of the in vivo effects of the ACE inhibition of Perindopril. *Endocrinology* 1988; **123**:50–55.
19. Chai SY, Mendelsohn FAO, Paxinos G. Angiotensin converting enzyme in rat brain visualized by quantitative in vitro autoradiography. *Neuroscience* 1987; **20**:615–627.
20. Ng KKF, Vane JR. Fate of angiotensin I in the circulation. *Nature* (London) 1968; **218**:144–150.
21. Bakhle YS. Conversion of angiotensin I to angiotensin II by cell-free extracts of dog lung. *Nature* (London) 1968; **220**:919–921.
22. Dorer FE, Kahn JR, Lentz KE, Levine M, Skeggs LT. Purification and properties of angiotensin-converting enzyme from hog lung. *Circ Res* 1972; **31**:356–366.
23. Das M, Soffer RL. Pulmonary angiotension-converting enzyme. Structural and catalytic properties. *J Biol Chem* 1975; **250**:6762–6768.
24. Oshima G, Gecse A, Erdos EG. Angiotensin I converting enzyme of the kidney cortex. *Biochim Biophys Acta* 1974; **350**:26–37.
25. Erdos EG, Sloane EM. An enzyme in human blood plasma that inactivates bradykinin and kallidin. *Biochem Pharmacol* 1962; **11**:585–592.
26. Erdos EG, Yang HYT. An enzyme in microsomal fraction of kidney that inactivates bradykinin. *Life Sci* 1967; **6**:659–662.
27. Yang HYT, Erdos EG. Second kininase in human blood plasma. *Nature* 1967; **215**:1402.
28. Yang HYT, Erdos EG, Levin Y. A dipeptidyl carboxypeptidase that converts angiotensin I and inactivates bradykinin. *Biochim Biophys Acta* 1970; **214**:374–376.
29. Yang HYT, Erdos EG, Levin Y. Characterization of dipeptide hydrolase (kininase II: angiotensin I converting enzyme). *J Pharmacol Exp Ther* 1971; **177**:291–300.
30. Elisseeva, YE, Orekhovich VN, Pavlikhina LV, Alexeenko LP. Carboxycathepsin: A key regulatory component of two physiological systems involved in regulation of blood pressure. *Clin Chim Acta* 1971; **31**:413–419.
31. Ferreira SH, Rocha e Silva M. Potentiation of bradykinin and eledoisin by BPF (bradykinin potentiating factor) from *Bothrops jararaca* venom. *Experentia* 1965; **21**:347–349.
32. Ferreira SH. A bradykinin-potentiating fact (BPF) present in the venom of *Bothrops jararaca*. *Br J Pharmacol* 1965; **24**:163–169.
33. Ferreira SH, Vane JR. The detection and estimation of bradykinin in the circulating blood. *Br J Pharmacol Chemother* 1967; **29**:367–377.
34. Ferreira SH, Vane JR. The disappearance of bradykinin and eledoisin in the circulation and vascular beds of the cat. *Br J Pharmacol Chemother* 1967; **30**:417–424.
35. Bakhle, YS, Reynard AM, Vane Jr. Metabolism of the angiotensins in isolated perfused tissues. *Nature* (London) 1969; **222**:956–959.
36. Ferreira SH, Bartelt DC, Greene, LJ. Isolation of bradykinin-potentiating peptides from *Bothrops jararaca* venom. *Biochemistry* 1970; **9**:2583–2593.
37. Greene LJ, Camargo ACM, Krieger EM, Stewart JM, Ferreira SH. Inhibition of the conversion of angiotensin I to II and potentiation of bradykinin by small peptides present in Bothrops jararaca venom. *Circ Res* 1972; **30**:62–71.
38. Krieger EM, Salgado HC, Assan CJ, Greene LJ, Ferreira SH. Potential screening test for detection of overactivity of renin-angiotensin system. *Lancet* 1971; **1**:269–271.
39. Ondetti MA, Williams NJ, Sabo EF, Pluscec J, Weaver ET, Kocy O. Angiotensin-converting enzyme inhibitors from the venom of *Bothrops jararaca* isolation, elucidation of structure and synthesis. *Biochemistry* 1971; **10**:4033–4039.
40. Laragh JH. Vasoconstriction-volume analysis for understanding and treating hypertension. The use of renin and aldosterone profiles. *Am J Med* 1973; **55**:261–274.
41. Byers LD, Wolfenden R. A potent reversible inhibitor of carboxypeptidase. *J Biol Chem* 1972; **247**:606–608.
42. Byers LD, Wolfenden R. Binding of the biproduct analog benzylsuccinic acid by carboxypeptidase. *Biochemistry* 1973; **12**:2070–2078.
43. Ondetti MA, Rubin B, Cushman DW. Design of specific inhibitors of angiotensin-converting enzyme: New class of orally active antihypertensive agents. *Science* 1977; **196**:441–444.

44. Ferguson RK, Brunner HR, Turini GA, Garvras H, McKinistry DN. A specific orally active inhibitor of angiotensin-converting enzyme in man. *Lancet* 1077; **1**:775–778.
45. Johnston CI, McGrath BP, Millar JA, Matthews PG. Long-term effects of captopril (SQ 14 225) on blood-pressure and hormone levels in essential hypertension. *Lancet* 1979; **2**:493–495.
46. Rubin B, Laffan RJH, Kotler DG, O'Keefe EH, DeMaio DA, Goldberg ME. SQ 14,225 (D-3-mercapto-2-methylpropanoyl-L-proline), a novel orally active inhibitor of angiotensin I converting enzyme. *J Pharmacol Exp Ther* 1978; **204**:271–280.

SUMMARY

This paper traces the history and phylogeny of the renin-angiotensin system (RAS). The background to the discovery of renin, the juxtaglomerular apparatus, and the vasoactive end-product, angiotensin, is described. Skeggs first discovered hypertensin-converting enzyme, which after isolation was renamed angiotensin converting enzyme (ACE). The discovery of kininase II—the enzyme that destroys bradykinin—was made through a completely different route, and only later was shown to be identical to ACE. The first ACE inhibitors were preceded by bradykinin-potentiating factor (BPF) found in the venom of the South American pit viper. Subsequently, these inhibitory substances were shown to be peptides which were then purified, sequenced, and synthesized. These synthetic peptides inhibited ACE. The goal was to design a potent, specific, orally-active ACE inhibitor. The development of the first and subsequent generations of ACE inhibitors is traced, and future areas of interest are discussed.

RÉSUMÉ

Cette étude retrace l'historique et la phylogénie du système rénineangiotensine. On décrit ce qui a amené à la découverte de la rénine, du mécanisme juxtaglomérulaire, et de l'élément vaso-acteur, l'angiotensine. Skeggs a été le premier à découvrir l'enzyme de conversion de l'hypertensine, qui, après isolation, a changé de nom et a pris celui d'enzyme de conversion de l'angiotensine (IEC). La découverte de la kininase, enzyme destructeur de la bradykinine, s'est faite de façon complètement différente et ce n'est que plus tard qu'on a prouvé qu'elle était identique à l'enzyme de conversion de l'angiotensine. Le facteur de potentialisation de la bradykinine, que l'on a découvert dans le venin de vipères en Amérique du Sud a donc précédé les premiers inhibiteurs de l'enzyme de conversion de l'angiotensine. Par la suite, on a montré que ces substances étaient des peptides qui ont alors été purifiés, mis en séquence, et synthétisés. Ces peptides synthétiques inhibaient l'enzyme de conversion de l'angiotensine. L'objectif était de créer un inhibiteur de l'enzyme de conversion de l'angiotensine qui soit puissant, spécifique et susceptible d'être administré par voie buccale. On retrace ici le développement des générations successives d'inhibiteurs de l'enzyme de conversion de l'angiotensine et on discute des voies à envisager pour l'avenir.

ZUSAMMENFASSUNG

Diese Veröffentlichung verfolgt die Geschichte und Phylogenie des Renin-Angiotensin-Systems (RAS). Beschrieben wird die Entdeckungsgeschichte des Renins, des juxta-glomerulären Apparates und des vasoaktiven Endprodukts Angiotensin. Skeggs entdeckte zunächst das Hypertensin-konvertierende Enzym, das nach seiner Isolierung umbenannt wurde in Angiotensin-konvertierendes Enzym (ACE). Die Entdeckung der Kininase II, dem Enzym, das Bradykinin zerstört, folgte hingegen einem völlig anderen Weg; und die Identität mit ACE konnte erst später gezeigt werden. Die ersten ACE-Inhibitoren folgten auf die Entdeckung des Bradykinin-potenzierenden Faktors (BPF) im Gift der südamerikanischen Höhlenviper. Später konnte gezeigt werden, dass diese inhibitorisch wirkenden Substanzen aus Peptiden bestehen, die dann gereinigt, sequentiert und synthetisiert wurden. Diese synthetischen Peptide wirkten inhibitorisch gegenüber ACE. Das Ziel war, einen potenten, spezifischen und oral aktiven ACE Inhibitor zu finden. Beschrieben wird die Entwicklung des ersten ACE Inhibitors und folgender Generationen, und zukünftige Interessengebiete werden diskutiert.

RIASSUNTO

Questo articolo ripercorre la storia e filogenia del sistema renina-angiotensina (SRA). Viene descritto il background della scoperta della renina, dell'apparato juxtaglomerulare e del prodotto vasoattivo finale, l'angiotensina. Skeggs scoperse l'enzima transformatore dell'ipertensina che, dopo essere stato isolato, venne ribattezzato enzima isomerizzante dell'angiotensina (EIA). La scoperta del chininase II I/M, l'enzima che distrugge la bradichinina I/M, venne fatta sequendo un percorso completamente diverso e solo in seguito si dimostrò essere identico all'EIA. I primi inibitori dell' EIA furono preceduti dal fattore di potenziamento della bradichinina, trovato nel veleno del crotalo sudamericano. In seguito tali sostanze inibitrici si dimostrarono essere dei peptidi che vennero quindi purificati, sequenziati e sintetizzati. Questi peptidi sintetici inibivano l'EIA. L'obiettivo era di realizzare un inibitore potente e specifico dell'EIA, attivo per via orale. Viene trattato lo sviluppo della prima e delle successive generazioni di inibitori dell'EIA e vengono discussi vari aspetti che interessano la ricerca futura.

SUMÁRIO

Traçam-se a história e a filogenia do sistema renina-angiotensina (RAS). Describem-se os antecedentes à descoberta da renina, o aparelho justaglomerular e o produto vasoativo final, a angiotensina. Skeggs foi o primeiro em descobrir a enzima convertidora da hipertensina, que após de islada se rebatizou "enzima convertidora da angiotensina" (ACE). A descoberta da quinin-asa II—a enzima que destrói a bradiquinina—efeituou-se através de uma ruta completamente diferente, e só mais tarde demonstrou-se que é idêntica à ACE. Os primeiros inibidores da ACE foram precedidos pelo fator potencia-dor da bradiquinina (BPF) encontrado no veneno de uma víbora sulameri-cana. Posteriormente, demonstrouse que estas substâncias inibidoras são peptídios, que em seguida foram purificados, seqüenciados e sintetizados. Estos peptídios sintéticos inibiam a ACE. O objetivo era de disenhar um inibidor da ACE potente, específico e de atividade oral. Discutem-se o desen-volvimento das gerações primeiras e posteriores dos inibidores da ACE, assim como as áreas de interesse no futuro.

RESUMEN

Este trabajo bosqueja la historia y filogenia del sistema renina-angiotensina (RAS). Se describen los antecedentes al descubrimiento de la renina, el apar-ato yuxtaglomerular y el producto vasoactivo, la angiotensina. Skeggs fue el primero en descubrir la enzima convertidora de la hipertensina, que después de aislada se rebautizó "enzima convertidora de la angiotensina" (ACE). El descubrimiento de la quininasa II—la enzima que destruye la bradiquinina—se efectuó a través de una ruta completamente diferente, y sólo más tarde se demostró que es idéntica a la ACE. Los primeros inhibidores de la ACE fueron precedidos por el factor de potenciación de la bradiquinina (BPF) encontrado en el veneno de una víbora sudamericana. Posteriormente se demostró que estas sustancias inhibidoras son péptidos, que a continuación se purificaron, estableciéndose su secuencia y efectuándose su síntesis. Estos péptidos sintéticos inhibían a la ACE. El objetivo era desarrollar un inhibidor de la ACE potente, específico y de actividad oral. Se discute el desarrollo de los primeros inhibidores de la ACE y las generaciones subsecuentes, así como futuras áreas de interés.

要約

本論文では，レニン-アンジオテンシン系（RAS）の発見・研究の経緯ならびに系統発生をたどる。レニンの発見の背景，傍糸球体装置，および血管作動性最終産物であるアンジオテンシンについて述べる。

Skeggs は初めてハイパーテンシン変換酵素を発見した。これは単離同定後，アンジオテンシン変換酵素（ACE）と改名された。一方，ブラディキニン分解酵素であるキニナーゼⅡは，まったく別の研究過程でみつけられ，のちに ACE と同一のものであることが判明した。

　最初の ACE 阻害薬は，南米産ガラガラヘビの毒液中に見出されたブラディキ
ニン増強因子(BPF)からつくられた。ついで，これらの阻害物質はペプチドであ
ることがわかり，分離精製，アミノ酸配列の決定，そして合成がなされた。これ
らの合成ペプチドは確かに ACE を阻害した。最終目標は強力で特異性の高い，経
口可能な ACE 阻害薬をつくりだすことであった。

　ここでは，ACE 阻害薬の最初のものから次世代のものまでの開発経緯をあとづ
け，将来の興味の焦点について考察する。

Cardiac and Renal Failure: An Expanding Role for ACE Inhibitors, edited by C. T. Dollery and L. M. Sherwood, Hanley & Belfus, Inc., Philadelphia.

Molecular Cloning of Human Vascular Angiotensin I-Converting Enzyme

Florent Soubrier, François Alhenc-Gelas, Christine Hubert, Jacqueline Allegrini and Pierre Corvol

The angiotensin I-converting enzyme (peptidyl dipeptidase A, EC 3.4.15.1) plays a key role in the control of blood pressure and water and salt metabolism by hydrolyzing angiotensin I (ANG I) into angiotensin II (ANG II). The same enzyme is able to inactivate bradykinin by the release of a C-terminal dipeptide and was originally called kininase II by Erdos.[1] Angiotensin I-converting enzyme (ACE) is not specific for ANG I and bradykinin. It can cleave many other substrates by releasing a C-terminal dipeptide from enkephalins, neurotensin, and substance P free acid.[1] More importantly, ACE is not a pure carboxy-dipeptidase since it can act as a peptidyl-tripeptidase by removing a C-terminal tripeptide from des-Arg[9] bradykinin. In fact, ACE can even be considered as an endopeptidase, since it can remove a C-terminal dipeptide or tripeptide from a protected C-terminal peptide, such as substance P.

ACE is a metallopeptidase with a zinc atom in its active center. Its activity can therefore be inhibited by metal chelating agents. In addition, the enzymatic activity of ACE depends strongly on the presence of chloride ions, its activity being abolished by extensive dialysis against chloride free buffer. In this regard, the chloride dependence of ACE activity is unique among the metallo-peptidase family.

ACE is a widely distributed peptidase occurring, for example, as a membrane-bound ectoenzyme on the surface of vascular endothelial cells and renal epithelial cells, and also as a circulating enzyme in plasma (Figure 1). The estimated molecular size for kidney ACE is 170 Kdaltons (170 K). A second type of ACE with a smaller molecular size (100 K) was found in the testis. This enzyme has the same enzymatic activity as endothelial and epithelial ACE. Although the physiological role of ACE in extravascular tissues

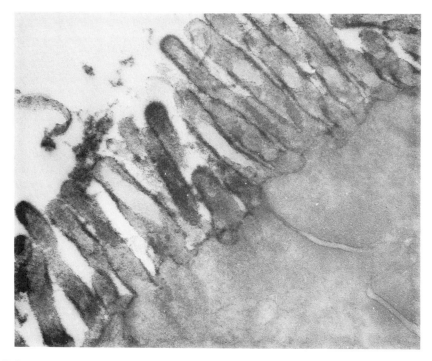

FIG. 1. Ultrastructural immunohistochemistry shows that the angiotensin I-converting enzyme is localized in the apical plasmallemal membrane, mainly in the brush border of human intestinal cells. Polyclonal antihuman renin antibody revealed with PAP technique. Normal human jejunum. Magnification × 90,000.

remains a matter of current debate, it is well established that the enzyme present in vascular endothelium and in plasma plays an essential role in circulatory homeostasis, because it activates ANG I into the potent vasopressor and aldosterone-stimulating peptide, ANG II.

For this reason, inhibitors of ACE have been recently designed as therapeutic agents and are widely used for the treatment of hypertension and cardiac failure. These inhibitors were designed on the basis of similarities of the enzymatic properties of ACE with those of carboxypeptidase A.[2] However, no structural information was available on ACE or on the nature of its active site. A recent paper by Bernstein *et al*[3] reported the isolation of a cDNA fragment of mouse kidney ACE. The present study summarizes the recent work published by our group[4] on the complete structure of human endothelial ACE as revealed by molecular cloning.

PURIFICATION AND PARTIAL SEQUENCING OF ACE

The cortex of fresh post-mortem kidneys was minced, suspended in potassium phosphate buffer 20 mM, pH 8, containing a mixture of protease inhibitors, and homogenized. The particulate fraction was then sedimented by centrifugation at 105,000 g for 1 hour; the pellet was then resuspended in potassium phosphate buffer and treated for 18 h with the detergent CHAPS 8 mM (Serva). The supernatant obtained after centrifugation at 105,000 g for 1 hour was dialyzed to remove CHAPS and then applied to a column of phenyl-Sepharose 4B (Pharmacia). The enzyme activity was retained and eluted as a single peak after applying a linear gradient of CHAPS up to 10 mM. The purification was completed by affinity chromatography on Lisinopril-Sepharose 4B, as described.[5] The protein isolated after this last step was analyzed by SDS polyacrylamide gel electrophoresis. The purified ACE migrated as a single species with an apparent molecular mass of 170 Kdaltons. Its enzymatic activity, determined with furanacryloyl-L-phenylalanyl-glycyl-glycine (FAPGG) as substrate, showed apparent kinetic constants equal to 136 μM for K_m and 22100 min^{-1} for k_{cat}, similar to those measured for the rabbit pulmonary enzyme.

The NH$_2$-terminal amino-acid sequence analysis, performed by M. John and G. Tregear at the Howard Florey Institute (Melbourne, Australia), revealed a high degree of similarity with NH$_2$-terminal sequences of the rabbit and calf pulmonary ACE, and of the pig and mouse renal enzymes.[4] Thirteen internal peptidic sequences were also obtained after cleavage of ACE by cyanogen bromide and purification of the peptide fragments by reverse phase HPLC. Among the thirteen sequences identified, the peptide sequence [Met]-Trp-Ala-Gln-Ser-Trp-Glu-Asn-Ile completed by the putative preceding methionine (in brackets) was selected to synthesize a 64-fold redundant mixed oligomer on an automated DNA synthesizer (Gene Assembler, Pharmacia).

SCREENING OF HUMAN ENDOTHELIAL cDNA LIBRARIES AND NUCLEOTIDE SEQUENCING

A human umbilical vein endothelial cell cDNA library primed with oligo (dT) and constructed in λgt11 (Clonetech Lab. Inc.) was screened with the above ^{32}P-labeled oligomer. Two different clones were obtained by screening this library. They overlapped on 2323 base pairs and span 3840 nucleotides of the ACE mRNA. In order to obtain the cDNA corresponding to the 5' end of the mRNA, another endothelial cell cDNA library was constructed in our laboratory, and primed with an oligomer complementary to a 17-base sequence located near the 5' extremity of the more 5' clone, and with oligo (dT). A 300 bp DNA restriction fragment, isolated in this laboratory from a human ACE gene clone, λ1915, was used to screen the cDNA library. Several independent positive clones were obtained; three of them were selected and found to have a similar size of around 250 bp and an identical sequence. They contained the 5′ end of the coding sequence of ACE mRNA together with a short nontranslated region.

For nucleotide sequencing, phage inserts were subcloned in both orientations into the EcoRI site of plasmid vector Bluescript (Stratagene). Single-strand DNA was prepared by infection of cultures with M13 helper phage KO7 and sequenced by the chain termination method. Both strands of all regions were sequenced using the modified T7 polymerase (Sequenase, US Biochemical). All the 13 internal peptidic sequences and the NH$_2$-terminal amino acid sequence were found in the protein sequence deduced from the clones.

GENERAL STRUCTURE OF HUMAN ACE

Primary structure

The nucleotide sequence of ACE cDNA obtained by sequencing the three overlapping clones comprises 4024 nucleotides. The 3′ end of the sequence does not extend to the polyadenylation signal. The open reading frame from the first ATG codon until the stop codon TGA encodes 1306 amino acids. The complete amino-acid sequence of human ACE has been published by Soubrier et al.[4] The NH$_2$-terminal amino acid leucine determined by protein sequencing is located after a signal peptide of 29 residues. The exact length of this signal peptide is known, since the NH$_2$-terminal of the mature kidney enzyme was determined in this study. There are 17 potential asparagine-linked glycosylation sites in the molecule, mostly grouped in the amino terminal region of the protein and in the region located at the junction between the two homologous domains. Glycosylation of the protein explains the apparent discrepancy between a calculated Mr of 146.6 K for the mature enzyme and the value of 170 K observed by gel electrophoresis.

Several interesting features emerge from the amino acid structure of ACE (Figure 2).

Internal Homology. Evidence For Gene Duplication and
For Two Putative Catalytic Centers.

One striking feature was the presence of a high degree of internal homology. Two domains could be delimited in the sequence that are surrounded by nonhomologous regions. At the amino acid level the overall similarity calculated on 356 residues is 67.7%. The identity is maximal in the central part of these two domains where, for example, a similarity of 89% is observed for

STRUCTURE OF HUMAN ACE

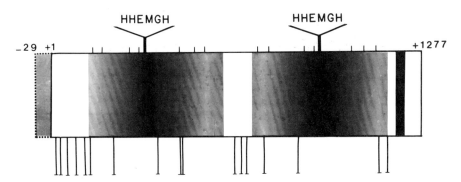

FIG. 2. Schematic structure of human ACE as revealed by molecular cloning and amino-acid sequencing. A signal peptide (29 amino-acids) is first encoded and rapidly cleaved off during maturation. The mature enzyme comprises two homologous domains symbolized by dark areas. Within each domain, a putative active center is able to coordinate the Zinc atom and to attack the peptide bond to be cleaved (indicated by the one-letter code). Near the carboxy-terminus is located a hydrophobic region (in dark) that likely inserts ACE into the plasma membrane. The position of cysteine residues and the potential asparagine-linked glycosylation sites are indicated by vertical bars above or below the diagram of ACE, respectively.

segments situated between amino acids 361-404 and 959-1002 and comprising essential residues of the putative active site (see below). The number and positions of the cysteine residues are the same in the two domains, indicating that possibilities for establishing intramolecular disulfide bridges are conserved.

A computer-assisted search revealed no clear significant homology with any other protein in the NBRF bank. However, short segmental identities were revealed when alignment was made with the regions involved in catalytic activity of thermolysin, another zinc protease.[6] From the x-ray structure analysis of this protein made by Kester and Mathews,[7] two histidine (142 and 146) and a glutamic acid residue (166) were found to coordinate the zinc atom. Corresponding residues are also found in the two domains of ACE. Another glutamic acid (Glu 143) located between histidine 142 and 146 of thermolysin, which acts as a general base in catalysis, is again found in the two domains of ACE. Finally, another possible homology is observed around histidine 231 of thermolysin, which stabilizes the transition state by formation of a hydrogen bond to the water molecule with the oxygen of the scissile bond to be cleaved. This histidine residue is conserved in the two domains of ACE (Figure 3). Similar short sequences were also observed in the corresponding regions of rat or rabbit neutral endopeptidase (NEP), a Zn-metalloendopeptidase able to hydrolyze enkephalins, kinins and several neuropeptides, like ACE, but with different efficiency and sensitivity to inhibitors.[8,9]

Analysis of ACE structure reveals that the region homologous to the cata-

hACE	T	V	H	H	E	M	G	H	365		E	A	I	391
hACE	V	A	H	H	E	M	G	H	963		E	A	I	989
THERM	V	V	A	H	E	L	T	H	146		E	A	I	168
rNEP	V	I	G	H	E	I	T	H	581/588					

hACE	H	L	H	K	-	I	-	G	409
hACE	H	L	H	S	-	L	-	N	1007
THERM	H	I	N	S	G	I	I	N	238
rNEP	H	L	N	-	G	I	-	N	635/643

FIG. 3. Homology between amino-acid sequence (one-letter notation) of human ACE (hACE), thermolysin from *Bacillus thermoproteolyticus* (THERM)[6] rat, or rabbit neutral endopeptidase (rNEP).[8,9] The first and second lines refer to the first and second domains of ACE. Numbers refer to the last amino-acid position in each protein segment. Identical residues are boxed. Gaps are indicated by dashes.

lytic sites of thermolysin and neutral endopeptidase is present twice in the molecule. These two putative catalytic centers are located within the most homologous part of the two domains of ACE. Whether both of these putative active sites of ACE are involved in catalysis cannot be determined from sequence analysis. It has, however, been reported that each molecule of enzyme contains only one atom of zinc, suggesting that only one domain is able to coordinate the metal.[10] Likewise binding studies with competitive ACE inhibitors suggest a single class of site.[11] These observations may indicate that, despite its repetitive structure, ACE has only one functional active site per molecule.

The sequence of ACE cDNA indicates that it most probably results from a gene duplication. Since other known mammalian ACEs are of a similar size, it is likely that they also result from a gene duplication that occurred before mammalian radiation. The high degree of similarity between the two domains could suggest that they both remained under selective pressure.

Anchoring of ACE to Plasma Membranes.
Relation with Soluble Circulating ACE

ACE is a membrane-bound ectoenzyme largely distributed on the endothelial surface of the pulmonary vessels. It is also bound to the cell membrane in structures specialized for reabsorption of water and solutes, such as brush borders of renal, intestinal and choroid epithelial cells. The mature enzyme is most probably anchored to the cell membrane by its carboxy-terminal hydrophobic segment. Indeed, a search for membrane associated helices indicates that only two regions have the highest probability of being involved in membrane insertion, one being the peptide signal which is cleaved off during maturation, the other being located near the C-terminus. Hooper *et al.*[12] have shown that membrane-bound pig kidney ACE can be solubilized by detergent or trypsin treatment, but not by phospholipases, and that the enzyme solubilized by either treatment has similar molecular weight and identical NH_2-terminal sequence, suggesting direct attachment by the carboxy-terminal part of the molecule. However an attachment through a glycosyl-phosphatidylinositol, as in the case of some other kidney microvillar ectoenzymes, cannot be excluded.[13]

The relationships between the anchored cellular enzyme and its circulating form have yet to be elucidated. The plasma enzyme probably originates from the vascular endothelium and is enzymatically and immunologically identical to the solubilized membrane bound enzyme.[14,15] Several hypotheses can be proposed: (1) No evidence for a second ACE mRNA was found in endothelial cells in culture, which seems to exclude that the circulating enzyme proceeds from a second mRNA generated by alternate splicing; (2) An enzymatic cleavage of the anchored enzyme could occur leading to the soluble enzyme. However, no consensus processing region close to the hydrophobic helix inserted into the membrane was detected from the primary amino acid sequence; (3) Finally, the soluble form of the enzyme might be released from the plasma membrane by passive linkage, a phenomenon that has been involved in the generation of some plasma enzymes from liver origin.

Presence of a Single ACE Gene in Human Genome.
Possible Alternate RNA Splicing of Testicular Enzyme

Soubrier et al.[4] found by Southern hydridization the presence of one ACE gene per human haploid genome encoding the different forms of ACE. Northern blot experiments showed that endothelial ACE mRNA is 4.3 kb long, whereas a shorter testicular ACE mRNA was detected (3kb). This observation is in agreement with the observation of El Dorry et al.[16] who found that testicular ACE is synthesized as a shorter polypeptide chain than the vascular endothelial enzyme. High level of sequence similarity was found by alignment with the seven internal tryptic peptide sequences of rabbit testicular ACE determined by Soffer et al.[17] The results of the present study suggest that the testicular ACE mRNA and the endothelial ACE mRNA result from differential splicing of the gene transcript.

The cloning of human testicular ACE cDNA will help to elucidate the relationship between the vascular and the testicular forms of ACE. It will also reveal which of the two catalytic sites might be functional, since testicular ACE should possess only one of the domains of vascular ACE, according to the size of its mRNA and of its gene product (100 K).

Basic and Clinical Implications from the Elucidation of ACE Structure

The discovery of two putative active centers in ACE structure deserves further study. Although only one mole of radiolabeled ACE inhibitor is bound with a high affinity per mole of enzyme, it is possible that the second site loosely binds captopril or other inhibitors. Another catalytic function, other than the formation of ANG II from ANG I, may also exist for the second putative catalytic site. It is possible that the second catalytic site is demasked or alters the function of the first catalytic center in certain conditions (circulating enzyme vs membrane-bound enzyme, different tissue localization of ACE, . . .). The mechanism of action of chloride ion on the activity of the enzyme is not known at the molecular level. Site-directed mutagenesis and ultimately crystallization of the enzyme will help in elucidating its mode of action.

The level of human plasma ACE is constant within a normal individual but varies from 1 to 5 between individuals (J. Richard, F. Alhenc-Gelas, *et al.*, unpublished results). Cambien *et al.*[18] have shown that there was a genetic determination of plasma ACE levels. It will be interesting to link plasma ACE levels with the different ACE genotypes, as determined by RFLP of the ACE gene.

REFERENCES

1. Erdös EG, Skidgel RA. The angiotensin I-converting enzyme (editorial). *Lab Invest* 1987; **56**:345–348.
2. Ondetti MA, Rubin B, Cushman DW. Design of specific inhibitors of angiotensin-converting enzyme: New class of orally active antihypertensive agents. *Science* 1977; **196**:441–444.
3. Bernstein KE, Martin BM, Bernstein EA, Linton J, Striker L, Striker G. The isolation of angiotensin-converting enzyme cDNA. *J Biol Chem* 1988; **263**:11021–11024.
4. Soubrier F, Alhenc-Gelas F, Hubert C, Allegrini J, John M, Tregear G, Corvol P. Two putative active centers in human angiotensin I-converting enzyme revealed by molecular cloning. *Proc Natl Acad Sci* 1988; **85**:9386–9390.
5. Bull HG, Thornberry NA, Cordes EH. Purification of angiotensin-converting enzyme from rabbit lung and human plasma by affinity chromatography. *J Biol Chem* 1985; **260**:2963–2972.
6. Titani K, Hermodson MA, Ericsson LH, Walsh KA, Neurath H. Amino-acid sequence of thermolysin. *Nature New Biol* 1972; **238**:35–37.
7. Kester WR, Matthews BW. Crystallographic study of the binding of dipeptide inhibitors to thermolysin: implications for the mechanism of catalysis. *Biochemistry* 1977; **16**:2506–2516.
8. Malfroy B, Schofield PR, Kuang WJ, Seeburg PH, Mason AJ, Henzel WJ. Molecular cloning and amino acid sequence of rat enkephalinase. *Biochem Biophys Res Commun* 1987; **144**:59–66.
9. Devault A, Lazure C, Nault C, Le Moual H, Seidah NG, Chretien M, Kahn P, Powell J, Mallet J, Beaumont A, Roques BP, Crine P, Boileau G. Amino acid sequence of rabbit kidney neutral endopeptidase 24.11 (enkephalinase) deduced from a complementary cDNA. *EMBO J* 1987; **6**:1317–1322.
10. Das M, Soffer RL. Pulmonary angiotensin converting enzyme structural and catalytic properties. *J Biol Chem* 1975; **250**:6762–6768.
11. Strittmatter SM, Snyder SH. Characterization of angiotensin converting enzyme by [H³] captopril binding. *Mol Pharmacol* 1986; **29**:142–148.
12. Hooper N, Keen J, Pappin DJC, Turner AJ. Pig kidney angiotensin converting enzyme: Purification and characterization of amphypathic and hydrophilic forms of the enzyme establishes C-terminal anchorage to the plasma membrane. *Biochem J* 1987; **247**:85–93.
13. Hooper NM, Turner AJ. Ectoenzymes of the kidney microvillar membrane. *Biochem J.* 1988; **250**:865–869.
14. Das M, Hartley JL, Soffer RL. Serum angiotensin-converting enzyme isolation and relationship to the pulmonary enzyme. *J Biol Chem* 1977; **252**:1316–1319.

15. Alhenc-Gelas F, Weare JA, Johnson RL Jr, Erdös EG. Measurement of converting enzyme level by direct radioimmunoassy. *J Lab Clin Med* 1983; **101**:83–96.
16. El-Dorry HA, Pickett CB, MacGregor JS, Soffer RL. Tissue-specific expression of mRNA for dipeptidyl carboxypeptidase isoenzymes. *Proc Natl Acad Sci* (*USA*) 1982; **79**:4295–4297.
17. Soffer RL, Berg T, Sulner J, Lai CY. Pulmonary and testicular angiotensin-converting isoenzymes. *Clin Exp Hypertens Theory Practice* 1987; **A9 (2 and 3)**: 229–234.
18. Cambien F, Alhenc-Gelas F, Herbeth B, Andre JL, Rakotovao R, Gonzales MF, Allegrini J, Bloch C. Familial resemblance of plasma angiotensin-converting enzyme level. *Am J Hum Genet* 1988; **43**:774–780.

SUMMARY

The primary amino-acid sequence of human vascular endothelial cell angiotensin I-converting enzyme (ACE) has been determined from molecular cloning of its cDNA. The mature enzyme is produced after cleavage of a signal peptide and its probably anchored to plasma membrane by an hydrophobic sequence located near its carboxy terminal. The most striking feature of ACE is the presence of a high degree of internal homology between two large domains, which suggests that the molecule is the result of a gene duplication. Each domain bears a putative active site, according to their close similarities, with short amino-acid sequences located around critical residues of the other endometallopeptidases. Since earlier experiments suggest the presence of a single zinc atom bound with each molecule of ACE, only one of the two domains should be catalytically active. Genomic DNA analysis with the cDNA probe is consistent with the presence of a single gene for ACE in the haploid human genome. Whereas the ACE gene is transcribed as a 4.3 kb mRNA species in vascular endothelial cells, a 3.0 kb transcript was detected in the testis where a shorter form of ACE is synthesized.

RÉSUMÉ

La séquence amino-acide de l'enzyme de conversion de l'angiotensine I de la cellule endothéliale vasculaire humaine a été déterminée à partir du cloning moléculaire de son acide désoxyribonucléique complémentaire (cADN). L'enzyme mûr est produit après le clivage d'un peptide témoin et est probablement ancré à la membrane plasmatique par une séquence hydrophobique située près de son extrêmité carboxyique. La caractéristique la plus frappante de l'enzyme de conversion de l'angiotensine est la présence d'un haut degré d'homologie interne entre deux domaines importants, ce qui suggère que la molécule résulte d'une duplication du gène. Chaque domaine a un site putatif actif, selon leurs étroites ressemblances, avec de courtes séquences amino-acides situées autour des résidus critiques des autres endometallopeptidases. Puisque des études antérieures suggèrent la présence d'un seul atome de zinc fixé à chaque molécule de l'enzyme de conversion de l'angiotensine, seul un des deux domaines devrait être catalytiquement actif. L'analyse génomique de l'acide désoxyribonucléique (ADN) avec la sonde d'un ADN complémentaire (cADN) est conforme à la présence d'un gène unique pour l'enzyme de conversion de l'angiotensine dans le génome humain haploïde. Tandis que le gène de l'enzyme de conversion de l'angiotensine est transcrit comme une espèce de mARN de 4,3 kb dans les cellules endothéliales vasculaires, on a détecté une transcription de 3,0 kb dans le testicule où une forme plus courte de l'enzyme de conversion de l'angiotensine est synthétisée.

ZUSAMMENFASSUNG

Die primäre Aminosäuresequenz des menschlichen Vaskular-Endothelialzellen-Angiotensin I konvertierenden Enzyms ACE ist bestimmt worden durch Cloning seiner cDNA. Das reife Enzym wird nach der Spaltung eines Signal-Peptids produziert und ist wahrscheinlich durch eine hydrophobe Sequenz in der Nähe seiner Carboxy Endgruppe mit der Plasma-Membran verbunden. Auffällig ist die Anwesenheit einer hochgradigen internen Homologie zwischen zwei grossen Teilsequenzen, was andeutet, dass das Molekül aus einer Genduplikation resultiert. Jede dieser Teilsequenzen trät eine wahrscheinlich aktive Gruppe, wenn man die Ähnlichkeit mit kurzen Aminosäuresequenzen in Betracht zieht, die in der Nachbarschaft kritischer Überreste der anderen Endometallopeptidasen lokalisiert sind. Nur eine der beiden Teilsequenzen sollte katalytisch aktiv sein, da frühere Experimente auf die Anwesenheit nur eines einzigen Zinkatoms pro ACE-Molekülbindung hinweisen. Die genome DNA-Analyse an der cDNA-Probe ist in Übereinstimmung mit der Anwesenheit eines einzigen Gens für ACE im haploiden menschlichen Genom. Während das ACE-Gen als eine 4,3 kb mRNA Spezies in vaskular-endothelialen Zellen beschrieben wird, wurde in den Hoden, wo eine kürzere ACE-Form synthetisiert wird, eine Transkription von 3,0 kb gefunden.

RIASSUNTO

La sequenza aminoacida primaria dell'enzima isomerizzante dell'angiotensina I (EIA) delle cellule vascolari endoteliali umane è stato ottenuto mediante clonazione molecolare del suo cDNA. L'enzima maturo viene prodotto in seguito a segmentazione di un peptide di segnalazione ed è probabilmente ancorato alla membrana plasmatica da una sequenza idrofobica situata vicino alla sua estremità carbossile. La caratteristica più interessante dell'EIA è la presenza di un alto grado di omologia interna fra due grandi settori, il che fa pensare che la molecola sia il risultato di una duplicazione genica. Ogni settore comporta un sito attivo putativo, secondo le loro strette somiglianze, con corte sequenze aminoacide situate attorno a residui critici degli altri endometallopeptidasi. Dato che precedenti esperimenti sembrano indicare la presenza di un unico atomo di zinco legato a ciascuna molecola di EIA, solo uno dei due domini dovrebbe essere cataliticamente ativo. L'analisi genomica del DNA mediante la sonda cDNA è coerente con la presenza di un unico gene per l'EIA nel genoma umano aploide. Benchè il gene EIA sia trascritto come una specie mRNA da 4,3 kb in cellule vascolari endoteliali, si è riscontrata una trascrizione di 3.0 kb nel teste, dove viene sintetizzata una forma più corta di EIA.

SUMÁRIO

A seqüência aminoácida primária da ACE (enzima convertidora da célula endotelial vascular humana angiotensina I) tem-se determinado a partir da duplicação molecular do seu cDNA. A enzima madura é produzida após da clivagem de um peptídio sinalizador e provavelmente é ancorada à membrana plasmática mediante uma seqüência hidrofóbica localizada cerca do seu terminal carboxi. A característica mais notável da ACE é a presença de um alto grau de homologia interna entre dois grandes domínios, o que sugere que a molécula é o resultado de uma duplicação de genes. Cada domínio mantém um sítio ativo putativo, de acordo com a sua verdadeira similaridade, com outras seqüências aminoácidas curtas localizadas nos arredores de restos cíticos endometalopeptidasas. Devido a que experimentos anteriores sugerem a presença de um átomo único de zinco ligado a cada molécula da ACE, só um dos dois domínios deve ser cataliticamente ativo. A análise genômica do DNA com uma sonda de cDNA indica a presença de um gene único para a ACE no genoma haplóide humano. Enquanto que o gene da ACE é transcrito como uma espécie mRNA de 4,3 kb nas células endoteliais vasculares, detectou-se uma transcrição de 3,0 kb no testículo, que sintetiza uma forma mais curta da ACE.

RESUMEN

La secuencia aminoácida primaria de la enzima convertidora de la angiotensina I (ACE) de la célula endotelial vascular humana se ha determinado a partir de la duplicación molecular de su cDNA. La enzima madura es producida después de la segmentación de un péptido señalador y probablemente es enclavada en la membrana plasmática mediante una secuencia hidrofóbica ubicada cerca de su carboxi-terminal. La característica más sorprendente de la ACE es la presencia de un alto grado de homología interna entre dos amplios dominios, lo que sugiere que la molécula es el resultado de una duplicación de genes. Cada dominio mantiene un supuesto sitio activo, de acuerdo a su verdadera similaridad, con otras secuencias aminoácidas cortas ubicadas en los alrededores de restos críticos de otras endometalopeptidasas. Debido a que experimentos anteriores sugieren la presencia de un átomo único de cinc ligado a cada molécula de la ACE, solo uno de los dos dominios debe ser catalíticamente activo. El análisis genómico del DNA con una sonda de cDNA indica la presencia de un gen único para la ACE en el genoma haploide humano. Mientras el gen de la ACE es transcrito como una especie mRNA de 4,3 kb en las células endoteliales vasculares, se detectó una transcripción de 3,0 kb en el testículo, que sintetiza una forma más corta de la ACE.

要約

　ヒト血管内皮細胞アンジオテンシン I 変換酵素（ACE）の一次構造アミノ酸配列が，その cDNA 分子クローニングによって決定された。シグナルペプチドの開裂後に，完成したかたちの酵素が産生され，これはおそらく，C 末端近傍の疎水性の部分によって細胞質膜につなぎ止められている。

　この ACE の最も注目すべき特徴は，分子内の 2 つの大きな領域が互いに高い相同性をもつということで，この事実は ACE 分子が遺伝子重複の結果生じたものであることを示唆している。いずれの領域とも推定上の活性部位を有している。というのは，他のエンドメタロペプチダーゼの必須残基部分にみられる短いアミノ酸配列と相同の配列がいずれにも存在するからである。以前の研究では，ACE1 分子当り 1 つの亜鉛原子結合しかないことが示唆されており，2 領域の一方しか触媒活性をもたないと考えられる。

　cDNA プローブを用いたゲノム分析の結果は，半数体のヒトゲノムにおいて ACE については 1 つの遺伝子が存在するという見解と一致する。この ACE 遺伝子は血管内皮細胞においては 4.3 kb の mRNA として複写されるが，より短いかたちの ACE が合成されるような実験においては，3.0 kb の複写物が検出された。

Cardiac and Renal Failure: An Expanding Role for ACE Inhibitors, edited by C. T. Dollery and L. M. Sherwood, Hanley & Belfus, Inc., Philadelphia.

DISCUSSION

DOLLERY: Have you any evidence for genetic polymorphism of ACE?

CORVOL: The phenotypic distribution is clearly in favor of a strong familial linkage for plasma ACE. We are studying the genotypic analysis.

GANTEN: How sure are you that there is only one gene coding for converting enzyme? Have you actually sequenced the genomic DNA?

CORVOL: This is clearly a single gene. We have sequenced a good part of the testicular ACE cDNA and it is clearly the result of an alternate gene splicing.

JOHNSTON: In general they all show the same binding characteristics in one site, but the kidney seems to be a bit different from the heart.

CORVOL: There is another way to approach this question of the activities of the two catalytic centers, which is the binding of the zinc atom. It is said that there is one zinc atom bound per mole of ACE. In some circumstances you might unmask the activity of the second center and therefore get different binding.

JOHNSTON: Do you think it may also have a different affinity for an inhibitor? This would make your suggestion that you might eventually design something to fit the second site better than the first site possible.

CORVOL: Yes, it is worth trying.

SONNENBLICK: Is it correct that most of the conversion of ANG I to ANG II takes place in the lungs? If that is so what is the enzyme doing in the other parts of the vascular system?

JOHNSTON: Vane's original suggestion was that the lung was an endocrine organ that produced ANG I. That is not true. In other tissues, destruction of ANG II is more or less balanced by the production of ANG I, whereas in the lung ANG II is not metabolized at all. The lung becomes the only real net exporter of ANG II. Some detailed metabolic clearance studies from the Howard Florey Institute have shown that a lot of tissues contribute to the circulating level of ANG II. For example, the contribution to plasma ANG II from the peripheral circulation of the leg was 15%.

IMURA: Have you studied the expression of the ACE gene in a variety of human tissues and did you find any difference in the size of mRNA except for the testes?

CORVOL: In the lung we found a very low level of mRNA with a 4.3 kb size. We were very surprised, because purifying ACE is quite easy, but detecting it by *in situ* hybridization is very difficult. I suppose that there is a very low turnover rate of this converting enzyme. We spent a year making libraries and were unable to detect the mRNA. The best source is a culture of endothelial cells as they produce a lot of converting enzyme.

SHERWOOD: Dr Corvol, have you had an opportunity to determine factors either *in vitro* or *in vivo* that regulate gene expression of ACE?

CORVOL: There are two very interesting factors. Glucocorticoids are able to increase ACE activity in isolated cells.[1]. We are presently studying this synthesis. Androgens are also able to increase the activity of ACE in testes.

SHERWOOD: Do you know yet whether glucocorticoids or androgens affect the transcription rate?

CORVOL: Not yet.

SCHWARTZ: Alternative splicing for some proteins is known to be a means of regulating the expression of different isoforms during ontogenic development. In addition to the tissue specificity, did you look at the expression of the enzyme during development in the different tissues?

CORVOL: No.

BEARN: May I follow up on Colin Dollery's question on polymorphisms? The observation of a positive correlation coefficient between sibs and not between parents and sibs is very suggestive evidence of a genetic influence. Whether there is a major gene or several major genes will be clarified in the future. For a long time we have been looking for a major molecular genetic influence on hypertension, and this is a very important observation. Moreover, it is not beyond the realm of possibility that in the future we may be able to predict whether patients will respond to any particular antihypertensive agent on the basis of genetic analysis at the molecular level.

CORVOL: Yes, it could be so.

BEARN: There are many examples where the amount of protein synthesized depends on the nature of the specific structural gene. This could be relevant to your data.

CORVOL: You are quite right. It is one of the things it would be wise to do now. It might be important in terms of clinical assessment of the efficacy of ACE inhibitors in some patients.

BEARN: You might be able to determine which patients are more likely to respond than others.

CORVOL: That is right.

MEZEY: Do you have any information regarding the age relationship to ACE content?

CORVOL: Yes we do. ACE appears to be present very early—at 3 months in the human fetus. The content of ACE decreases with age; it is higher in children than in their parents. There is a negative correlation between ACE and age until the age of 20 years.

Cardiac and Renal Failure: An Expanding Role for ACE Inhibitors, edited by C. T. Dollery and L. M. Sherwood, Hanley & Belfus, Inc., Philadelphia.

Mechanisms of Action of ACE Inhibitors

H. R. Brunner, B. Waeber, J. Nussberger

It has been 15 years since angiotensin-converting enzyme (ACE) inhibitors were introduced into clinical research and, in many countries, it has been more than 8 years since the first orally active ACE inhibitor, captopril, was made available for general therapeutic use.[1-4] Today, there are at least four ACE inhibitors marketed worldwide, and several more are soon to be launched. This growing number of new ACE inhibitors reflects their acceptance by physicians as an important therapy for the treatment of clinical hypertension and congestive heart failure.

ACE inhibitors are designed to dissociate the generation of angiotensin II (ANG II) from renin activity. They markedly reduce ANG II levels, by inhibiting the conversion of angiotensin I (ANG I) to ANG II, while actually stimulating renin secretion. Several methods were developed to measure the plasma activity of ACE. However, it was discovered that most conversion of ANG I to ANG II is carried out by converting enzyme in the endothelial cells, primarily in the pulmonary vascular bed.[5] This raises the question of whether or not ACE activity measured in plasma reflects global, *in vivo* conversion. To assess the effect of ACE inhibitors, we must measure ANG II rather than plasma ACE or renin activity.

ACE is chemically identical to kininase II. Thus, it has always been tempting to speculate that ACE inhibition not only reduces ANG II levels but also leads to bradykinin accumulation. While measuring circulating bradykinin is extremely difficult, measuring tissue bradykinin is even harder. Therefore, we cannot be certain if changes in bradykinin (and possibly prostaglandin) levels contribute to the antihypertensive effect of ACE inhibitors.

Rather than attempting to present an exhaustive discussion of all postulated mechanisms of action of ACE inhibitors, which have been reviewed elsewhere,[6] this discussion presents our current understanding of the effects of short- and long-term ACE inhibition on plasma ANG II.

41

IMMUNOREACTIVE "ANGIOTENSIN II" DURING ACE INHIBITION

In 1981, once the efficacy of the converting-enzyme inhibitor, enalapril, had been established in normal volunteers,[7] it was administered to 19 hypertensive patients.[8] When evaluating the data obtained from the measurement of immunoreactive "angiotensin II" (ir-ANG II) and of plasma renin activity, an interesting relationship was observed. Prior to the administration of enalapril, plasma ir-ANG II levels in the 9 patients in whom they were measured correlated very well with plasma renin activity. These results are illustrated in panel A of Figure 1. In all four panels, the initial ir-ANG II to plasma renin activity relationship is depicted as a solid line. Also shown in all panels are two parallel dotted lines that represent the relationship (regression line ± 1 SD from regression) observed previously in normal volunteers 4 and 10 hours after 10 mg of enalapril or lisinopril.[7] Results obtained 4 hours after administration of enalapril are illustrated in panel B of Figure 1. They fall within the range determined in the normal volunteers. Interestingly, even at peak ACE inhibition, there was still a clear and statistically significant correlation between plasma ir-ANG II and plasma renin activity, although the slope of this correlation is shifted considerably compared with that observed prior to the administration of enalapril. In panel C of Figure 1, data obtained 12 to 16 hours following administration of 10 or 20 mg of enalapril are depicted. Plasma ir-ANG II levels tended to increase in some patients (values above the dotted lines), suggesting a tendency for the blockade to wear off. In panel D of Figure 1, plasma ir-ANG II levels after 24 hours of enalapril treatment returned to baseline. However, the normal relationship determined before blockade is still not reached, since the return to baseline of ir-ANG II levels has occurred in the face of a still markedly elevated plasma renin activity. These data suggest that, even during peak ACE inhibition, ir-ANG II levels were influenced by plasma renin activity and ANG I. Two important conclusions can be drawn from these observations: that blockade of ANG II generation by ACE inhibition was not complete even at peak effect, and therefore that the renin and ANG I levels existing during ACE inhibition are more important than originally thought.

In a more recent study using a new ACE inhibitor, trandolapril, similar observations were made (unpublished data on file). This compound was administered to groups of normal volunteers for 10 days at three oral dosage levels, 0.5, 2, and 8 mg once a day. On days 1 and 10, various components of the renin angiotensin system were measured in the plasma before and 2, 4 and 6 hours after drug administration. The results of the measurement of plasma ACE activity clearly correlated with the dose of drug given, indicating a definite dose/inhibition response relationship. This measurement confirmed global ACE inhibition as seen by the ratio of plasma ir-ANG II to ANG I, which was also reduced in a dose-dependent fashion. On day 1, however, and even more so on day 10, the increasing dose of ACE inhibitor induced marked, dose-dependent increases in plasma ANG I levels. Plasma ir-ANG II levels were significantly reduced with the 0.5 mg dosage, but more so on day 10 than on day 1. In contrast, ir-ANG II levels were also reduced with the 8 mg dose, but tended to be higher on day 10 than on day 1. Overall, plasma levels of ir-ANG II on day 10, at peak effectiveness of the drug, were the same with both the 0.5 mg and 8 mg dosages. Thus, once again the prevailing ANG I level appears to determine the plasma ir-ANG II level. Clearly, any therapeutic gain that would have resulted from an increased dose of the ACE inhibitor was offset by the compensatory increase in renin secretion and, consequently, ANG I levels. Assuming that ACE inhibitors reduce blood pressure by reducing plasma ANG II, what is the optimal dose of an ACE inhibitor? It has always seemed doubtful that for any ACE inhibitor increasing the dose, which provides biochemical maximal ACE-inhibition once a day, results in a net therapeutic gain. For the first time, these observations suggesting that increasing doses do not produce lower and lower plasma ANG II levels may provide an explanation for the lack of therapeutic benefit derived from excessive dose increases.

DISSOCIATION BETWEEN ACE INHIBITION AND BLOOD PRESSURE

In the late 1970s, when captopril was still being administered at very high doses, a clear dissociation was observed between the time ACE inhibition occurred and the time blood pressure was reduced.[9] In patients treated for several weeks with captopril, no ACE inhibition could be detected 12 hours after the last dose of 200 mg, though blood pressure remained reduced. The same phenomenon has been observed with enalapril. If administered once a day, it clearly controls blood pressure for 24 hours, despite a return to baseline of plasma ir-ANG II before the next dose of the drug.[8,10] Based on this dissociation, it has been postulated that ACE inhibitors reduce blood pressure by some mechanism that is independent of ANG II, perhaps through the accumulation of bradykinin[11] or an increase in vasodilating prostaglandins.[12] Another explanation for the phenomenon is that, because ACE inhibition may last longer in tissues, ACE inhibitors might reduce blood pressure by inhibiting the conversion of ANG I to ANG II in the vascular wall rather than in plasma.[13-15] While this is a fascinating concept, it is still unclear why, if the theory is true, the ANG II, which reappears in plasma, cannot reach the vascular, or even the intracellular ANG II receptor, when it is known that ANG I and ANG II diffuse easily between plasma and tissues.[16]

Considering this dissociation, it is important to remember how the other antihypertensive drugs work. It is widely recognized that there is no definitive relationship between the plasma half-life of any antihypertensive drug and the duration of its antihypertensive action. It is also widely accepted that there is no apparent correlation between plasma levels after discontinuation of an antihypertensive drug and an increase in blood pressure.[17] Often, it takes

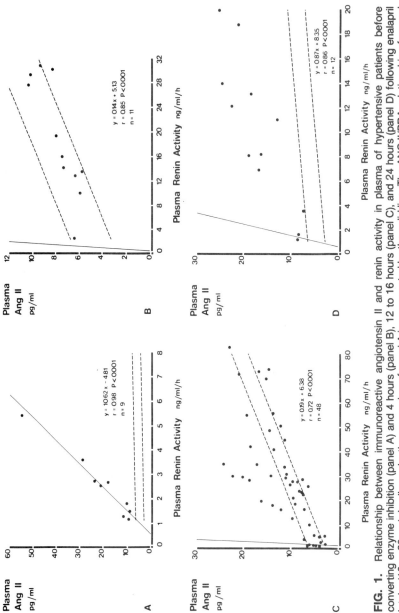

FIG. 1. Relationship between immunoreactive angiotensin II and renin activity in plasma of hypertensive patients before converting enzyme inhibition (panel A) and 4 hours (panel B), 12 to 16 hours (panel C), and 24 hours (panel D) following enalapril intake (10 or 20 mg). In all panels, the regression of panel A is represented by the solid line. The ANG II/PRA-relationship of normal volunteers during peak ACE inhibition (4 and 10 hours following 10 mg enalapril) is represented by the area between the dotted lines (regression ± 1 SD). Recovering from ACE inhibition, ir-ANG II reaches pretreatment levels when PRA is still markedly increased. From Biollaz et al.,[8] with permission.

weeks or months after the drug is stopped before an increase in blood pressure can even be detected. Therefore, this dissociation phenomenon seems to apply not only to ACE inhibitors but to all antihypertensive drugs.

THE MEASUREMENT OF TRUE ANGIOTENSIN-(1-8)OCTAPEPTIDE

The octapeptide, ANG II, along with its precursor decapeptide, ANG I, its C-terminal nonapeptide, and breakdown fragments consisting of 7, 6, 5, and fewer amino-acids circulate in plasma. Chemically, ANG I differs from ANG II in the two amino-acids at the C-terminal. The sequence of reduction to the breakdown fragments of ANG II begins with the N-terminal. Consequently, in order to specifically measure ANG II by radioimmunoassay alone, antibodies are needed which can simultaneously identify the N- and C-terminals.[18] So far, antisera with such properties are not available, and the antisera used most often are only selective for the C-terminal of angiotensin. While these readily differentiate ANG I from ANG II they exhibit considerable cross-reactivity with the smaller fragments. When using such antisera, it is necessary to separate the different angiotensins prior to the radioimmunoassay to improve specificity. This separation can be achieved by high-performance liquid chromatography (HPLC). Detection limits of conventional HPLC procedures are several orders of magnitude higher than the *attomols* measured when calculating the level of ANG II during ACE inhibition. By combining the almost absolute specificity of HPLC with the extreme sensitivity of a radioimmunoassay, it is now possible to specifically measure angiotensin-(1-8)octapeptide with a limit of detection of 0.1 fmol/ml and an overall recovery rate of 80% or more.[19] Moreover, this methodology permits the measurement of the various metabolites of ANG II in plasma. Using this method it was observed that ir-ANG II in plasma does not fall to zero after short-term ACE inhibition because of the presence of cross-reacting angiotensin fragments in plasma.[20]

Even with these vastly improved measurement techniques, there were persistent problems that needed solving. For example, conventional inhibitor cocktails containing EDTA and other peptidase inhibitors did not stop renin activity after blood sampling.[20] To solve the problem of angiotensin generation *in vitro*, Waite introduced the method of whole-blood precipitation, which, if performed immediately after drawing blood, allowed an accurate measurement of circulating ANG I.[21] A similar difficulty arises when attempting to measure ANG II, especially after ACE inhibition. Substantial amounts of renin present in plasma continue to produce enormous amounts of ANG I *in vitro*. The combination of renin and ANG I generates ir-ANG II, albeit at a reduced rate, due to the presence of EDTA and the ACE inhibitor. It has been shown *in vivo* and *in vitro* that ANG II can be generated even in the presence of potent ACE inhibition. Addition of a synthetic renin inhibitor to the sampling tube prevents *in vitro* generation of ANG I and ANG II, thereby allowing a more accurate measurement of circulating ANG II.[22]

With this markedly improved, though somewhat tedious, methodology, the investigation of the precise role of ANG II in blood pressure regulation, especially before and during ACE inhibition, has become feasible and reproducible. Considering all of the difficulties in attempting to measure plasma ANG II, it is not surprising that its role in blood pressure homeostasis remains to be established. Today, it seems inappropriate to expect to determine the mechanisms of ACE inhibition and the role of ANG II using an inferior methodology or by relying solely on the measurement of immunoreactive "angiotensin II."

TRUE ANGIOTENSIN II DURING ACE INHIBITION

In a pilot study, when ramipril was administered to normotensive volunteers, it reduced ir-ANG II by only 46%.[19] In comparison, true ANG II or angiotensin-(1-8)octapeptide fell from 5.2 ± 1.2 fmol/ml to undetectable levels (<0.4 fmol/ml). Thus it was demonstrated for the first time that plasma ANG II was virtually reduced to zero with initial administration of an ACE inhibitor.

A similar experiment was performed in which plasma-converting enzyme and renin activity, as well as blood angiotensin I, plasma aldosterone levels, and immunoreactive and true ANG II levels were measured. The behavior of these different components was followed over a 24-hour period. One hour after ramipril was administered, plasma ACE activity was reduced by more than 90%, plasma angiotensin-(1-8)octapeptide had fallen from 3.8 ± 1.0 fmol/ml to undetectable levels, while ir-ANG II had only decreased by 44%. Plasma renin activity and blood ANG I levels had hardly changed. By 4 hours after drug administration, plasma angiotensin-(1-8)octapeptide was again detectable and, by 8 hours, when plasma renin activity and ANG I levels had increased five-fold, it had reached 1.5 fmol/ml. Based on the measurement of true ANG II in plasma containing EDTA and phenanthroline, these results strongly suggest that this hormone is influenced by circulating renin, even at peak blood levels of an ACE inhibitor. Preliminary data of similar experiments with a renin inhibitor in blood sampling tubes support this conclusion and suggest that we are dealing with an *in vivo* phenomenon rather than with an *in vitro* artifact.[22]

In yet another study, plasma ANG II and ACE activity were measured in nine patients treated for at least 8 months with enalapril[10] (Figure 2). Blood samples were drawn in EDTA with phenanthroline on the morning before and 2 hours after the administration of enalapril. Plasma-converting enzyme activity fell from 17 ± 5.4 to 0.9 ± 0.3 nmol/ml/hr. At the same time, plasma ir-ANG II fell by only 17%, while angiotensin-(1-8)octapeptide decreased from 2.7 ± 0.9 to 0.9 ± 0.3 fmol/ml ($p < 0.05$). These results once

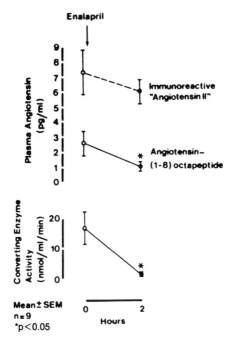

FIG. 2.   Effect of the enalapril morning dose in nine hypertensive patients treated for at least 8 months with the converting-enzyme inhibitor enalapril. Plasma ANG-(1-8)octapeptide, but not immunoreactive "ANG II", decreased significantly (paired t test) 2 hours after drug administration (1 pg ANG II = 0.96 fmol ANG II). From Nussberger *et al.*,[19] with permission.

more confirm that, probably due to renin stimulation, angiotensin-(1-8)octapeptide remains present in the plasma of patients receiving long-term ACE inhibitor therapy. The results also confirm that there is no tachyphylaxis to the converting enzyme inhibitory effect of enalapril, nor to the blockade of ANG II generation in plasma, despite some claims to the contrary.

EFFECT OF ACE INHIBITION ON ANGIOTENSIN II IN PATIENTS WITH PRIMARY ALDOSTERONISM

Patients with elevated plasma renin activity, and many with what appear to be normal or even low renin levels, have experienced a reduction in blood pressure while being treated solely with an ACE inhibitor. This phenomenon has been cited repeatedly to support the belief that ACE inhibitors have an ANG II-independent antihypertensive effect. It is argued that low plasma renin activity does not affect vascular tone, and if ANG II levels are already low, ACE inhibitors will not reduce them further. It seems appropriate, therefore, to investigate whether or not ACE inhibitors can reduce circulating

Acute Converting-Enzyme Inhibition in Primary Aldosteronism

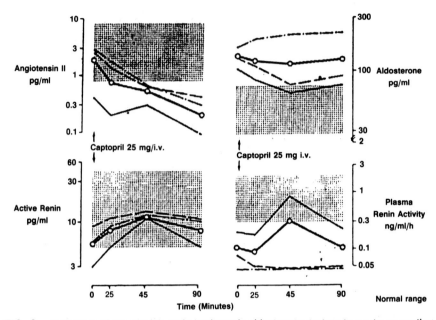

FIG. 3. Response of the plasma renin-angiotensin-aldosterone system to acute converting-enzyme inhibition in three patients with primary aldosteronism. The heavy line with the circles represents the mean values. Shaded areas represent the normal range (mean ± 2 SD) obtained in 15 supine healthy subjects. The lower end of the logarithmic scales indicates the detection limit of our methods. Low initial angiotensin-(1-8)octapeptide concentrations further decrease after treatment with captopril, while aldosterone levels remain abnormally high and renin values extremely low. From Nussberger et al.,[23] with permission.

ANG II in patients who start with very low levels to begin with, such as those with primary aldosteronism.

Figure 3 illustrates the effect of converting-enzyme inhibition on the components of the renin-angiotensin systems in three patients with primary aldosteronism.[23] The shaded areas represent the normal range of the variables measured (mean ± 2 SD in supine normal volunteers), the lower end of the logarithmic scale represents the detection limit, and the heavy line represents the mean value. Pre-drug low renin activity and abnormally high plasma aldosterone levels confirmed the diagnosis of primary aldosteronism in the study patients. Patients arrived at the outpatient facility 1 hour before starting the study and were installed comfortably in a supine position. After blood sampling had been performed to establish pre-drug baseline, patients received an intravenous injection of the ACE inhibitor, captopril. Following the captopril injection, plasma ANG II, which was low to begin with at 1.80 ± 0.70 fmol/ml (mean ± SEM), fell markedly to 0.17 ± 0.09 fmol/ml within 90 minutes.

These results clearly demonstrate that, even in patients with the lowest possible ANG II levels, ACE inhibition substantially reduces circulating ANG II. It is therefore unfair to assume that ACE inhibition does not reduce plasma ANG II in patients with low renin hypertension. True, blood pressure of *these* patients with primary aldosteronism does not fall significantly after treatment with captopril, but response or nonresponse of blood pressure to substantial reduction of ANG II has nothing to do with the inhibitory effect of the drug *per se*. Rather, it depends upon the set-point of the pressure/response curve to existing ANG II levels, which are known to fluctuate significantly from patient to patient, and even within a given patient.

ACE INHIBITION VERSUS RENIN INHIBITION

Renin inhibition, like ACE inhibition, reduces the production of ANG II. Therefore, by measuring ANG II in plasma we can assess the efficacy and potency of renin inhibitors. In a recent study, two renin inhibitors were given to normal volunteers.[24] Both compounds reduced plasma angiotensin-(1-8) octapeptide, in a dose-dependent fashion, to very low levels, comparable with those observed during ACE inhibition. Because renin inhibitors reduce plasma levels of ANG II with efficacy similar to that of ACE inhibitors, without affecting parameters such as bradykinin degradation, a comparison of the effects of renin and ACE inhibitors should indicate whether or not ACE inhibitors exert their effects primarily by reducing ANG II formation.

A classic experiment performed by Hofbauer *et al.* illustrates this technique.[25] Salt-depleted marmosets were treated with a renin inhibitor, to which the effect of an ACE inhibition was superimposed using the inverse sequence of therapy (Figure 4). Results showed that adding the ACE inhibitor to the renin inhibitor did not enhance the antihypertensive effect obtained with renin inhibitor alone. Hofbauer concluded that because it did not produce an enhanced effect, the ACE inhibitor must reduce blood pressure by blocking the generation of ANG II. This study seems to leave little hope for those suspecting that the effects of ACE inhibitors are independent of ANG II. However, we must remember that this was a short-term experiment performed under well-controlled conditions in an experimental prototype. The conclusions cannot, therefore, rule out the possibility of an ANG II-independent effect of ACE inhibitors in patients with essential hypertension. Only an orally-active renin inhibitor, which will enable us to treat hypertensive patients for a long period of time, will tell us if the results of Hofbauer's classic experiment reflects the usual clinical situation.

STUDIES WITH ANGIOTENSIN II ANTAGONISTS

To investigate the potential role of non-angiotensin II-dependent mechanisms of the antihypertensive effect of ACE inhibitors, experiments were performed in which an ACE inhibitor (teprotide) was added to a competitive

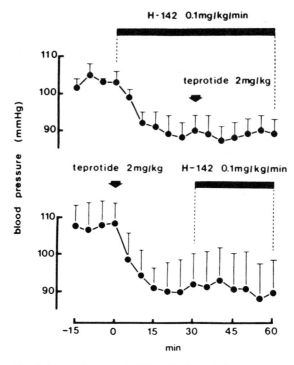

FIG. 4. Interaction between the renin inhibitor H-142 and the converting-enzyme inhibitor teprotide in conscious, mildly sodium-depleted marmosets. Effects of i.v. injection of teprotide on blood pressure during infusion of H-142 (upper panel). Effects of i.v. infusion of H-142 on blood pressure after i.v. injection of teprotide (lower panel). Means ± SEM, number = 3. From Hofbauer et al.,[25] with permission.

ANG II antagonist, saralasin, in normotensive and hypertensive rats on low to normal sodium intake.[26]

In this setting, the ACE inhibitor had no further antihypertensive effect. In another set of animal experiments, ANG II was infused for several days using osmotic minipumps. Thus, a model of pure ANG II-induced hypertension was created in which an ACE inhibitor was not expected to reduce ANG II generation. Indeed, blood pressure remained the same whether the animals received ANG II along with the ACE inhibitor or with placebo. Furthermore, saralasin normalized blood pressure equally in both groups.[27] The investigators could not, therefore, prove that the antihypertensive effect of ACE inhibitors was not influenced by ANG II. Once again we must consider that the design of this experiment makes it impossible to correlate its findings to the general clinical situation.

STUDIES WITH BRADYKININ ANTAGONISTS

A few years ago, Vavrek and his colleagues synthesized a new specific, competitive bradykinin antagonist.[28] This new tool provided a way to investigate the possible role of bradykinin accumulation following ACE inhibition. In this uncontrolled experiment, spontaneously hypertensive rats were given an ACE inhibitor followed by a bolus injection of the bradykinin antagonist.[29] An increase in blood pressure of >12 mmHg proved that the antihypertensive effect induced by the ACE inhibitor was partially reversed by the bradykinin antagonist. These results seem to suggest that bradykinin does contribute to the antihypertensive effect of ACE inhibitors. However, in a controlled experiment blood pressure in spontaneously hypertensive rats was reduced after the administration of the competitive ANG II antagonist, saralasin, before the bradykinin antagonist was administered. Surprisingly, as after ACE inhibition, following saralasin the bradykinin antagonist increased blood pressure equally. Thus, taking the two observations together, they do not support the concept that the ACE inhibition-induced blood pressure reduction is partly bradykinin-mediated but rather that bradykinin may take an active part in blood pressure regulation in hypertensive states. Again, these experiments were short-term studies of hypertensive animals. Long-term inhibition of bradykinin should yield more interesting data, and clinical experiments are needed to settle the question of whether or not bradykinin plays any role in the antihypertensive effect of ACE inhibitors.

CONCLUSION

Because ANG II appears to be the primary vasoactive component of the renin-angiotensin system, any assessment of drugs designed to inhibit this system, and thereby reduce vasomotor tone, should be based on the accurate measurement of the octapeptide, ANG II. The measurement of this hormone in plasma has presented considerable difficulties in the past, but now precise methods are available for determining ANG II in plasma with high degrees of specificity and sensitivity. With these methods, it has been clearly demonstrated that ACE inhibitors reduce circulating ANG II without tolerance development with prolonged use. Studies show that, even though there is some dissociation in time between the antihypertensive effect and the ANG II-reducing action of ACE inhibitors, there is little evidence that ACE inhibitors lower blood pressure without reducing plasma ANG II levels — if only for a short period during the day. Even during peak blockade, ANG II levels are probably still under the influence of circulating active renin. Accordingly, ACE inhibitors should still be used in a way that provides maximal ANG II reduction with minimal increase in active renin.

Increasing the dose of ACE inhibitors does not seem to increase therapeutic benefit in patients with normal plasma ANG II levels. However, in patients with very low plasma renin activity, as seen in those with primary aldosteronism, plasma ANG II is markedly reduced by ACE inhibition. Hence, there is little doubt that short-term as well as long-term treatment with ACE inhibitors at recommended dosages markedly reduces ANG II in plasma. Whether this reduction causes any change in blood pressure depends upon the setpoint of the pressure response to ANG II within each patient.

Although it is yet to be conclusively proven, studies using specific renin inhibitors and bradykinin antagonists suggest that ANG II-independent mechanisms are probably of secondary — not primary — importance to the antihypertensive effect of ACE inhibitors.

In our studies, we have only measured ANG II in plasma; measuring ANG II in tissue presents an even greater challenge. Studies completed to date do not answer the question of whether a local tissue renin-angiotensin system, rather than the components circulating in plasma, is the main determinant of blood pressure. They do suggest that, using current techniques, there is much more to be learned by the accurate measurement of the octapeptide, ANG II in plasma. The concept that tissue, rather than plasma ANG II, may determine vascular tone is intriguing and deserves thorough investigation.

REFERENCES

1. Ferreira SH, Bartelt DC, Greene J. Isolation of bradykinin-potentiating peptides from *Bothrops jararaca* venom. *Biochemistry* 1970; **9**:2583–2593.
2. Engel SL, Schaeffer TR, Waugh MH, Rubin B. Effects of the nonapeptide SQ 20.881 on blood pressure of rats with experimental renovascular hypertension. *Proc Soc Exp Biol Med* 1973; **143**:483–487.
3. Colier JG, Robinson BF, Vane JR. Reduction of pressor effects of angiotensin I in man by synthetic nonapeptide (B.P.P.9A or SQ20.881) which inhibits converting enzyme. *Lancet* 1973; **1**:72–74.
4. Gavras H, Brunner HR, Laragh JH, Sealey JE, Gavras I, Vukovich RA. An angiotensin converting enzyme inhibitor to identify and treat vasoconstrictor and volume factors in hypertensive patients. *N Engl J Med* 1974; **291**:817–821.
5. Ng KKF, Vane JR. Conversion of angiotensin I to angiotensin II. *Nature* 1967; **216**:762–766.
6. Waeber B, Nussberger J, Brunner HR. Angiotensin converting enzyme inhibitors in hypertension. In Laragh JH, Brenner BM, eds. *Hypertension: Pathophysiology, Diagnosis and Management*, New York, Raven Press, 1989 (in press).
7. Brunner DB, Desponds G, Biollaz J, Keller I, Ferber F, Gavras H, Brunner HR, Schelling JL. Effect of a new angiotensin converting enzyme inhibitor MK421 and its lysine analogue on the components of the renin system in healthy subjects. *Br J Clin Pharmacol* 1981; **11**:461–467.
8. Biollaz J, Brunner HR, Gavras I, Waeber B, Gavras H, Antihypertensive therapy with MK 421: Angiotensin II-renin relationships to evaluate efficacy of converting enzyme blockade. *J Cardiovasc Pharmacol* 1982; **4**:966–972.
9. Waeber B, Brunner HR, Brunner DB, Curtet AL, Turini GA, Gavras H. Discrepancy between antihypertensive effect and angiotensin converting enzyme inhibition by captopril. *Hypertension* 1980; **2**:236–242.
10. Hodsman GP, Zabludowski JR, Zoccali C, Fraser JR, Morton JJ, Murray GD, Robertson JIS. Enalapril (MK 421) and its lysine analogue (MK 521): a comparison of acute and chronic effects on blood pressure, renin-angiotensin system and sodium effects in normal man. *Br J Clin Pharmacol* 1984; **17**:233–241.

11. Swartz SL, Williams GH, Hollenberg NK. Converting enzyme inhibition in essential hypertension: The hypotensive response does not reflect only reduced angiotensin II formation. *Hypertension* 1979; I:106–111.

12. Zusman RM. Renin- and non-renin-mediated antihypertensive actions of converting enzyme inhibitors. *Kidney Int* 1984; 25:969–983.

13. Asaad MM, Antonaccio MJ. Vascular wall renin in spontaneously hypertensive rats: potential relevance to hypertension maintenance and antihypertensive effect of captopril. *Hypertension* 1982; 4:487–493.

14. Dzau VJ. Vascular renin-angiotensin: a possible autocrine or paracrine system in control of vascular function. *J Cardiovasc Pharmacol* 1984; 6:S377–S382.

15. Unger T, Ganten D, Lang RE. Tissue converting enzyme and cardiovascular actions of converting enzyme inhibitors. *J Cardiovasc Pharmacol* 1986; 8 (Suppl.10):S75–S81.

16. Campbell DJ. Circulating and tissue angiotensin systems. *J Clin Invest* 1987; 79:1–6.

17. Jennings G, Korner P, Esler M, Restall R. Redevelopment of essential hypertension after cessation of longterm therapy: preliminary findings. *Clin Exp Hypertens* 1984; A6:493–505.

18. Nussberger J, Bühler K, Waeber B, Brunner HR. Identification and quantitation of angiotensins. *J Cardiovasc Pharmacol* 1986; 8 (Suppl.10):S23–S28.

19. Nussberger J, Brunner DB, Waeber B, Brunner HR. True versus immunoreactive angiotensin II in human plasma. *Hypertension* 1985; 7 (Suppl.I):I1–I7.

20. Nussberger J, Brunner DB, Waeber B, Brunner HR. Specific measurement of angiotensin metabolites and in vitro generated angiotensin II in plasma. *Hypertension* 1986; 8:476–482.

21. Waite MA. Measurement of concentration of angiotensin I in human blood by radioimmunoassay. *Clin Sci* 1973; 45:51–64.

22. Nussberger J, Brunner DB, Waeber B, Brunner HR. In vitro renin inhibition to prevent generation of angiotensins during determination of angiotensin I and II. *Life Sci* 1988; 42:1683–1688.

23. Nussberger J, Waeber B, Brunner HR. Plasma angiotensin II and the antihypertensive action of angiotensin converting enzyme inhibition. *Am J Hypertens* 1989 (in Press)

24. Nussberger J, Waeber B, Brunner HR. ACE inhibition and renin inhibition. *J Hypertens* 1988 (in Press)

25. Hofbauer KG, Fuhrer W, Heusser Ch, Wood JM. Comparison of different drug interference with the renin-angiotensin system. *J Cardiovasc Pharmacol* 1985; 7 (Suppl.4):562–568.

26. Jaeger P, Ferguson RK, Brunner HR, Kirchertz EJ, Gavras H. Mechanism of blood pressure reduction by teprotide (SQ 20881) in rats. *Kidney Int* 1978; 13:289–296.

27. Textor SC, Brunner HR, Gavras H. Converting enzyme inhibition during chronic angiotensin II infusion in rats. Evidence against a non-angiotensin mechanism. *Hypertension* 1981; 3:269–276.

28. Vavrek RJ, Stewart J. Competitive antagonists of bradykinin. *Peptides* 1985 6:161–164.

29. Waeber B, Aubert JF, Flückiger JP, Nussberger J, Vavrek R, Stewart J, Brunner HR. Role of endogenous bradykinin in blood pressure control of conscious rats. *Kidney Int* 1988; 34 (Suppl 26):63–68.

ACKNOWLEDGMENTS

This work was supported by grants from the Cardiovascular Research Foundation and the Swiss National Science Foundation. The authors thank Ms A.F. Stalé and Mrs A. Dinkel for secretarial assistance.

SUMMARY

An assessment of the effects of ACE inhibitors depends on an accurate measurement of angiotensin II levels, rather than on plasma ACE or renin activity. Until recently, measurement of true angiotensin-(1-8)octapeptide has been hampered by cross-reactivity of the smaller breakdown fragments of angiotensin I (ANG I) and angiotensin II (ANG II). Combined use of high-performance liquid chromatography and radioimmunoassay now allow specific measurement of angiotensin-(1-8)octapeptide at levels of 0.1 fmol/ml. A comparison of the effects of renin inhibition and ACE inhibition, studies with ANG II antagonists, and, more recently, the use of bradykinin antagonists, have contributed towards the understanding of the mechanisms of action of ACE inhibitors. Experimental evidence suggests that ACE inhibitors cannot lower blood pressure without reducing plasma ANG II levels. Both long- and short-term treatment with ACE inhibitors at the appropriate dosages markedly reduces ANG II in plasma. Whether this reduction causes any blood pressure changes depends on the set-point of the pressure response to ANG II in each patient. Measurement of ANG II in tissue presents an even greater challenge than measurement of plasma ANG II. The intriguing question of whether a local tissue renin-angiotensin system, rather than the components circulating in plasma, is the main determinant of blood pressure, remains to be answered.

RÉSUMÉ

Une évaluation des effets des inhibiteurs de l'enzyme de conversion de l'angiotensine dépend d'une mesure exacte des niveaux d'angiotensine II, plutôt que de l'enzyme de conversion de l'angiotensine dans le plasma ou de l'activité rénine. Jusqu'à présent, la mesure du (véritable 1-8)octapeptide de l'angiotensine a été entravée par la réactivité croisée de plus petits fragments de l'angiotensine I et de l'angiotensine II. L'utilisation à la fois de la chromatographie liquide à haute performance et de l'analyse radioimmunologique permettent des mesures plus précises de l'octapeptide(1-8) de l'angiotensine à des niveaux de 0,1 fmol/ml. Une comparaison des effets de l'inhibition rénine et de l'inhibition de l'enzyme de conversion de l'angiotensine, des études avec des antagonistes de l'angiotensine II, et, plus récemment, l'utilisation des antagonistes de la bradykinine, ont contribué à une meilleure compréhension des mécanismes d'action des inhibiteurs de l'enzyme de conversion de l'angiotensine. Les résultats expérimentaux indiquent que les inhibiteurs de l'enzyme de conversion de l'angiotensine ne peuvent pas entraîner une baisse de la pression artérielle sans réduire les niveaux d'angiotensine II dans le plasma. Que cette réduction amène des changements de la pression artérielle dépend de la base déterminée de la réponse de la pression à l'angiotensine II chez chaque patient. La mesure de l'angiotensine II dans les tissus présente un plus grand défi que la mesure de l'angiotensine II dans le plasma. Reste à savoir si le système angiotensine-rénine d'un tissu localisé, plutôt que les composantes qui circulent dans le sang est le principal facteur déterminant de la pression artérielle.

ZUSAMMENFASSUNG

Die Messung der Effekte von inhibitoren des angiotensinkonvertierenden Enzyms ACE hängt ab von genauen Messungen der Angiotensin II (ANGII)-Konzentrationen, weit mehr als von Plasma-ACE oder Renin-Aktivität. Bis vor kurzem war die Messung des wahren Angiotensin-(1-8)-oktapeptids behindert durch Nebenreaktionen der kleineren Teilfragmente des Angiotensins I (ANGI) und des ANGII. Heute erlaubt die kombinierte Anwendung von Hochleistungs-Flüssigkeitschromatographie und Radio-Immunanalyse eine spezifische Messung von Angiotensin-(1-8)-oktapeptid in Konzentrationen von O,1 fMol/ml. Ein Vergleich der Effekte der Renin-Inhibition und der ACE-Inhibition, Studien mit ANGII-Antagonisten, und kürzlich auch die Verwendung von Bradykinin-Antagonisten haben zum Verständnis der Aktionsmechanismen von ACE-Inhibitoren beigetragen.

Experimentelle Ergebnisse zeigen, daß ACE-Inhibitoren den Blutdruck nicht verringern können, ohne den Gehalt an ANGII im Plasma zu erniedrigen. Sowohl Langzeit als auch Kurzzeitbehandlung mit ACE-Inhibitoren in angemessener Dosierung reduziert den ANGII-Gehalt im Plasma beträchtlich. Ob diese Reaktion Blutdruckveränderungen hervorruft, hängt in jedem individuellen Patienten von dem Punkt ab, an dem der Blutdruck auf ANGII reagiert.

Eine noch größere Herausforderung als die Messung des ANGII-Gehalts im Plasma stellt die Messung des ANGII im Gewebe dar. Eine faszinierende Frage bleibt bestehen in dem Problem, ob ein örtliches Gewebe-Renin-Angiotensin-System in der Hauptsache den Blutdruck bestimmt, oder ob die zirkulierenden Plasma-Inhaltsstoffe ausschlaggebend sind.

RIASSUNTO

Una valutazione degli effetti dell'enzima isomerizzante dell'angiotensina (EIA) dipende da una misurazione accurata dei livelli di angiotensina II (ANG II) piuttosto che dell'EIA del plasma o dell'attivita della renina. Fino a poco tempo fa la misurazione del vero ottapeptide dell'angiotensina (1–8) veniva ostacolata dalla reattivita incrociata dei frammenti più piccoli di angiotensina I (ANG I) e angiotensina II (ANG II). L'uso combinato di cromatografia liquida e di metodi radioimmunologici ad alto rendimento consentono adesso la misurazione specifica dell'ottapeptide dell'angiotensina (1-8) a livelli di 0,1 fmol/ml. Un paragone degli effetti dell'inibizione della renina e dell'inibizione dell'EIA, studi sugli antagonisti dell'ANG II e, più recentemente, l'uso di antagonisti della bradichinina, hanno contribuito alla comprensione del meccanismo attivo degli inibitori dell'EIA. Prove sperimentali suggeriscono che gli inibitori dell'EIA non possono abbassare la pressione sanguigna senza ridurre i livelli di ANG II nel plasma. La terapia, sia a lungo che a breve termine, con inibitori dell'EIA in dosi adatte riduce notevolmente l'ANG 2 nel plasma. Se questa riduzione causi dei cambiamenti nella pressione sanguigna dipende dalla soglia della reazione delle pressione all'ANG II in ciascun paziente. La misurazione dell'ANG II nel tessuto presenta una sfida ancora maggiore della misurazione dell'ANG II nel plasma. L'interessante domanda se il principale determinante della pressione sanguigna sia un sistema renina-angiotensina nel tessuto locale piuttosto che i componenti che circolano nell'organismo rimane tuttora senza risposta.

SUMÁRIO

A avialiação dos efeitos dos inibidores da enzima convertidora da angiotensina (ACE) depende de uma medição exata dos níveis da angiotensina II (ANG II) ao invés da atividade da renina ou dos níveis da ACE no plasma. Até muito recentemente, a medição do verdadeiro octapeptídio (1-8) da angiotensina tem-se visto dificultada pela reatividade cruzada de fragmentos mais pequenos da angiotensina I (ANG I) e a ANG II. O uso combinado de cromatografia líquida de alto rendimento e radioimunoensaio permite agora a medição específica do octapeptídio (1-8) da angiotensina a níveis de 0,1 fmol/ml. A comparação dos efeitos da inibição da renina e da ACE, os estudos com antagonistas da ANG II e, mais recentemente, o uso dos antagonistas da bradiquinina têm contribuído ao entendimento dos mecanismos de ação dos inibidores da ACE. A evidência experimental sugere que os inibidores da ACE não podem diminuir a pressão arterial sem reduzir os níveis plasmáticos da ANG II. Tanto o tratamento a largo como a curto prazo com inibidores da ACE às doses apropriadas reduzem marcadamente os níveis plasmáticos da ANG II. Se esta redução ocasionar mudanças na pressão arterial depende do ponto particular de resposta à pressão da ANG em cada paciente. A medição dos níveis da ANG II nos tecidos presenta um desafio ainda superior à da medição dos níveis plasmáticos da ANG II. A intrigante qüestão de se for o sistema renina-angiotensina do tecido local, ao invés dos componentes circulantes no plasma, o que primordialmente determina a pressão arterial ainda está por ser esclarecida.

RESUMEN

La determinación de los efectos de los inhibidores de la enzima convertidora de la angiotensina (ACE) depende de una medida exacta de los niveles de la angiotensina II (ANG II), en lugar de la actividad de la renina o los niveles de la ACE en el plasma. Hasta muy recientemente, la medición del verdadero octapéptido (1-8) de la angiotensina se ha visto dificultada por la reactividad cruzada de fragmentos más pequeños de la angiotensina I (ANG I) y la ANG II. El uso combinado de cromatografía líquida de alto rendimiento y radioinmunoensayo permite ahora la medición específica del octapéptido (1-8) de la angiotensina a niveles de 0,1 fmol/ml. La comparación de los efectos de la inhibición de la renina y de la ACE, los estudios con antagonistas de la ANG II y, más recientemente, el empleo de los antagonistas de la bradiquinina han contribuido a la comprensión de los mecanismos de acción de los inhibidores de la ACE. La evidencia experimental sugiere que los inhibidores de la ACE no pueden disminuir la presión arterial sin reducir los niveles plasmáticos de la ANG II. Tanto el tratamiento a largo como a corto plazo con inhibidores de la ACE a las dosis apropiadas reducen marcadamente los niveles plasmáticos de la ANG II. El hecho de si esta reducción causa cambios en la presión arterial depende del punto particular de respuesta a la presión de la ANG II en cada paciente. La medición de los niveles de la ANG II en los tejidos constituye un reto aún superior a la medición de los niveles plasmáticos de la ANG II. Todavía no hay respuesta a la intrigante cuestión de si es el sistema renina-angiotensina del tejido local, en vez de los componentes circulantes en el plasma, el que primordialmente determina la presión arterial.

要約

　アンジオテンシン変換酵素（ACE）阻害薬の効果の評価は，血漿 ACE または レニン活性よりもむしろアンジオテンシン II 濃度の測定によってなされる。最近 まで，真のアンジオテンシン-(1-8)オクタペプチドの測定は，アンジオテンシン I および II の分解された小断片との交差反応によって妨げられていた。しかし現 在では，高速液体クロマトグラフィーとラジオイムノアッセイ（RIA）とを組み合 わせることにより，アンジオテンシン-(1-8)オクタペプチドを 0.1 fmol/ml レ ベルまで特異的に測定できるようになった。そして，レニン阻害と ACE 阻害との 効果の比較や，アンジオテンシン II 拮抗薬を用いた研究，さらに最近のブラディ キニン拮抗薬の使用などが，ACE 阻害薬の作用機序の解明に役立っている。

　これらの実験成績から，ACE 阻害薬は血漿アンジオテンシン II 濃度の低下な しには，血圧を低下させないことが示唆されている。適量の ACE 阻害薬の長期お よび短期治療のいずれにおいても血漿中のアンジオテンシン II を著明に減少さ せる。この減少がなんらかの血圧変化をひき起こすかどうかは，各患者ごとのア ンジオテンシン II に対する血圧反応の set-point に依存している。

　組織中のアンジオテンシン II の測定は，血漿アンジオテンシン II の測定より もさらに期待が寄せられている。血漿中の循環成分よりむしろ，局所組織のレニ ン-アンジオテンシン系が血圧の主要な決定因子であるか否かという興味深い疑 問が，答えるべき課題として残っている。

Cardiac and Renal Failure: An Expanding Role for ACE Inhibitors, edited by C. T. Dollery and L. M. Sherwood, Hanley & Belfus, Inc., Philadelphia.

Application of the New Biology to Hypertension Research: The Renin-Angiotensin Paradigm

D. Ganten, K. Lindpaintner, Th. Unger, J. Mullins

Hypertension develops as a secondary complication of another treatable disorder, such as renal artery stenosis, in only a small percentage of cases. In the great majority of patients, no such underlying cause can be identified, and these cases have been classified as "primary hypertension." Although the precise etiology of primary hypertension remains obscure, there is strong and convincing evidence that genetic factors together with environmental effects play a key role in its pathogenesis. Clinicians will continue to be limited to treatment approaches that are essentially palliative rather than curative until the pathogenesis of this disorder is much more clearly understood. Thus, efforts to understand the pathogenesis of primary hypertension have as their common goal the eventual development of specific therapeutic modalities aimed at curing or preventing this disease.

Physiologic, endocrinologic, pharmacologic, and neurobiologic studies have identified a number of systems that affect circulatory regulation and may, in certain forms of secondary hypertension, cause the abnormal elevation of blood pressure. Historically, one of the first attempts to develop animal models for hypertension research was that of Tigerstedt and Bergman,[1] who injected kidney extract (renin) into rabbits and observed a sustained increase of blood pressure. Subsequently, several models of experimental hypertension have been developed by placing a lesion on vasculature, kidney, or other organs of otherwise healthy animals. The resulting hypertensionogenic dysfunction resembles in many instances specific hypertensive diseases in humans. Surgical manipulation of the kidney or of the renal artery, for example, results in renal hypertension. Along similar lines, major advances in hypertension research have accompanied the development of genetically hypertensive rats.[2] Recently a single-gene defect has been successfully introduced into a hypertensive rat model.[3] Genetic modeling of animals is likely to expand in the future and will include recombinant DNA techniques.

GENETIC HYPERTENSION IN RATS

The major difficulty in developing animal models for primary hypertension resides in the disease itself. Human primary hypertension may be considered a single entity from a clinical point of view. With respect to pathophysiology, natural history, response to treatment, and complications, however, it is a heterogeneous disease, and no uniform abnormality apart from the elevated blood pressure has been defined. In its early stages, even the classifications "normotensive" and "hypertensive" pose major problems, because blood pressure is a quantitative trait and the dividing line between normal variations and disease is arbitrary.

Genetically hypertensive rats have been obtained by genetic selection.[2-9] Inbred hypertensive strains provide a homogeneous population of hypertensive animals. The onset of high blood pressure occurs early, and complications occur at a predictable age if the environment is controlled. This is not the case in human primary hypertension, where onset occurs at various ages and other factors are uncontrolled; its course, therefore, is much less predictable with respect to severity and complications. Thus, the homogeneity of inbred hypertensive rats has advantages for scientific investigations, but caution must be exercised in extrapolating research results to humans because of the etiological heterogeneity of human hypertension.

The obvious and undisputed similarity of the hypertensive disease process in patients and in rats is its spontaneous, idiopathic development in genetically predisposed subjects. The pathophysiological heterogeneity in humans finds its counterpart in the different strains of spontaneously hypertensive rats. *A priori*, it is almost certain that the various inbred strains of hypertensive rats have trapped (i.e., genetically fixed), different, but overlapping subsets of specific genetic abnormalities causing high blood pressure. Thus, one expects differences between strains as well as similarities. The individual patient presenting with primary hypertension may have single or combined defects in salt sensitivity, renal electrolyte handling, cellular cation exchange, mineralocorticoid sensitivity, cellular calcium regulation, vascular reactivity, sympathetic tone, or neurogenic factors. Each strain of genetically hypertensive rats displays unique pathophysiological features linked to the development of hypertension that often resemble disorders found in subgroups of hypertensive patients. Thus, the cause of hypertension in an individual hypertensive patient may closely resemble the disturbances found in one or more of the rat strains.

ESTABLISHMENT OF TRANSGENIC RATS

The limitation of rats with genetic, spontaneous hypertension resides in the polygenetic nature of the hypertensive disease and the complexity of primary and secondary interactions. Using molecular biological techniques it is now possible to specifically manipulate the genome of hypertensive and normotensive rats, and to selectively and specifically test the contribution of individual genes and regulatory elements for the development and maintenance of high blood pressure. The availability of these methodologies to generate transgenic animals enables for the first time discrete and purposeful genetic manipulation to be carried out. Animals bred in this way offer entirely new possibilities for studying the influence of a variety of factors or intact, non-pharmacologically treated organisms. These techniques open new avenues in hypertension research, in particular through their potential for allowing dissection of the extremely complex interactions among the different organ systems that together regulate the circulation. In principle, transgenic technology can be applied to all animal species.[10]

The following considerations support the use of the rats as an experimental animal model in hypertension research: The rat, more often than any other species, has been used in basic pathophysiological and therapeutic hypertension research. Therefore, we have at our disposal a wealth of physiologic data. Even more importantly, genetically determined models of primary hypertension have been thoroughly studied in the rat. Mice are poorly or not at all suited for this type of experimentation, and bigger animals would be impracticable. In contrast to mice, the molecular biological and genetic studies in rats can easily be complemented by extensive pathophysiological, hemodynamic, electrophysiological, endocrinological, and pharmacological investigations using well established, reliable methods.

As a first approach the renin-angiotensin system (RAS) represents a particularly promising area of application for this new technology. The RAS is one of the most important systems for cardiovascular homeostasis; the genes for both renin and angiotensinogen have been sequenced and are well-characterized. Furthermore, the system has gained additional interest due to the newly-recognized relationships between circulating and local tissue systems. Through transgenic modification of the RAS, important new insights into the pathogenesis of hypertension may be possible, which may result in major advances in the clinical management of hypertension. This technique can be applied to virtually all blood-pressure regulating systems, enzymes, peptides, and receptors, as long as the respective genes are available. The establishment of transgenic rat models will combine the precision of this new biology with the versatility of the rat as an experimental animal for hypertension research. A most promising area of application is, for example, the transfection of rats with human genes, allowing the development of specific inhibitors of human enzymes or receptors in transgenic rats as one application. This would considerably facilitate drug development and reduce the ethical and financial problems involved in primate experimentation. Thus, transgenic animal techniques will provide research and industry with a new set of valuable and specific models for pathophysiological and therapeutic research. Transgenic techniques will also help us to understand the increasingly complex hormonal and tissue renin-angiotensin system as a target for novel therapeutic approaches.

THE RENIN-ANGIOTENSIN PARADIGM

The development of inhibitors of the renin-angiotensin system as antihypertensive agents began about 15 years ago, with some scepticism because it had been assumed that they would be effective only in pathophysiological conditions, such as renal arterial stenosis, in which a stimulated plasma RAS contributes to the elevation and maintenance of high blood pressure. Despite the expected limited therapeutic spectrum of inhibitors of the RAS, the converting enzyme (CE) inhibitor captopril was developed as the prototype of this new class of antihypertensive drugs. Several other inhibitors are presently being developed or are already on the market (e.g., enalapril, ramipril, cilazapril, perindopril, lisinopril, fosinopril, zofenopril and others).

Initially, the antihypertensive mechanism of CE inhibitors was believed to depend on a reduction of circulating angiotensin II (ANG II) levels, leading to an inhibition of the direct effects of angiotensin on vascular smooth muscle contraction, aldosterone release, and sodium retention. However, evidence accumulated from studies in hypertensive patients, as well as in animals with various types of experimental hypertension, showing that blood pressure could be lowered by CE inhibitors independently of whether the plasma RAS was stimulated or not. It thus became increasingly difficult to reconcile the antihypertensive effects of CE inhibitors with the original concepts about their mechanism of action. Several other pharmacodynamic effects had to be considered, because CE is identical with the bradykinin degrading enzyme, kininase II,[11] CE inhibitors can also potentiate the vasodepressor effects of bradykinin. Moreover, actions of CE inhibitors possibly unrelated to CE inhibition, such as alterations of vascular smooth muscle permeability to sodium[12] and interactions with the prostaglandin systems via the stimulatory effects of kinins, and different pharmacokinetic properties had to be considered to explain the blood pressure lowering effects on these drugs.[13-22]

Most of the early clinical pharmacological studies on CE inhibitors focussed on acute effects of the drugs on blood pressure and parameters of the RAS. In these studies it has been repeatedly demonstrated that, upon CE administration, the expected changes of the blood parameters of the RAS did occur: ANG II was lowered, angiotensin I (ANG I) increased, CE activity was inhibited, renin activity increased due to the withdrawal of the negative feedback inhibition by ANG II, and aldosterone levels in plasma or urine were decreased. More careful analysis, especially in cases following chronic treatment with CE inhibitors, revealed that this simple scheme had to be reconsidered. In fact local angiotensin synthesis in cardiovascular organs, such as the vasculature, the heart, the adrenal gland and the brain, may be more important.

THE VASCULAR RENIN-ANGIOTENSIN SYSTEM

The argument that vascular renin may contribute locally to blood pressure regulation and hypertension independently of the plasma RAS[23-26] has been supported in recent years through findings of studies that have demonstrated the presence of the components of the RAS and of the genetic materials required for local angiotensin production in the vascular wall.[27-30] In addition, it has been found that renin is synthesized in cultured aortic smooth muscle cells,[31] and renin gene expression has been discovered in vascular endothelial cultured cells.[32] Moreover, the capability of the vascular RAS to synthesize the effector peptide ANG II, independently of the hormonal RAS, has been demonstrated in cultured bovine aortic endothelial cells[33] and in isolated mesenteric vessel preparations.[34]

Locally generated angiotensin may act in many ways to influence vascular tone and distensibility. These include a direct vasoconstriction by stimulation of angiotensin receptors on the smooth muscle cells of the vascular media,[35] facilitation of adrenergic transmission leading to vasoconstriction by increased vascular tone,[36,37] and stimulation of Na^+ and Ca^{2+} transport systems across the cell membrane, as recently demonstrated in cultured vascular smooth muscle cells.[38] In addition, ANG II may even exert vasodilatory effects through stimulation of endothelial prostacyclin synthesis,[39] although the functional significance of this effect is still unclear.

Evidence pointing to a pathophysiological role of a stimulated vascular RAS in hypertension has been provided by several groups. In addition to the studies cited above, which report on stimulated vascular RAS in spontaneously hypertensive rat (SHR) animals with hypertension of renal origin, Okamura et al.[40] demonstrated increased vascular CE activity and an enhanced vasoconstrictor response to ANG I in arteries isolated from one-clip, two-kidney hypertensive rats. Interestingly, both the CE inhibitor enalapril and an ANG II receptor antagonist lowered blood pressure in these animals, despite the fact that the plasma RAS was not stimulated. This finding supports the idea that vascular, rather than plasma RAS stimulation, helps to maintain high blood pressure in some forms of hypertension.

A number of studies have shown that CE inhibition can antagonize pre- and postsynaptic action of noradrenaline (for review see Refs. 41, 42). In line with these findings are those by Schölkens et al.[43] which demonstrated that, in isolated vascular preparations (pulmonary artery from guinea pigs, thoracic aorta from rabbits and rat mesentery), CE inhibitors attenuated the vasoconstrictor responses to noradrenaline but not to potassium chloride. It is important to note that in this study local ANG II generation and sympathetic neurotransmission were not only inhibited by CE inhibitors *in vitro*, but also by oral CE inhibitor pretreatment prior to removal of vascular tissue (*ex vivo*).

More recently, Nakamura et al.[34] demonstrated, that ANG II can be released from isolated mesenteric arteries upon β-adrenergic stimulation with isoproterenol. Further study results by the same authors together with those by Kwasaki et al.[44] and Götheret et al.[45] suggest that in isolated rat mesenteric vessels, the β-adrenoceptor mediated enhancement of vascular noradrenergic transmission is caused by a stimulation of local vascular ANG II synthesis, an effect blocked by CE inhibitors in these studies.

Results indicating that local vascular ANG II generation can also be reduced by CE inhibitors in man have been obtained by Webb and Collier.[46] The authors reported that during an infusion of ramiprilat (the active parent diacid of ramipril) into the brachial arteries of hypertensive and normotensive patients, the intrabrachially infused doses of ANG I had to be increased by a factor of 20 to obtain the same vasoconstriction as was found before ramipril administration, whereas the vasoconstrictor responses to ANG II were not affected by the CE inhibitor.

Although the data discussed above suggest that CE inhibitors may antagonize the vascular RAS when acting locally, it is important to realize that interference of these drugs with vascular CE may lead to reduced vascular ANG II synthesis, but may also have an impact on other local peptide systems such as kinins, and might even alter vascular texture by mechanisms unrelated to CE inhibition. The following examples may suffice to illustrate these possible important aspects of local CE inhibitor action.

Scherf et al.[47] reported on a stimulation of prostacyclin synthesis in isolated aortic preparations from rats treated orally with the CE inhibitor ramipril (*ex vitro*), and in aortic tissue exposed to ramiprilat *in vitro*. Since aprotinin, a kallikrein inhibitor, attenuated the effect of ramiprilat, the increase in prostacyclin production was thought to be caused by a CE inhibitor-induced accumulation of vascular kinins. On the other hand, Oshima et al.[48] observed a decrease in aortic prolyl-hydrolase, the rate-limiting enzyme of collagen synthesis, following prolonged oral treatment of SHR with hypotensive doses of captopril. Since the authors were unable to demonstrate this effect after single oral captopril administration in SHR or when aortic tissue from untreated normotensive rats was exposed to captopril *in vitro*, they concluded that the reduction in prolyl-hydrolase could be due to the hypotensive, rather than to direct vascular action, of the CE inhibitor. In previous morphometric experiments designed to investigate the effects of antihypertensive treatment on vascular hypertrophy, we observed that in normotensive six-month-old spontaneously hypertensive rats of the stroke-prone substrain (SHRSP) whose mothers had been treated with an antihypertensive dose of captopril during pregnancy, and who had been kept on captopril until sacrifice, the renal arteries, their branches, and their resistance vessels did not exhibit any signs of media hypertrophy.[49] As in the study by Oshima et al.,[48] the lack of development of vascular hypertrophy could be explained hemodynamically (i.e., by the failure of these animals to develop hypertension), but it is also possible that captopril exerted some direct effect on the vascular texture. Thus, it remains to be seen in more detailed experiments if chronic CE inhibitor treatment alters vascular texture independently of hemodynamic changes and whether this alteration is due to the CE inhibition (e.g., suppressed proliferative actions of ANG II) or to an unspecific effect of these drugs unrelated to CE inhibition.

In conclusion, there is accumulating experimental and clinical evidence that inhibition of vascular CE in resistance vessels, large arteries, and veins may contribute to the beneficial actions of CE inhibitors in cardiovascular diseases. However, much remains to be learned about the exact localization and regulation of vascular ANG II synthesis and the various actions that vascular ANG II and locally generated CE-dependent vasodilator peptides may exert on vascular function and texture.

THE CARDIAC RENIN-ANGIOTENSIN SYSTEM

Renin activity in dog hearts was first demonstrated by Hayduk et al.[50] Although nephrectomy showed no effects, sodium depletion resulted in enhanced enzyme activity. We, too, were able to measure renin in different parts of the heart,[51] and recently other investigators found renin-like activity in isolated myocytes from rats[52] and mice.[53] The latter study also confirmed that cardiac renin is influenced by sodium balance through observation of increased activity of cardiac renin found after dietary sodium depletion.

A requirement for the demonstration of local synthesis of proteins and peptides is expression of their gene in the tissue. We have recently been successful in identifying and quantitating renin and angiotensin mRNA expression in a number of extra-renal tissues,[54] including the heart,[55] thus confirming previous reports. In these studies, we used a 760 base-pair fragment of the renin gene containing exon 9, which we had previously isolated from a rat genomic clone bank. This DNA fragment was cloned into the poly-linker site of plasmid pSPT18, flanked by promotors for T7 and SP6 polymerase, respectively. Thus, synthesis of renin cRNA and mRNA from the T7 and SP6 promotor was possible by *in vitro* transcription after linearization with EcoRI or HindIII. RNA was prepared from the four chambers of rat hearts by lithium chloride/urea extraction and ethanol precipitation,[56,57] and we were able to demonstrate expression of the renin gene in all four chambers of the heart by Northern blotting and liquid hybridization assay.

Relative signal strength was greatest in the right atrium, followed by the right and left ventricle. Similarly, angiotensinogen mRNA expression was demonstrated in the atria and ventricles using a probe prepared from a 712 base-pair BamHI cDNA fragment cloned into pSPT18. The demonstration that the genes for both renin and angiotensinogen are expressed in cardiac tissues establishes the potential for synthesis of these proteins in the mammalian heart.

To correlate these findings with direct protein measurements, we measured angiotensin in five regions of the rhesus monkey heart. Concentration per gram of wet tissue weight ranged between 100 and 500 fmol for ANG II and 30 and 150 fmol for ANG I.[58] For both peptides, concentrations were highest in the right atrium, followed by the right ventricle, the left atrium, the interventricular septum, and the left ventricle. In a subsequent experiment, we obtained additional evidence for the cardiac origin of these peptides by documenting that CE inhibition lowered cardiac ANG II in nephrectomized rabbits. Because circulating angiotensin levels in these animals are undetectable, the effect of CE inhibition must be presumed to be caused by their action on locally generated peptides. This was further studied in experiments designed to investigate intracardiac generation of ANG II.

Indirect evidence for the intracardiac activation of ANG I to ANG II was first presented by Needleman et al.[59] and Nakashima et al.,[60] who used bioassay systems to show activation of exogenously infused ANG I after passage through the coronary circulation. The presence of angiotensin converting enzyme in the heart was also later confirmed by biochemical measurements.[61]

The possible physiologic significance of locally generated ANG II suggested indirectly by the cardio-protective effect of CE inhibitors in regional myocardial ischemia is documented by several authors. Angiotensin II has a pronounced vasoconstrictor effect on coronary arteries,[62] and exogenously administered angiotensin II is known to be a potent inotropic agent acting through both direct and indirect myotropic mechanisms. These effects may further jeopardize an already compromised myocardium. Because of the effect of the renin-angiotensin system on a number of effector systems involved in cardiovascular homeostasis (i.e., arterial and venous vascular smooth muscle, adrenal cortex, central nervous system), the elucidation of its specific cardiac effects has usually been approached with experimental designs that use isolated heart or muscle strip preparations.

Angiotensin II has been found, with rare exceptions,[63] to exert a positive inotropic influence on myocardial function. When sympathetic facilitation was carefully avoided, dose-dependent direct positive inotropic effects of angiotensin II were shown in isolated atria and papillary muscle strips of rabbits,[62] dogs,[64] cats,[65,66] and guinea pigs.[62] Different investigators have found that the magnitude of this response to sympathetic nerve stimulation,[67] to a 15-fold increase in developed tension.[68] In addition, data from our laboratory[69] suggest that myotropic actions of angiotensins are species-specific. Ramipril, enalapril, or a vehicle was given to groups of rats, guinea pigs, and rabbits. One hour later, the animals were killed, their hearts were mounted in a Langendorff apparatus, and the effects of adding ANG I and ANG II to the perfusate were evaluated. In control hearts, both peptides decreased coronary flow in all species, whereas contractile force was increased in rats, decreased in guinea pigs, and unchanged in rabbits after treatment with each agent. Pretreatment with angiotensin CE inhibitors inhibited the effect of ANG I perfusion but had no effect on the action of ANG II.

There is general consensus that facilitation of sympathetic nervous influences on the heart by ANG II contributes greatly to its inotropic actions. The majority of studies conclude that this facilitation is based primarily on an increase in the amount of neurotransmitter released from presynaptic nerve terminals,[67,68,36] although ANG II has also been shown to decrease prejunctional re-uptake,[70] stimulate sympathetic ganglia,[71] increase catecholamine biosynthesis,[72] release catecholamines from the adrenal medulla,[73] and sensitize post-junctional structures.[74] We have recently reported on experiments in which the physiologic relevance of this interaction with the sympathetic nervous system was tested in the heart. Isolated perfused heart preparations with sympathetic cardiac nerves left intact[75] were prepared from rabbits that had been pretreated orally, one hour before they were killed, with either vehicle (control) or ramipril. Sympathetic nerve stimulation increased heart rate and contractility and decreased coronary flow. These effects were significantly reduced in animals pretreated with CE inhibitor. A similar attenuation was observed when the active diacid moiety of ramipril was added to the perfusate prior to electrical stimulation. These experiments are of particular importance to the proposed cardiac renin-angiotensin system, because the observed effects must be presumed to be caused by the inhibition of locally generated ANG II in the absence of exogenous angiotensins.

The potential physiologic role of the cardiac renin-angiotensin system is emphasized by studies demonstrating a cardio-protective effect of CE inhibitors in subjects with regional myocardial ischemia. Ertl *et al.*[76] demonstrated a reduction in infarct size after coronary artery ligation in dogs treated with CE inhibitors. Their observation that the area at risk and the infarcted area were smaller than would have been expected from the concomitant augmentation of coronary flow afforded by CE indicates additional effects of these agents, possibly on myocardial metabolism. This has been confirmed by examining the effects of CE inhibitors in isolated, perfused rat hearts subjected to a 15-minute period of regional ischemia by occluding the left anterior descending artery.[77] During the subsequent reperfusion phase, lactate dehydrogenase and creatine kinase activities in the coronary effluent were significantly lower when the CE inhibitor ramiprilat was added to the perfusion medium or had been administered orally before the animal was killed. In addition, CE inhibitor administration was associated with preservation of myocardial stores of glycogen and high-energy phosphates, which were both markedly depleted in untreated hearts. These effects were accompanied by a significant reduction in the incidence and duration of ventricular arrhythmias during the reperfusion period. All effects associated with CE inhibition could be abolished by addition of angiotensin II to the perfusate. Significantly, an isolated heart preparation was used instead of the *in situ* preparation used in other studies; thus, the effects of CE inhibition are presumed to be caused by their action on local, intracardiac generation of ANG II. Of course, this does not rule out a possibly equally important role of kinins, which would be expected to accumulate after CE-inhibitor treatment.

The results of these animal studies complement the clinical observations of a decreased incidence of arrhythmias in subjects treated with angiotensin CE inhibitors.[78,79] Given the important role of malignant ventricular arrhythmias in morbidity and mortality associated with ischemic heart disease, the suggested influence of the cardiac renin-angiotensin system assumes major clinical importance.

THE BRAIN RENIN-ANGIOTENSIN SYSTEM

The existence of an active RAS in the brain is now well documented.[80] Intracerebroventricular (ICV) application of different CE inhibitors lowered blood pressure in SHRSP,[81-84] as well as in renal hypertensive rats[85] and in DOCA-salt hypertensive rats,[86] suggesting an involvement of the brain in the antihypertensive action of CE inhibitors. However, whether these drugs gain access to the central nervous system (CNS) upon systemic administration is still controversial. Although some earlier studies suggested that the CE inhibitor captopril does not penetrate the blood-brain barrier following acute systemic application,[87,88,89] other groups have reported on an inhibition in CE in brain tissue homogenates after systemic treatment with CE inhibitors.[61,90-92] Results obtained with brain tissue homogenates must be interpreted with caution, because this method does not allow differentiation between CE activity derived from neuronal and vascular structures. It is difficult, therefore, to decide whether the marked inhibition seen in some brain areas after oral CE inhibitor treatment is due to an inhibition of neuronal CE activity, or whether it reflects CE inhibition in the brain vasculature, or in contaminating blood plasma. A better approach for determining access of orally applied CE inhibitors of the CNS is the measurement of CE inhibition in the cerebrospinal fluid (CSF), because interferences with blood plasma and brain vasculature can be ruled out by appropriate sampling techniques.

Indirect evidence for an inhibition of CE in CSF following systemic CE-inhibitor administration suggested by *in vivo* studies demonstrating that the dipsogenic and pressor effects of ICV-injected renin or angiotensin I (ANG I) were decreased following a single oral dose of captopril.[41,93] More recently, Geppetti *et al.*[94] showed a substantial inhibition of CE in the CSF, as determined by a fluorometric assay, after acute oral captopril treatment in man.

CONCLUSION

Recent investigations have revealed that, in addition to the hormonal plasma renin-angiotensin system, there is an autocrine or paracrine endogeneous tissue renin-angiotensin system. This may be even more important to the chronic therapeutic effects of CE inhibitors than interference with the hormonal plasma renin-angiotensin system. The plasma renin-angiotensin system is considered an acute regulator of vascular tone and electrolyte and volume homeostasis; the tissue renin-angiotensin system probably serves more chronic long-term functions.

Molecular biological studies of gene expression of renin, angiotensinogen, and CE in different target tissues, combined with pathophysiological and pharmacological studies in hypertensive animals and man, can lead to new considerations in understanding the pharmacokinetics and pharmacodynamics of the drug, improved therapeutic use, and to the possibility of the development of new, more specific target directed drugs. In the past, investigations using genetically hypertensive rats and other animal models have allowed major advances in our understanding of the pathophysiology of hypertension. These valuable research resources will continue to assist us in finding the source of human hypertension and ultimately preventing this disease. In the future, the application of the "new biology" to hypertension research using recombinant DNA technology and, in particular, the establishment of transgenic rats, will provide powerful and specific new animal models for hypertension research. It is through this type of basic research, and the responsible use of all available *in-vitro* and *in-vivo* methods, that new and better treatment modalities for hypertension will be designed.

ACKNOWLEDGEMENT

This work was supported in part by grants from the Deutsche Forschungsgemeinschaft (DFG), SFB 317, and National Institute of Health (NIH) USA 1RO HL 35821-01. The competent secretarial help of Daniela Wirth is gratefully acknowledged.

REFERENCES

1. Tigerstedt R, Bergman PF. Niere und Kreislauf. *Scand Arch Physiol* 1989; **8**:223–279.
2. Rascher W, Clough D, Ganten D, eds. *Hypertensive Mechanisms: the Spontaneously Hypertensive Rat as a Model to Study Human Hypertension.* Stuttgart, Schauttauer Verlag, 1982; 777–802.

3. Ganten U, Rascher W, Lang RE, et al. Development of a new strain of spontaneously hypertensive rats homozygous for hypothalamic diabetes insipidus. *Hypertension* 1983; **5(Suppl I)**:I119–I128.
4. Yamori K, Okamoto K. Zymogram analyses of various organs from spontaneously hypertensive rats. *Lab Invest* 1970; **22**:206–211.
5. Rapp JP, Dahl LK. Mendelian inheritance of 18- and 11β-steroid hydroxylase activities in the adrenals of rats genetically susceptible or resistant to hypertension. *Endocrinology* 1972; **90**:1435–1446.
6. Tanase H. Genetic control of blood pressure in spontaneously hypertensive rats (SHR). *Exp Animals* 1979; **28**:519–530.
7. Rapp JP. A genetic locus (Hyp-2) controlling vascular smooth muscle response in spontaneously hypertensive rats. *Hypertension* 1972; **4**:459–467.
8. Okamoto K, Yamori Y, Ooshima A, park C, Haebara H, Matsumoto M. Establishment of the inbred strain of the spontaneously hypertensive rat and genetic factors involved in hypertension. In Okamoto K, ed. *Spontaneous Hypertension: Its Pathogenesis and Complications*. Tokyo, Igaku Shoin, 1972; 1–8.
9. Undenfriend S, Bumpus FM, Foster HL, et al. Spontaneously hypertensive rats: guidelines for breeding, care and use. *ILAR News* 1976; **19**:G1–G20.
10. Palmiter RP, Brinster RL. Germline transformation of mice. *Ann Rev Genetics* 1966; **20**:465–499.
11. Yang H-YT, Erdös EG, Levin YA. A dipeptidyl carboxypeptidase that converts angiotensin I and inactivates bradykinin. *Biochem Biophys Acta* 1970; **214**:374–376.
12. Ito K, Koike H, Miyamoto M, Ozaki H, Kishimoto T, Urakawa N. Long-term effects of captopril on cellular sodium content and mechanical properties of aortic smooth muscle from spontaneously hypertensive rats. *J Pharmacol Exp Ther* 1981; **19**:520–525.
13. Thurston H, Swales JD. Converting enzyme inhibitor and saralasin infusion in rats. Evidence for an additional vasodepressor property of converting enzyme inhibitor. *Circ Res* 1978; **42**:588–592.
14. Sweet CS, Arbegast PT, Gaul SL, Blaine EH, Gross DM. Relationship between angiotensin I blockade and antihypertensive properties of single doses of MK421 and captopril in spontaneous and renal hypertensive rats. *Europ J Pharmacol* 1986; **76**:167–176.
15. Unger Th, Yukimura T, Marin-Grez M, Lang RE, Rascher W, Ganten D. SA446, a new orally active converting enzyme inhibitor: Antihypertensive action and comparison with captopril in spontaneously hypertensive rats. *Europ J Pharmacol* 1982; **78**:411–420.
16. Crantz FR, Swartz SL, Hollenberg NK, Moore ThJ, Williams GH. Differences in response to the peptidyldipeptide hydrolase inhibitor SQ20881 and SQ14225 in normal-renin essential hypertension. *Hypertension* 1980; **2**:604–609.
17. Boomsma F, De Bruyn JHB, Derkx FHM, Schalekamp MADH. Opposite effects of captopril on angiotensin-I—converting enzyme "activity" and "concentration"; relation between enzyme inhibition and long-term blood pressure response. *Clin Sci* 1981; **60**:491–498.
18. Schalekamp MADH, Wenting GJ, De Bruyn JHB, Man in t'Veld AJ, Derkx FHM. Hemodynamics of captopril in essential and renovascular hypertension: correlation with plasma renin. In *ACE Inhibition in Hypertension: From Principle to Practice*. Symposium, Dallas, Nov 1981. New York, Biomedical Information Corp 1982; 19–39.
19. Giudicelli JF, Richer C, Mattei A. Pharmacokinetics and biological effects of captopril and hydrochloroazide after acute and chronic administration either alone or in combination in hypertensive patients. *Br J Clin Pharmacol* 1987; **23**:51S–63S.
20. Schoenberger JA, Wilson DJ. Once-daily treatment of essential hypertension with captopril. *J Clin Hypertens* 1986; **4**:379–387.
21. De Cesaris R, Ranieri G, Salzano EV, Liberatore SM. Once daily treatment with angiotensin converting enzyme inhibitor in mild hypertension: a comparison of captopril and enalapril. *J Hypertens* 1987; **5**:S595–S597.
22. Garanin G. A comparison of once-daily antihypertensive therapy with captopril and enalapril. *Current Therap Res* 1986; **40**:567–575.
23. Rosenthal J, Boucher R, Rojo Ortega JM, Genest J. Renin activity in aortic tissue of rats. *Can J Physiol Pharmacol* 1969; **47**:53.
24. Ganten D, Hayduk K, Brecht HM, Boucher R, Genest J. Evidence of renin release or production in splanchnic territory. *Nature* 1970; **226**:551.

25. Thurston H, Swales JD. Blood pressure response of nephrectomized hypertensive rats to converting enzyme inhibition: evidence for persistent vascular renin activity. *Clin Sci Mol Med* 1977; **52**:299:304.
26. Thurston H, Swales JD, Bing RF, Hurst BC, Marks ES. Vascular renin-like activity and blood pressure maintenance in the rat: studies of the effect of changes in sodium balance, hypertension and nephrectomy. *Hypertension* 1979; **1**:643–649.
27. Campbell DJ, Habener JF. Angiotensinogen gene is expressed and differentially regulated in multiple tissues of the rat. *J Clin Invest* 1986; **78**:31–39.
28. Dzau VJ. Vascular angiotensin pathways: a new therapeutic target. *J Cardiovasc Pharmacol* 1987; **10**:S9–S16.
29. Swales JD, Heagerty AM. Vascular renin-angiotensin system: The unanswered questions. *J Hypertens* 1987; **5**:S1–S5.
30. Darby I, Aldred P, Crawford RJ, Fernley RT, Niall HD, Penschow JD, Ryan GB, Coghlan JP. Gene expression in vessels of the ovine cortex. *J Hypertens* 1985; **3**:9–12.
31. Re R, Fallon JT, Dzau VJ, Quay SC, Haber E. Renin synthesis by canine aortic smooth muscle cells in culture. *Life Sci* 1982; **30**:99–106.
32. Lilly LS, Pratt RE, Alexander RW. Renin expression by vascular endothelial cells in culture. *Circ Res* 1984; **57**:312–318.
33. Kifor I, Dzau VJ. Endothelial renin-angiotensin pathway: evidence for intracellular synthesis and secretion of angiotensins. *Circ Res* 1987; **60**:422–428.
34. Nakamura M, Jackson EK, Inagami T. Beta adrenoceptor-mediated release of angiotensin II from mesenteric arteries. *Am J Physiol* 1986; **250**:H144–H148.
35. Oliver JA, Sciacca RR. Local generation of angiotensin II as a mechanism of regulation of peripheral vascular tone in the rat. *J Clin Invest* 1984; **74**:1247–1251.
36. Malik KU, Nasjletti A. Facilitation of adrenergic transmission by locally generated angiotensin II in rat mesenteric arteries. *Circ Res* 1976; **38**:26–30.
37. Zimmermann BG. Adrenergic facilitation by angiotensin: does it serve a physiological function? *Clin Sci* 1981; **60**:343–348.
38. Kuriyama S, Nakamura A, Hopp L, Fine BP, Kino M, Cragoe E Jr, Aviv A. Angiotensin II effect on $^{22}Na^+$ transport in vascular smooth muscle cells. *J Cardiovasc Pharmacol* 1988; **11**:139–146.
39. Toda N. Endothelium-dependent relation induced by angiotensin II and histamine in isolated arteries of dog. *Br J Pharmacol* 1984; **81**:301–307.
40. Okamura T, Myazaki M, Inagami T, Toda N. Vascular renin-angiotensin system in two-kidney, one clip hypertension. *Hypertension* 1986; **8**:560–565.
41. Unger Th, Ganten D, Lang RE. Pharmacology of converting enzyme inhibitors: New aspects. *Clin Esp Hypertens* 1983; **A5**:1333–1354.
42. Ball SG. ACE inhibitors and the nervous system. *J Card Vasc Pharm* (in press).
43. Schölkens BA, Xiang JZ, Tilly H. Influence of the converting enzyme inhibitors Hoe 498, enalapril and captopril on vascular reactivity of isolated arterial preparations. *Clin Exp Hypertens* 1984; **A6**:1807–1813.
44. Kawasaki H, Cline WH Jr, Su C. Involvement of the vascular renin-angiotensin system in beta adrenergic receptor-mediated facilitation of vascular neurotransmission in spontaneously hypertensive rats. *J Pharmacol Exp Ther* 1984; **231**:23–32.
45. Göthert M, Kollecker P. Subendothelial β_2-adrenoceptors in the rat vena cava: facilitation of the release via local stimulation of angiotensin II synthesis. *Naunyn-Schmiedeberg's Arch Pharmacol* 1986; **334**:156–165.
46. Webb DJ, Collier JG: Vascular angiotensin conversion in humans: *J Cardiovasc Pharmacol* 1986; **8**:S40–S44.
47. Scherf H, Pietsch R, Landsberg G, Kramer HJ, Düsing R. Converting enzyme inhibitor ramipril stimulates prostacyclin synthesis by isolated rat aorta: evidence for a kinin-dependent mechanism. *Klin Wochenschr* 1986; **64**:742–745.
48. Oshima T, Matsushita Y, Miyamoto M, Koike H. Effect of long-term blockade of angiotensin converting enzyme with captopril on blood pressure and aortic prolyl hydroxylase activity in spontaneously hypertensive rats. *Europ J Pharmacol* 1983; **91**:283–286.
49. Henrichs KJ, Unger Th, Berecek KH, Ganten D. Is arterial media hypertrophy in spontaneously hypertensive rats a consequence of or a cause for hypertension. *Clin Sci* 1980; **59**:331s–333s.
50. Hayduk K, Boucher R, Genest J. Renin activity and content in various tissues in dogs under

different pathophysiological states. *Proc Soc Exp Biol Med* 1970; **134**:252–255.
51. Ganten D, Ganten U, Granger O, Boucher R, Genest J. Renin in heart muscle and arterial tissue (abstr.). *Verh Dtsch Ges Kreislaufforsch* 1972; **38**:268.
52. Re RN, Michalik RJ, Dzau VJ. Cardiac myocytes contain renin (abstr.). *Clin Res* 1983; **31**:845A.
53. Dzau VJ, Ellison KE, Brody T, Ingelfinger J, Pratt RE. A comparative study of the distributions of renin and angiotensinogen messenger ribonucleic acids in rat and mouse tissues. *Endocrinology* 1987; **120**:2334–2338.
54. Suzuki F, Hellmann T, Murakami K, Ludwig G. Expression of the genes for renin and angiotensinogen in tissues of rats (abstr.). *Naunyn Schmiedeberg's Arch Pharamacol* 1987; **335**:R66.
55. Ganten D, Ludwig G, Hennhoefer C. Genetic control of renin in the tissues of different strains of mice (abstr.). *Naunyn Schmiedeberg's Arch Pharmacol* 1986; **332**:R59.
56. Auffray C, Rougeon F. Purification of mouse immunoglobulin heavy chain mRNAs from total myeloma tumor RNA. *Eur J Biochem* 1980; **107**:303–314.
57. Le Muer M, Glanville N, Mandel JL, Gerlinger P, Palmiter R, Chambon P. The ovealbumin gene family: hormonal control of X- and Y-gene transcription and mRNA accumulation. *Cell* 1981; **23**:561–571.
58. Lindpaintner K, Wilhelm M, Jin M, Unger Th, Lang RE, Ganten D. Tissue renin-angiotensin systems: focus on the heart. *J Hypertens* 1987; **5**:S33–S38.
59. Needleman P, Marshall GR, Sobel BE. Hormone interactions in the isolated rabbit heart. *Circ Res* 1975; **37**:802–808.
60. Nakashima A, Angus JA, Johnston CI. Chronotropic effects of angiotensin I, angiotensin II, bradykinin and norepinephrine in guinea pig atria. *Eur J Pharmacol* 1982; **81**:479–485.
61. Unger Th, Ganten D, Lang RE, Schölkens BA. Is tissue converting enzyme inhibition a determinant of the antihypertensive efficacy of converting enzyme inhibitors? Studies with two different compounds, Hoe-498 and MK-421, in spontaneously hypertensive rats. *J Cardiovasc Pharmacol* 1984; **6**:872–880.
62. Heeg E, Meng K. Die Wirkung des Bradykinins, Angiotensins und Vasopressins auf Vorhof, Papillarmuskel, und isoliert durchströmte Herzpräparate des Meerschweinschens. *Naunyn Schmiedeberg's Arch Pathol* 1965; **250**:35–47.
63. Freer RJ, Pappano AJ, Pech MJ, et al. Mechanisms for the positive inotropic effect of angiotensin II on isolated cardiac muscle. *Circ Res* 1976; **39**:178–183.
64. Kobayashi M, Furukawa Y, Chiba S. Positive chronotropic and inotropic effects of angiotensin II in the dog heart. *Eur J Pharmacol* 1978; **50**:17–25.
65. Dempsey PJ, McCallum ZT, Kent KM, Cooper T. Direct myocardial effects of angiotensin II. *Am J Physiol* 1971; **220**:477.
66. Koch-Weser J. Myocardial actions of angiotensin. *Circ Res* 1964; **14**:337–344.
67. Starke K, Werner U, Schuermann HJ. Wirkungen von Angiotensin auf Funktion und Noradrenalinabgabe isolierter Kaninchenherzen in Ruhe und bei Sympathikusreizung. *Naunyn Schiederberg's Arch Pharmacol* 1966; **265**:170–186.
68. Blumberg AL, Acherly JA, Peach MJ. Differentiation of neurogenic and myocardial angiotensin II receptors in isolated rabbit atria. *Circ Res* 1976; **36**:719–726.
69. Xiang J, Linz W, Becker H, et al. Effects of converting enzyme inhibitors ramipril and enalapril on peptide actions and sympathetic neurotransmission in the isolated heart. *Eur J Pharmacol* 1984; **113**:215–223.
70. Khairallah PA. Action of angiotensin on adrenergic nerve endings. *Fed Proc* 1972; **31**:1351–1357.
71. Swartz SL, Williams GH, Hollenberg NK, Levine L, Denk JR, Moore TJ. Captopril-induced changes in prostaglandin production. *J Clin Invest* 1980; **65**:1257–1264.
72. Roth RH. Action of angiotensin on adrenergic nerve endings. *Fed Proc* 1972; **31**:1358–1364.
73. Westfall TC. Local regulation of adrenergic neurotransmission. *Physiol Rev* 1977; **57**:659–728.
74. Clough DP, Mulroy SC, Angell D, Hatton R. Interference by inhibitors of the renin-angiotensin system with neurogenic vasoconstriction. *Clin Exp Hypertens* 1983; **5**:1287–1299.
75. Xiang JZ, Schoelkens BA, Ganten D, Unger Th. Effects of sympathetic nerve stimulation are attenuated by the converting enzyme inhibitor Hoe-498 in isolated rabbit hearts. *Clin Exp Hypertens* 1984; **6**:1853–1857.

77. Ertl G, Kloner RA, Alexander RW, Braunwald E. Limitation of experimental infarct size by an angiotensin converting enzyme inhibitor. *Circulation* 1982; **65**:40–48.
77. Linz W, Schoelkens BA, Han YE. Beneficial effects of the converting enzyme inhibitor, ramipril, in ischemic rat hearts. *J Cardiovasc Pharmacol* 1986; **8**:S91–S99.
78. Cleland JGF, Dargie HJ, Hodsman GJP, et al. Captopril in heart failure. A double-blind controlled trial. *Br Heart J* 1984; **52**:530–535.
79. Webster MWI, Fitzpatrick MA, Nicholls MG, Ikram H, Wells JE. Effect of enalapril on ventricular arrhythmias in congestive heart failure. *Am J Cardiol* 1985; **5**:566–569.
80. Ganten D, Lang RE, Lehmann E, Unger Th. Brain angiotensin: on the way to becoming a well-studied neuropeptide system. *Biochem Pharmacol* 1984; **33**:3523–3528.
81. Stamler JF, Brody MJ, Phillips MI. The central and peripheral effects of captopril (SQ 14225) on the arterial pressure of the spontaneously hypertensive rat. *Brain Res* 1980; **186**:499–503.
82. Hutchinson JS, Mendelsohn, FAO, Doyle AE. Blood pressure responses of conscious normotensive and spontaneously hypertensive rats to intracerebroventricular and peripheral administration of captopril. *Hypertension* 1980; **2**:546–550.
83. Unger Th, Kaufmann-Bühler I, Schölkens B, Ganten D. Brain converting enzyme inhibition: a possible mechanism for the antihypertensive action of captopril in spontaneously hypertensive rats. *Eur J Pharmacol* 1981; **70**:467–478.
84. Phillips MI, Kimura B. Converting enzyme inhibitors and brain angiotensin. *J Cardiovasc Pharmacol* 1986; **8(suppl 10)**:82–90.
85. Suzuki H, Kondo K, Handa M, Saruta T. Role of the brain isorenin-angiotensin system in experimental hypertension in rats. *Clin Sci* 1981; **61**:175–180.
86. Pochiero M, Nicoletta P, Losi E, Bianchi A, Caputi AP. Cardiovascular responses of conscious DOCA-salt hypertensive rats to acute intracerebroventricular and intravenous administration of captopril. *Pharmacol Res Comm* 1983; **15**:173–182.
87. Vollmer RR, Boccagno JA. Central cardiovascular effects of SQ 14225, an angiotensin converting inhibitor in chloralose anesthetized cats. *Eur J Pharmacol* 1977; **45**:117–125.
88. Mann JFE, Rascher W, Dietz R, Schömig A, Ganten D. Effects of an orally-active converting enzyme inhibitor, SQ 14255, on pressor responses to angiotensin administered into brain ventricles of spontaneously hypertensive rats. *Clin Sci* 1979; **56**:585–589.
89. Hutchinson JS, Hooper R, Jarrott B, Mendelsohn FAO, Louis WJ. Captopril does not cross the blood cerebrospinal fluid barrier in the spontaneously hypertensive rat after a single, intravenous injection. In Rascher W, Clough D, Ganten D (eds). *Hypertensive mechanisms.* Stuttgart Schattauer Verlag 1982;691–694.
90. Cohen ML, Kurz KD. Angiotensin converting enzyme inhibition in tissues from spontaneously hypertensive rats after treatment with captopril or MK-421. *J Pharmacol Exp Ther* 1982; **220**:63–69.
91. Norman JA, Lehmann M, Goodman FR, Barclay BW, Zimmermann MB. Central and peripheral inhibition of angiotensin converting enzyme (ACE) in the SHR: Correlation with the antihypertensive activity of the inhibitors. *Clin Exp Hypertens* 1987; **A9 (2&3)**:461–468.
92. Nakata K, Nishimura K, Takada T, Ikuse T, Yamauchi H, Iso T. Effects of an angiotensin-converting enzyme (ACE) inhibitor, SA446, on tissue ACE activity in normotensive, spontaneously hypertensive, and renal hypertensive rats. *J Cardiovasc Pharmacol* 1987; **9**:305–310.
93. Evered MD, Robinson MM, Richardson MA. Captopril given intracerebroventricularly, subcutaneously or by gavage inhibits angiotensin converting enzyme activity in the rat brain. *Eur J Pharmacol* 1980; **68**:443–449.
94. Geppetti P, Spillantini MG, Frilli S, Pietrini U, Fanciullacci M, Sicuteri F. Acute oral captopril inhibits angiotensin converting enzyme activity in human cerebrospinal fluid. *J Hypertens* 1987; **5**:151–154.

SUMMARY

Hypertension represents one of the most serious public health problems, both in terms of the number of people affected or at risk and because of its long-term sequelae, which are a major cause of morbidity and mortality in our societies. Despite continued research efforts, primary hypertension, which accounts for the vast majority of cases, remains poorly understood and is thus far amenable only to palliative treatments. Based on epidemiologic and experimental data, however, one can be fairly certain that primary hypertension is a genetically transmitted, inheritable disease.

Studies directed at clinical problems such as hypertension are limited by the fact that neither *in vitro* or *in vivo* test systems nor computer simulation are able to provide a precise experimental counterpart for a human disease. Meaningful generalizations from experimental models to human disease are, therefore, difficult. Evidence suggests, however, that several models of experimental hypertension, in particular the genetically hypertensive rat, share a number of important features with primary hypertension in humans. Thus, use of these models, in conjunction with proper scientific questions and appropriate research methodology, has improved our understanding of the disease and the possibilities for its treatment and prevention.

The introduction of transgenic animals into hypertension research represents a powerful new approach to the study of this disease and is expected to lead to significant advances in its understanding. To be put to use appropriately and productively, implementation of this technique calls for a concerted effort involving scientists working in different areas and on different aspects of hypertension. The renin-angiotensin system is particularly suited to the application of this new biology in hypertension research.

RÉSUMÉ

L'hypertension représente un des problèmes les plus graves de la santé publique, à la fois de par le nombre de gens qui en sont atteints ou sous risque, et à cause de ses séquelles à long terme, qui sont une des causes principales de morbidité et mortalité dans nos sociétés. En dépit des efforts permanents de la recherche, l'hypertension essentielle qui représente la vaste majorité des cas, demeure pratiquement incomprise, et n'a été jusqu'à présent soumise qu'à des traitements palliatifs. D'après les données épidémiologiques et expérimentales, on peut, cependant, affirmer que l'hypertension essentielle est une maladie génétiquement transmissible à ses descendants. Des études portant sur les problèmes cliniques tels que l'hypertension sont limitées par le fait que ni les systèmes de tests *in vitro* ou *in vivo* ni la simulation sur ordinateur ne peuvent fournir une contrepartie expérimentale précise de la maladie humaine. Il est donc difficile de généraliser à partir de modèles expérimentaux de la maladie humaine. On constate, cependant, que plusieurs modèles d'hypertension expérimentale, surtout chez le rat génétiquement hypertensif, partagent un certain nombre de caractéristiques avec l'hypertension essentielle chez l'homme. C'est ainsi que, l'utilisation de ces modèles, de concert avec les questions scientifiques appropriées et une méthodologie de recherche bien choisie, ont réussi à améliorer notre compréhension de la maladie et d'envisager les possibilités thérapeutiques et la prévention de la maladie.

L'introduction d'animaux transgéniques dans le domaine de la recherche sur l'hypertension représente une nouvelle approche intéressante pour l'étude de cette maladie et devrait mener à une plus grande compréhension de la maladie. Pour être utilisée convenablement et avec profit, l'application de cette technique exige un effort concerté de tous les chercheurs qui travaillent dans différents domaines et sur différents aspects de l'hypertension. Le système rénine-angiotensine convient particulièrement à l'application de cette nouvelle biologie dans la recherche de l'hypertension.

ZUSAMMENFASSUNG

Hypertonie stellt eins der ernstesten Probleme des öffentlichen Gesundheitswesens dar; und zwar sowohl in Hinsicht auf die Zahl der betroffenen Personen als auch im Hinblick auf die damit verbundenen Spätschäden, die eine grosse Auswirkung auf die Krankheitsziffern und Mortalitätsraten in unseren Gesellschaften haben. Trotz fortgesetzter Bemühungen der Forschung bleibt die primäre Hypertonie, die für die Mehrzahl der Fälle verantwortlich ist, relativ wenig erforscht und ist damit nur lindernder Behandlung zugänglich. Epidemiologische und experimentelle Daten geben jedoch einen ziemlich sicheren Hinweis darauf, dass primäre Hypertonie eine genetisch übertragbare, erbliche Krankheit ist.

Studien, die sich mit klinischen Problemen wie der Hypertonie befassen, scheitern an der Tatsache, dass weder in vitro- noch in vivo-Testsysteme, noch Computersimulationen in der Lage sind, ein präzises experimentelles Modell für eine menschliche Krankheit zu liefern. Daher sind bedeutsame Verallgemeinerungen aus experimentellen Modellen auf menschliche Krankheiten mit Schwierigkeiten verbunden. Es liegen jedoch Hinweise dafür vor, dass verschiedene Modelle für experimentelle Hypertonie — insbesondere die genetisch hypertonische Ratte — einige wichtige Eigenschaften mit der primären Hypertonie in Menschen teilen. So hat die Verwendung dieser Modelle, zusammen mit angemessenen wissenschaftlichen Fragen und Forschungsmethoden, unser Verständnis der Krankheit und der Behandlungs- und Vorsorgemöglichkeiten verbessert.

Die Verwendung von transgenen Tieren in der Hypertonie-Forschung stellt einen wichtigen neuen Zugang zum Studium dieser Krankheit dar und sollte erwartungsgemäss zu bedeutungsvollen Fortschritten in ihrem Verständnis führen. Um eine angemessene und produktive Verwendung zu gewährleisten, muss diese Technik in einem konzertierten Programm angewendet werden, das die Bemühungen von Wissenschaftlern verschiedener Richtungen vereinigt und sich auf verschiedene Aspekte der Hypertonie konzentriert. Besonders geeignet für die Anwendung dieser neuen Biologie in der Hypertonie-Forschung ist das Renin-Angiotensin-System.

RIASSUNTO

L'ipertensione rappresenta uno dei problemi di salute pubblica più gravi, sia in termini del numero di persone afflitte o a rischio sia a ragione delle sue lunghe sequele che sono una causa importante di stati patologici e mortalità nelle nostre società. Malgrado continui sforzi di ricerca, l'ipertensione primaria, che è responsabile della stragrande maggioranza dei casi, rimane mal compresa ed è finora oggetto solo di cure palliative. Sulla base di dati epidemiologici e sperimentali, si può essere tuttavia alquanto certi che l'ipertensione primaria è una malattia trasmessa geneticamente e quindi ereditabile.

Studi rivolti verso problemi clinici quali l'ipertensione sono limitati dal fatto che né i sistemi di test in vitro néquelli in vivo né la simulazione su computer sono in grado di fornire una precisa controparte sperimentale ad un morbo umano. Le generalizzazioni significative da modelli sperimentali a malattie umane sono quindi difficili. I fatti tuttavia suggeriscono che vari modelli di ipertensione sperimentale, in particolar modo il topo geneticamente ipertensivo, hanno varie caratteristiche in comune con l'ipertensione primaria negli esseri umani. Quindi l'uso di tali modelli, assieme alle domande scientifiche adatte al caso e ad un'idonea metodologia di ricerca, hanno migliorato la nostra comprensione della malattia e le possibilità di curarla e prevenirla.

L'introduzione di animali transgenici nella ricerca sull'ipertensione rappresenta un nuovo poderoso modo di affrontare lo studio di questa malattia e ci si aspetta che porti a significativi passi avanti nella sua comprensione. Per poter essere messa in uso correttamente e produttivamente, l'attuazione di questa tecnica richiede uno sforzo concertato di scienziati che lavorano in campi diversi e su diversi aspetti dell'ipertensione. Il sistema renina-angiotensina è particolarmente adatto all'applicazione di questa nuova biologia nella ricerca sull'ipertensione.

SUMÁRIO

A hipertensão representa um dos problemas mais sérios da saúde pública, tanto em termos do número de pessoas afetadas ou sob risco de hipertensão, como em termos das seqüelas a largo prazo, as quais são uma causa importante da morbidade e da mortalidade em nossas sociedades. Apesar dos contínuos esforços de pesquisa, a hipertensão essencial, que representa a grande maioria dos casos, ainda não é bem entendida e até agora só existem tratamentos de alívio. Contudo, com base nos dados epidemiológicos e experimentais, há bastante certeza de que a hipertensão essencial é uma doença herdável e genéticamente transmitida. Os estudos dirigidos aos problemas clínicos, tais como a hipertensão, são limitados pelo fato que nem os sistemas de teste *in vitro* ou *in vivo*, nem as simulações de computador são capazes de proporcionar um modelo experimental exato da doença humana. Protanto, é difícil estabelecer generalizações significativas dos modelos experimentais que são aplicáveis à doneça humana. Contudo, a evidência sugere que vários modelos de hipertensão experimental, particularmente o rato genéticamente hipertenso, compartilham várias características importantes com a hipertensão essencial nos humanos. É assim que o uso destos modelos, em conjunção com investigações científicas adequadas e a metodologia apropriada de pesquisa, têm melhorado nosso entendimento da doença e as possibilidades para seu tratamento e prevenção. A introdução de animais transgênicos na pesquisa da hipertensao representa um enfoque poderoso encaminhado ao estudo desta doença e espere-se que conduza a avanços significativos no entendimento da hipertensão. Para que se ponha no uso de maneira apropriada e produtiva, a implementação desta técnica requer um esforço conjunto de científicos que trabalham em diferentes áreas e aspectos da hipertensão. O sistema renina-angiotensina é particularmente adequado para a aplicação desta nova biologia na pesquisa da hipertensão.

RESUMEN

La hipertensión representa uno de los problemas más serios de salud pública, tanto en términos del número de personas que se ven afectadas o enfrentan riesgo de hipertensión, como en términos de las secuelas a largo plazo, que son una de las principales causas de morbilidad y mortalidad en nuestra sociedad. A pesar de los continuos esfuerzos de investigación, la hipertensión esencial, que representa la gran mayoría de casos, todavía no se entiende cabalmente y hasta ahora solo existen tratamientos de alivio. Sin embargo, en base a los datos epidemiológicos y experimentales, hay bastante certeza de que la hipertensión esencial es una enfermedad heredable y genéticamente transmitida. Los estudios dirigidos a los problemas clínicos, tales como la hipertensión, se ven limitados por el hecho de que ni los sistemas de ensayo *in vitro* o *in vivo,* ni las simulaciones de computadora son capaces de proporcionar un modelo experimental preciso de la enfermedad humana. Por lo tanto, es difícil establecer generalizaciones significativas de los modelos experimentales que se apliquen a la enfermedad humana. Sin embargo, las evidencias dan a entender que varios modelos de hipertensión experimental, en particular la rata genéticamente hipertensa, comparten varias características importantes con la hipertensión esencial en los humanos. Es así que el empleo de estos modelos, en conjunción con investigaciones científicas adecuadas y la metodología apropiada de investigación, han mejorado nuestro entendimiento de la enfermedad y las posibilidades para su tratamiento y prevención. La introducción de animales transgénicos en la investigación de la hipertensión representa un enfoque poderoso encaminado al estudio de esta enfermedad y se espera que lleve a avances significativos en el entendimiento de la hipertensión. Para que se ponga en uso de manera apropiada y productiva, la implementación de esta técnica requiere un esfuerzo conjunto de científicos que trabajan en diferentes áreas y aspectos de la hipertensión. El sistema renina-angiotensina es particularmente adecuado para la aplicación de esta nueva biología en la investigación de la hipertensión.

要約

　高血圧は，患者数あるいは今日の社会ではその長期予後において主要な疾病および死因に結びつくという点でも，最も重要な公衆衛生上の問題となっている。長年の研究努力にもかかわらず，患者の大多数を占める本態性高血圧症については，まだ不明な点が多く対症療法に頼るしかない。しかし，疫学調査や実験データによると，本態性高血圧症は遺伝的に伝わる疾患であることが明らかにされつつある。

　In vitro や *in vivo* での実験系，またはコンピュータシミュレーションのいずれにおいても，ヒトの疾患に対する正確な実験的対照物をつくりだせないために，高血圧のような臨床的課題についての研究には限界がある。実験モデルでの成績をヒトの疾患に意味のあるかたちであてはめることには無理がある。実験データによれば，いくつかの実験的高血圧モデル，とくに遺伝性高血圧ラットは，ヒトの本態性高血圧症の重要な特徴を有していることが示唆されている。そこで，これらのモデルを用いて，適切な科学的設問と方法論を組み合わせて研究することによって，この疾患の理解を深め，治療と予防の可能性も広がることになろう。

　遺伝的動物の高血圧研究への導入は，本疾患研究の新しい有力なアプローチ手段となり，その理解を深めるのに大いに役立つと期待される。この技法を適切かつ生産的に実施するには，異なった分野や異なった角度で高血圧を研究している科学者たちを包含した共同研究が必要である。高血圧研究において，レニン-アンジオテンシン系はこの新しい生物学研究法を適応するのにとくに適している。

Cardiac and Renal Failure: An Expanding Role for ACE Inhibitors, edited by C. T. Dollery and L. M. Sherwood, Hanley & Belfus, Inc., Philadelphia.

DISCUSSION

PETERS: Dr Ganten, what are the effects of ACE inhibitors on embryonic growth?

GANTEN: We have treated female rats before pregnancy with various converting-enzyme inhibitors including SH-containing and non-SH containing compounds. We did not find any obvious effects on the litter size or on other parameters of the offspring. At the present time we have no real evidence that there are any detrimental effects in the rat. However Dr Broughten-Pipkin in the UK reported important effects on litter size and stillbirth rate in the sheep. I am not sure whether these are experimental differences or species differences and I think the problem needs further investigation.

LANGMAN: I wanted to ask about the generalized data on growth. Are there effects on other tissues — for example wound healing and colonic growth. Colonic hypertrophy is a disease of old age and of considerable importance, in relation to the almost ubiquitous occurrence of diverticulosis.

GANTEN: The data I am aware of concern 3T3 cells, which I mentioned in my presentation. There is also an effect on growth in zona glomerulosa cells of the rat adrenal gland and on the growth of vascular smooth muscle.

CORVOL: Human hepatocarcinoma cells also respond to angiotensin II [ANG II] by an increase in radiolabeled thymidine incorporation. There is also an increase in cell numbers. The doses of ANG II which had to be given to show this effect were quite high. What doses did you use in the experiment you just mentioned.

GANTEN: We established dose response curves. The lowest dose we used was the 100 ng per 5 ml Petri dish, which is not unreasonably high. I would like to mention in this context a recent report from the Charlottesville Group by Peach and colleagues. They did not see an effect of angiotensin on aortic smooth cell number *in vitro*. They reported an increase in protein synthesis but no mitogenic effects. I would also like to add that 3T3 cells can be transformed to SV40 3T3 cells by infection with simian virus 40; these transformed cells are tumor cells. They can be transplanted into hamsters and tumor growth is observed in these animals. In this *in vivo* study we found the reverse: angiotensin inhibited rather than stimulated growth. We therefore have to be careful with the interpretation of these data and with extrapolation from *in vitro* to *in vivo* conclusions.

MORGAN: Dr Brunner, if you show that ANG II rises back to normal at 24 hours, what do you think is the cause of the rise in renin that persists? Do you think that some of your observations are the result of using a drug that does not work for 24 hours? If you use a drug with a half-life of 24 hours perhaps you wouldn't see these changes. When we give ANG II chronically in rats and mice, it does not return to normal levels at all, it stays at zero.

BRUNNER: We gave the ACE inhibitor in a dose of 20 mg, once daily. Usually plasma ANG II levels return to normal within 24 hours. However, as you point out, we don't see plasma renin activity coming back to normal. I am still not clear what this means. Of course, ACE activity, however it is measured, does not return to normal for 2 or 3 days. My interpretation is that renin secretion is driven by ANG II, because of this partial inhibition of ACE, but I don't know the precise answer. It is a fact that plasma renin activity stays high much longer than angiotensin levels are reduced.

LEDINGHAM: I wanted to comment on the capacity of angiotensin to promote cell growth. Is there not evidence that in renal proximal convoluted tubule cells in culture mitogenesis induced by epidermal growth factor is enhanced in the presence of angiotensin? This was published in the *American Journal of Physiology* last year.

There have been suggestions that among the very large number of different converting-enzyme inhibitors there may be some with specific penetration, and therefore activity in specific vascular beds. Could you say how many different chemical structures you have looked at in relation to your question about where in the heart ACE inhibitor might prevent reperfusion arrhythmia? Might there be different access to vascular endothelium, myocyte or even cardiac fatty tissue?

GANTEN: We did not see any major difference between the various compounds we used: enalapril, captopril, ramipril and cilazapril all worked similarly.

I would like to add that some of these experiments were done in collaboration with the group in Frankfurt, Dr Schölhens, and colleagues. Treatment has been given both *in vitro* with the addition of converting enzyme inhibitors to the perfusate, but also *in vivo* with antihypertensive doses, 10 mg/Kg of enalapril or equivalent ACE inhibitor in the rat. Similar effects were seen on the isolated heart. I don't think we are dealing with merely experimental, *in vitro* pharmacology.

COHN: I wanted to ask Dr Brunner about the time course of the reactive rise in renin and angiotensin I [ANG I]. There has been some suggestion that this does not persist during chronic therapy. I wonder what your concept is of the persistence of that reactive response?

BRUNNER: I would not agree that it goes away with long-term treatment. Over a long period of time, of course, it is very difficult to keep all conditions equal. Renin still responds to salt depletion even during ACE inhibition. To compare renin measurements over a long period we would have to keep all other conditions equal, which is extremely difficult.

POOLE-WILSON: I would like to come back to the question of the localization of ACE in the heart. We were unable to find any ACE in cell membranes from isolated sheep myocytes. We concluded that most of the ACE was in the endothelial cells. This leads to the idea that most of the results reported on ischemic preparations are due to a reduced heterogeneity of flow through the ischemic tissue at the time of reperfusion. I would put it to you that that is the explanation for your experiment.

GANTEN: Did you say that these were myocyte membranes not cells?

POOLE-WILSON: Yes.

GANTEN: We have done similar experiments using cultures of cardiomyocytes. We did find enzyme activity but it was much lower than in the endothelium.

POOLE-WILSON: We were very sure on that point. The cell membranes were obtained from isolated sheep myocytes.

SCHWARTZ: Dr Ganten, you have shown that giving ACE inhibitors at low dosage reverses cardiac growth induced by pressure overload. Did you try, or do you know if, pretreating the rats before doing the aortic stenosis prevents cardiac hypertrophy?

GANTEN: Yes, it does, although it has not been done with low doses of converting-enzyme inhibitors.

BRUNNER: I like the experiment using induced aortic stenosis. Riegger and his co-workers got the same results. What is the evidence that you need cardiac tissue renin for the explanation for this result? As you have pointed out, ANG I and II and renin are taken up by tissues, and I am not convinced that you need to imply renin and ANG II from cardiac tissue origin since ANG II from the circulation could have been responsible for the observed effect.

GANTEN: Cardiac tissue and circulating angiotensin are probably both involved in the same events, possibly using, at least in part, the same receptors. The argument for local angiotensin is still indirect. Angiotensin clearly is a growth factor, and at a low dose of converting enzyme inhibitor the plasma angiotensin is high as seen in the untreated hypertensive animals. It is much higher than in normotensive animals and yet cardiac hypertrophy has returned to normal. This surprised us and must indicate that there is a further element in addition to circulating angiotensins. It may be both, circulating and local peptide.

JOHNSTON: Is tissue angiotensin too low?

BRUNNER: If plasma angiotensin is not low, then why is tissue angiotensin low?

GANTEN: I agree with you that there are many unanswered questions and we will continue to study them.

Cardiac and Renal Failure: An Expanding Role for ACE Inhibitors, edited by C. T. Dollery and L. M. Sherwood, Hanley & Belfus, Inc., Philadelphia.

Worldwide Use of Pharmacologic Agents in Hypertension and Heart Failure

Errol S. McKinney

Over the past few decades there have been many changes worldwide in the treatment of hypertension and of congestive heart failure (CHF). As many as 10 to 20% of the adult population are found to have mild elevations of blood pressure from time to time,[1] but by no means should all of them be treated with antihypertensive drugs. On the other hand, patients with mild hypertension are at greater risk of cardiovascular disease. Trials of drug therapy have shown that treatment prevents progression of hypertension to the accelerated or malignant phase, reduces the incidence of stroke and CHF, and may prevent or reverse left ventricular hypertrophy (LVH).[2-6] Despite these benefits, the approach to pharmacologic intervention in the treatment of this disease has evolved only slowly over the last two decades. Recently published guidelines of the Joint National Committee on Detection Evaluation, and Treatment of High Blood Pressure (JNC 4) complement recent recommendations by the World Health Organization and International Society of Hypertension[1] which favor "individualized" or patient-directed care as a replacement for the old stepped-care approach to antihypertensive therapy. It is now recommended that first-step treatment may be initiated with either diuretics, beta-adrenergic blocking agents (beta-blockers), angiotensin-converting enzyme (ACE) inhibitors, or calcium entry blockers. Factors such as demographics, concomitant disease, biochemical evaluations, and special populations with management problems (for example: LVH, coronary vascular disease, cerebral vascular disease)[7] should be taken into account when selecting initial therapy.

Congestive heart failure (CHF) is a condition reportedly affecting 1% of the population, with an annual incidence of approximately 3 in 1000.[8] Although the prognosis of Class IV CHF is poor (annual mortality is in excess of 50% in well-recognized cases),[9] ACE inhibitors may be associated with both hemodynamic and symptomatic improvements in the disease with long-term use.[10] In fact, the recently published CONSENSUS trial study results show that the addition of enalapril to conventional therapy in patients with severe CHF reduces mortality.[10] These findings may have a significant effect on the future direction of treatment for this disease.

HYPERTENSION PRESCRIBING PATTERNS

United States

By far the largest of the markets reviewed in terms of prescription volume, total hypertension prescriptions in the U.S. increased from 1984 to 1987 by 8%, from 88 million to 95 million (Figure 1). From 1986 to 1987, however, prescriptions declined from 100 million to 95 million. These two years saw significant declines of older therapies: synthetic hypotensives, diuretics, and beta blockers. This may reflect the changing approaches in hypertension treatment from multi-therapy to monotherapy. During this time, the market

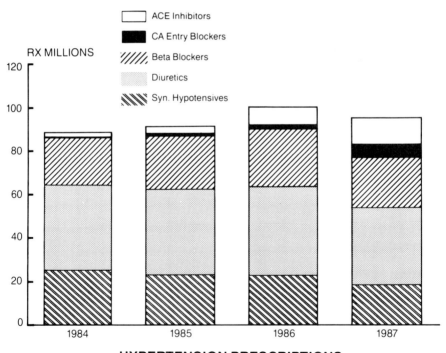

FIG. 1. Hypertension prescriptions in the United States (1984 through 1987).

was also undergoing a dramatic restructuring with the use of ACE inhibitors and calcium-entry blockers increasing from 10% to 20% of the total.

United Kingdom

The prescribing patterns in Europe are somewhat different from those in the U.S. (Figure 2). In the U.K., for example, total hypertension prescriptions were 26 million in 1987, an increase of 9% per year from 1984. Use of synthetic hypotensives and diuretics was virtually unchanged, with 2% and 1% growth, respectively, during the same time period. Beta blockers continued to grow from eight million to ten million prescriptions. However, due to expansion of the entire market, this volume growth still resulted in a slight

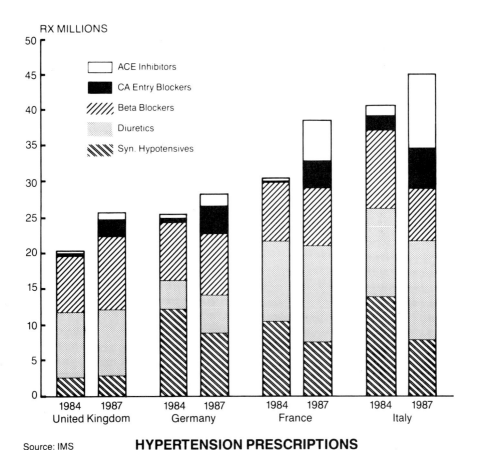

Source: IMS   **HYPERTENSION PRESCRIPTIONS**

FIG. 2. Hypertension prescriptions in Europe: United Kingdom, Germany, France, and Italy (1984 and 1987).

decline in market share from 38.6% in 1984 to 38.4% in 1987. Nonetheless, the older, more traditional therapies, beta-blockers and diuretics combined, still represent 74% of the market in 1987. In the U.K., new therapies have historically been accepted more slowly than in France or Italy, and as yet ACE inhibitors and calcium entry blockers occupy a smaller share of the market. Although they represented only 10% of total prescriptions in 1987, these two therapeutic classes were the fastest growing. ACE inhibitors have grown steadily to capture approximately 7% of the market.

In the U.K., most prescribed products are single entity drugs. As a result, fixed-ratio combination products, with the exception of beta-blockers, represent less than 3% of each therapeutic class. In the case of beta-blockers, combination products represent 29% of all prescriptions in this class.

Germany

In Germany, the pattern is somewhat different. Total hypertension prescriptions increased by 4% per year to 28 million in 1987. The only class of medication with declining prescriptions was synthetic hypotensives — down from 12 million in 1984 to 8.5 million in 1987, which still represented 30% of the market. Beta-blockers, with 31% of the total prescriptions, were the largest therapy class. This figure represented a growth of 3% to 8.7 million from 7.9 million prescriptions in 1984. Calcium-entry blockers and ACE inhibitors were the fastest growing therapies. The calcium blockers exhibited the largest increase, with market share up from 3% in 1984 to 13% in 1987. ACE inhibitors increased from 2% to 7% of the market during these years. Combination products accounted for more than 40% of the total for each therapeutic class, with the exception of calcium-entry blockers. Combinations accounted for only 17% of the calcium entry blocker prescriptions.

France

A very different picture can be seen in France, where the market is growing very rapidly. Here, beta-blockers have never been prescribed to the same degree as in other countries and ACE inhibitors are the most rapidly growing class for the treatment of hypertension. Total hypertension prescriptions increased by 8% per year from 1984 to 38 million in 1987. This expansion was fueled by the tremendous growth of ACE inhibitors as well as the calcium-entry blockers. As in the U.S., the use of ACE inhibitors has increased extremely rapidly to capture 16% of the antihypertensive market with six million prescriptions in 1987. Calcium-entry blockers represented 9% of the hypertension market in 1987 with 3.3 million prescriptions. Synthetic hypotensives declined in volume by 11% from ten million prescriptions in 1984 to seven million in 1987. Diuretics and beta-blockers had average growths of 5%

and 3%, respectively. Despite their positive growth, diuretics and beta-blockers, as well as synthetic hypotensives, have lost prescription share to ACE inhibitors and calcium-entry blockers.

Italy

In Italy, the picture was much the same, with ACE inhibitors capturing 22% of the hypertension prescription market in 1987. Total prescriptions increased by 3% to 45 million in 1987. Synthetic hypotensives and beta-blockers declined in 1987 by 18% and 6%, respectively. Diuretics leveled off, with an average 1% growth. Calcium-entry blockers grew from two million to six million prescriptions in 1987, which represented a 13% share. ACE inhibitors had an even greater increase in usage, having increased from two million in 1984 to ten million in 1987, which represented a change from 5% to 22% market share. This growth made ACE inhibitors the second largest therapeutic class after diuretics, which had a 31% share.

A Recent Trend

The recent hypertension treatment guidelines recommend increasing "individualization" of antihypertensive therapy. Inclusion of ACE inhibitors and calcium-entry blockers with traditional agents such as diuretics and beta-blockers as first-line therapy options is expected to further the emergence of these therapeutic classes in the treatment of hypertension.

PHYSICIAN PERCEPTION OF ANTIHYPERTENSIVE THERAPY

Increasingly, physicians perceive that they are treating multiple cardiovascular conditions rather than simply hypertension alone. This is due, in part, to the recognition of the concomitant nature of many cardiovascular diseases and to the availability of newer classes of antihypertensive therapy, which have broader or multiple cardiovascular uses. In a large physician diary study in the U.K., it was found that primary care physicians reported that more than half of their office-based cardiovascular patients have hypertension. In addition, 48% have ischemic heart disease and 25% have both ischemic heart disease and hypertension. Further, 37% have CHF, 18% of those with concomitant hypertension, and 26% of those with concomitant ischemic heart disease. Finally, 14% of office-based cardiovascular patients have all three conditions (Figure 3). The perception that a large percentage of their patients have multiple cardiovascular conditions increasingly influences the physicians' selection of therapy.

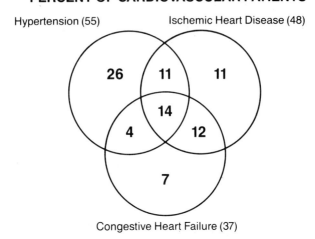

PERCENT OF CARDIOVASCULAR PATIENTS

Hypertension (55) Ischemic Heart Disease (48)

26 11 11

14

4 12

7

Congestive Heart Failure (37)

Source: MSDI Market Research

FIG. 3. Cardiovascular patients in the United Kingdom: percentage of patients with hypertension, ischemic heart disease, and congestive heart failure.

Another study involving nearly 400 one-on-one interviews with physicians in the U.K., Germany, and France took the results of the diary study a step further. It sought to obtain physician perceptions of antihypertensive therapies in relation to six categories of hypertensive patients as summarized in Table I. The results of the interview study were analyzed to prepare perceptual (joint space) maps that would visually portray physician perceptions of therapies on a wide variety of product features. These perceptions were listed using 7-point bipolar scales. This analysis highlights the perceived strengths and weaknesses of each antihypertensive class through three sets of relationships: (1) those among classes—the nearer the classes fell together in the perceptual space, the greater the perceived similarity among them; (2) those among attributes—the closer the attributes were to each other the greater association among them; and (3) interrelationships among classes and attributes—the further a class was in the direction indicated by the attribute factor, the more the brand was perceived to deliver that attribute. Figure 4 illustrates the perceptual map comparing beta-blockers, calcium-entry blockers and ACE inhibitors. Thus, the beta-blockers were perceived as particularly effective in younger patients, being closer to the arrowhead of the younger hypertensive vector, as well as in the hypertensive patient at risk, and less useful for the treatment of the elderly or the patient with heart failure. Calcium-entry blockers, on the other hand, were perceived as more appropriate than beta-blockers for the older hypertensive patient, roughly equal to the treatment of the hypertensive patient with angina, but they were perceived as

TABLE I. *Hypertensive patient categories*

Patient Type 1: Uncomplicated Hypertensive, Younger

Younger blue collar male with mildly elevated hypertension. No cardiovascular disease or risk factor other than hypertension.

Patient Type 2: Uncomplicated Hypertensive, Older

Elderly female with mild-to-moderate hypertension. There are no complicating cardiovascular risk factors.

Patient Type 3: Complicated Hypertensive, Angina

Retired male with mild-to-moderate hypertension. Has complained of some degree of exertional angina and can't function as he did in the past. There are no additional risk factors/conditions.

Patient Type 4: Complicated Hypertensive, Heart Failure

50-60-year-old female with severely elevated hypertension. Diagnosed as having heart failure (NY Heart Association Class II); lifestyle is somewhat restricted.

Patient Type 5: Complicated Hypertensive, Diabetes

50-60-year-old male with moderate hypertension diagnosed as having adult onset diabetes and mild proteinuria.

Patient Type 6: Hypertensive at Risk

Executive with mild-to-moderate hypertension who works, smokes, and drinks a bit too much. This patient has a history of known noncompliance and often breaks appointments with the physician. There are no other cardiovascular disease conditions.

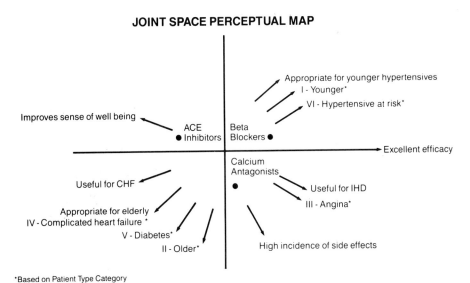

FIG. 4. Joint space perceptual map based on nearly 400 one-on-one interviews with physicians in France, Germany, and the United Kingdom.

having a distinctly higher incidence of adverse effects. Finally, the ACE inhibitors were most uniquely associated with an improved sense of well-being and improved quality of life. In addition, they were perceived as having a low incidence of side effects. ACE inhibitors were perceived as appropriate for elderly patients as well as for the treatment of hypertension with concomitant heart failure.

TREATMENT OF HEART FAILURE

Trends in the use of pharmacologic agents in the treatment of heart failure have broadly mirrored those in hypertension.

United States

In the U.S., although the number of prescriptions written for the treatment of CHF is still about one-third of those for hypertension, total prescriptions for CHF grew by 11% per year from 26 million in 1984 to 35 million in 1987. These data are summarized in Figure 5.

In terms of choice of treatment, diuretics and cardiac therapy (cardiac

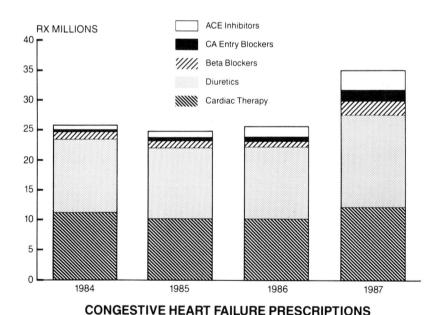

FIG. 5. Congestive heart failure prescriptions in the United States (1884 through 1987).

glycosides, nitrates, positive inotropes) were still the leading classes of drugs used for CHF, with 44% and 35%, respectively, in 1987. There have, however, been significant increases in the number of prescriptions for calcium entry blockers and ACE inhibitors between 1986 and 1987, with ACE inhibitors and calcium entry blockers roughly doubling their prescriptions for CHF to more than three million and two million, respectively. By 1987, ACE inhibitors held 9.2% of the total CHF prescription market.

United Kingdom

In the U.K., a different pattern emerges (Figure 6). The total prescriptions for CHF increased by 7% per year from 1984 to reach 10 million in 1987 in the U.K. In the U.K. cardiac therapy totaled 17.3% of CHF prescriptions in 1987, compared with 43.6% in the U.S. In 1987, diuretics were the predominant therapy for CHF in the U.K., accounting for 77% of total prescriptions, followed by cardiac therapy with 18%. In the U.K., ACE inhibitors have made a significantly smaller impression than in the U.S., capturing only 1.1% of total heart failure prescriptions. However, calcium-entry blockers and ACE inhibitors represent a rapidly growing treatment segment.

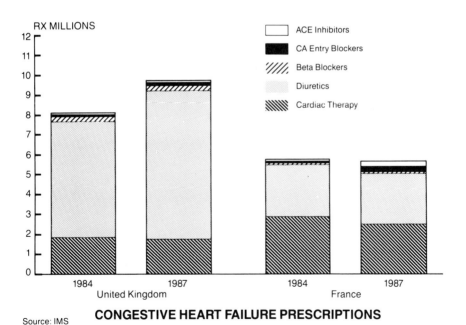

FIG. 6. Congestive heart failure prescriptions in the United Kingdom and France (1984 through 1987).

Germany

The different approaches between countries to the treatment of CHF can be highlighted by looking at the trends in Germany (Figure 7). Although Germany has the largest number of CHF prescriptions of the four European countries studied, the total number has decreased by 4% per year to 23 million in 1987. In Germany, cardiac therapy, predominantly cardiac glycosides, is still the largest class of drugs used to treat CHF (69% in 1987), despite the fact that the number of prescriptions has declined by 8% per year from 20 million to 16 million. Diuretics were in second place with a 15% share, having increased by 9% per year to 3.36 million prescriptions in 1987. Calcium-entry blockers increased by 6% to 2.4 million prescriptions, which represented 10% of the total CHF prescriptions. ACE inhibitor use increased to 400,000 prescriptions, which was about a 2% share in 1987.

France

The situation in France was somewhere between that in the U.K. and Germany (Figure 6), with ACE inhibitors accounting for 4.3% of prescriptions. Total prescriptions remained about 5.7 to 5.6 million between 1984 and

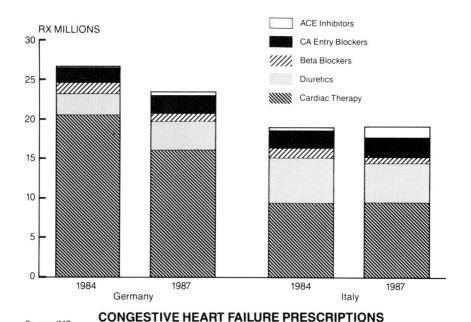

CONGESTIVE HEART FAILURE PRESCRIPTIONS

Source: IMS

FIG. 7. Congestive heart failure prescriptions in Germany and Italy (1984 and 1987).

1987. Cardiac therapy and beta-blockers declined by 4%, while diuretic usage remained little changed with a negative 1% growth. Diuretic and cardiac therapy were still the largest classes of CHF therapy, accounting for 89% of all prescriptions. Calcium-entry blockers and ACE inhibitors were the only classes of therapy with positive growth. They represented 5% and 4% share, respectively.

Italy

In Italy, there was a greater acceptance of ACE inhibitors and calcium-entry blockers in heart failure in 1987 (Figure 7). Total prescriptions remained level at 19 million with no growth over the past 4 years. Cardiac therapy, the leading class, had no growth. Diuretics and beta-blockers, which accounted for 30% share, had negative growth rates of 5% and 13%, respectively. Calcium-entry blockers and ACE inhibitors both increased to 1.3 million prescriptions in 1987, for 7% of the total CHF market each.

The dynamic changes seen in the hypertension market have been slower to take root in the treatment of the more severely ill heart failure patient. However, with the potential for decreased mortality associated with enalapril treatment that was reported by the CONSENSUS trial study group, there may well be an increased use of ACE inhibitors in the treatment of heart failure in the future.

REFERENCES

1. 1986 Guidelines for the Treatment of Mild Hypertension. Memorandum from the WHO/ISH. *Hypertension* 1986; **8**:957–961.
2. Australian National Blood Pressure Management Committee: The Australian therapeutic trial in mild hypertension. *Lancet* 1980; **1**:1261–1267.
3. Helegeland A: Treatment of mild hypertension. A five-year controlled drug trial. The Oslo Study. *Am J Med* 1980; **69**:725–732.
4. Hypertension Detection and Follow-up Program Cooperative Group: Five-year Findings of the Hypertension Detection and Follow-up Program. 1. Reduction in mortality of persons with high blood pressure, including mild hypertension. *JAMA* 1979; **242**:2562–2577.
5. Hypertension Detection and Follow-up Program Cooperative Group: Five-year Findings of the Hypertension Detection and Follow-up Program. Prevention and reversal of left ventricular hypertrophy with antihypertensive drug therapy. *Hypertension* 1985; **7**:105–112.
6. Veterans Administration Cooperative Study Group on Antihypertensive Agents: Effects of Treatment on Morbidity in Hypertension. I. Results in patients with diastolic blood pressures averaging 115 through 129 mm H. *JAMA* 1967; **213**:1143–1152.
7. The 1988 Report of the Joint National Committee on Detection, Evaluation, and Treatment of High Blood Pressure. *Arch Intern Med* 1988; **148**:1023–1038.
8. McFate Smith W: Epidemiology of Congestive Heart Failure. *Am J Cardiol* 1985; **55 (suppl A)**:3A–8A.
9. Appelfold MM: Chronic congestive heart failure: Where have we been? Where are we heading? *Am J Med* 1986; **80 (suppl 2B)**:73–77.
10. The CONSENSUS Trial Study Group: Effects of enalapril on mortality in severe congestive heart failure. Results of the Cooperative North Scandinavian Enalapril Survival Study (CONSENSUS). *N Engl J Med* 1987; **316**:1429–1435.

SUMMARY

This paper reviews the trends in the use of pharmacologic agents in hypertension and heart failure, in the United States, The United Kingdom, France, Germany and Italy. The data used have been derived from several sources, including IMS Hospital and Pharmacy audits and Merck Sharp & Dohme International (MSDI) market research involving a physician diary study of GPs in the UK, Germany and France, as well as physician interviews and focus groups conducted in these countries. Although older therapies (synthetic hypotensives, diuretics and beta-blockers in hypertension and diuretics and cardiac therapy in CHF) represent the bulk of the prescriptions, ACE inhibitors and calcium-entry blockers have made small but highly significant in-roads into the prescription markets in both these disease areas. The market trends are compared and contrasted in the five countries under review, and some of the similarities between the trends in the use of pharmacologic agents in heart failure and hypertension are highlighted. The trend towards increasing use of "individualized" antihypertensive therapy by adding an ACE inhibitor or a calcium-entry blocker to traditional forms of first-line antihypertensive therapy is discussed. Physician perception of current antihypertensive therapy is also reviewed.

RÉSUMÉ

Cette étude fait le point sur les interventions pharmacologiques utilisées actuellement pour traiter l'hypertension et l'insuffisance cardiaque aux Etats-Unis, en Grande Bretagne, en France, en Allemagne et en Italie. Les données proviennent de plusieurs sources: audits (IMS) des pharmacies et hôpitaux, études de marché de Merck Sharp & Dohme International (MSDI) comprenant une étude d'agenda médical de médecins de médecine générale en Grande Bretagne, en Allemagne et en France, entrevues avec des médecins, groupes focalisés dans les pays mentionnés. Bien que les traitements thérapeutiques plus anciens (hypotenseurs synthétiques, diurétiques et bétabloquants pour l'hypertension, et diurétiques et thérapie cardiaque pour les insuffisances cardiaques congestives) représentent la majorité des prescriptions, il faut quand même noter que les inhibiteurs de l'enzyme de conversion de l'angiotensine et les bloquants calciques ont fait leur entrée sur le marché dans le traitement de ces deux maladies. On compare et on contraste les tendances du marché dans les cinq pays étudiés, et on souligne quelques-unes des ressemblances concernant l'utilisation des agents pharmaceutiques utilisés dans le traitement des insuffisances cardiaques et de l'hypertension. L'activité de prescription de deux inhibiteurs de l'enzyme de conversion de l'angiotensine, l'enalapril et le captopril, est évaluée. L'adjonction d'inhibiteurs de l'enzyme de conversion de l'angiotensine ou de bloquants calciques sont des médicaments hypertenseurs d'utilisation croissante. On discute ici de cette nouvelle stratégie thérapeutique "individualisée" par rapport à la thérapeutique classique. On discute de l'attitude des médecins vis-à-vis des nouveaux traitements antihypertenseurs.

ZUSAMMENFASSUNG

Diese Veröffentlichung befaßt sich mit den Trends in der Verwendung pharmakologischer Mittel für Hypertonie und Herzinsuffizienz in den Vereinigten Staaten, dem Vereinigten Königreich, Frankreich, Deutschland und Italien. Die verwendeten Daten entstammen verschiedenen Quellen, einschließlich IMS Krankenhaus- und Apothekenrevisionen und MSDI-Marktforschung. Zu Rate gezogen wurden außerdem eine Studie über Praxistagebücher praktischer Ärzte in dem Vereinigten Königreich, Deutschland und Frankreich, zusammen mit interviews mit Ärzten und Zielgruppen in diesen Ländern. Obwohl ältere Therapiemethoden (wie synthetische blutdrucksenkende Mittel, Diuretika und Beta-Rezeptoren-blocker für Hypertonie und Diuretika und Herztherapien für hyperhämische Herzinsuffizienz) die meisten Rezepte ausmachen, haben ACE-Inhibitoren und Kalzium-Rezeptorenblocker einen kleinen, aber trotzdem sehr bedeutenden Vorstoß in den pharmazeutischen Markt dieser beiden Krankheiten zu verzeichnen. Die Markttendenzen in den fünf Ländern dieser Studie werden verglichen und kontrastiert; und diverse Ähnlichkeiten in den Trends der Verschreibung pharmakologischer Mittel für Herzinsuffizienz und Hypertonie werden hervorgehoben. Der Text betrachtet auch die Verschreibungsaktivität zweier ACE-Inhibitoren, Enalapril und Captopril; und der Trend zu erhöhter Verwendung von "individualisierter" antihypertonischer Therapie durch Zufügen eines ACE-Inhibitors oder eines Kalzium-Rezeptorenblockers zu traditionellen Therapieformen wird diskutiert. Besprochen wird außerdem die Haltung der Ärzte zu neueren antihypertonischen Therapieformen.

RIASSUNTO

Questo articolo esamina le tendenze nell'uso di agenti farmacologici nell'ipertensione e nell'insufficienza cardiaca negli Stati Uniti, in Gran Bretagna, Francia, Germania ed Italia. I dati sono stati tratti da varie fonti, compresi esami degli archivi di ospedali e farmacie IMS e un'indagine di mercato MSDI comprendente uno studio quotidiano di medici generici in Gran Bretagna, Germania e Francia come pure interviste con medici e inchieste di gruppo condotte in questi paesi. Benché terapie più antiquate (ipertensivi sintetici, diuretici e beta-bloccanti per l'ipertensione, diuretici e terapia cardiaca per l'insufficienza cardiaca congestiva) rappresentino il grosso delle ricette, gli inibitori dell'EIA ed i bloccanti dell'ingresso del calcio si sono guadagnati una piccola ma significativa quota dei mercati delle prescrizioni per entrambe queste malattie. Le tendenze del mercato vengono messe a confronto e contrasto nei clique paesi sotto esame ed alcune delle somiglianze fra le tendenze nell'uso di agenti farmacologici per l'insufficienza cardiaca e l'ipertensione vengono messe in risalto. Viene esaminata l'attività prescrittiva di due inibitori dell'EIA, enalapril e catopril e viene anche discussa la tendenza all'aumento nell'uso di terapie antiipertensive individualizzate mediante l'aggiunta di un inibitore dell'EIA o di un bloccante dell'ingresso del calcio nelle forme terapeutiche tradizionali.

SUMÁRIO

Revisam-se as tendências no uso de agentes farmacológicos para o tratamento da hipertensão e a insuficiência cardíaca nos Estados Unidos, no Reino Unido, no França, na Alemanha e na Itália. Os dados utilizados têm sido derivados de várias fontes, inclusive a auditoria de hospitais e de farmácias efetuada pelo IMS e a pesquisa de mercados realizada pela MSDI consistente num estudo dos diários de médicos gerais no Reino Unido, na Alemanha e na França, assim como entrevistas e grupos focais realizados com médicos nestos países. Ainda que os métodos terapêuticos mais antigos (hipotensivos sintéticos, diuréticos e betabloqueadores para a hipertensão, e diuréticos e terapia cardíaca para a insuficiência cardíaca congestiva) representam a maioria das receitas, os inibidores da ACE e os bloqueadores da entrada do cálcio têm conseguido um avanço pequeno, mas altamente significativo, no mercado de receitas para ambas doenças. Comparam-se e contrastam-se as tendências mercadológicas nos cinco países envolvidos, e ressaltam-se algumas das semelhanças entre as tendências no uso de agentes farmacológicos no tratamento da insuficiência cardíaca e a hipertensão. Revisa-se a atividade de receita de dois inibidores da ACE, enalapril e captopril, e discute-se a tendência atual para o aumento de uma terapia antihipertensiva "individualizada" mediante a adição de um inibidor da ACE ou um bloqueador da entrada de cálcio às formas tradicionais de terapia. Também revisa-se a percepção do médico quanto à terapia antihipertensiva atual.

RESUMEN

Este trabajo hace un análisis de las tendencias en el empleo de agentes farmacológicos para el tratamiento de la hipertensión y la insuficiencia cardíaca en los Estados Unidos, el Reino Unido, Francia, Alemania e Italia. Los datos empleados se han derivado de varias fuentes, incluyendo la auditoria de hospitales y de farmacias efectuados por IMS y la investigación de mercados realizada por Merck, Sharp & Dohme International consistente en un estudio de los diarios de médicos generales en el Reino Unido, Alemania y Francia, así como entrevistas y grupos focales realizados con médicos en estos países. Aunque los métodos terapéuticos más antiguos (hipotensores sintéticos, diuréticos y betabloqueadores para la hipertensión, y diuréticos y terapia cardíaca para la insuficiencia cardíaca congestiva) representan la mayor parte de las recetas, los inhibidores de la ACE y los bloqueadores de los canales del calicio han logrado posiciones pequeñas pero altamente significativas en el número de recetas para ambas enfermedades. Se compara y hace el contraste entre las tendencias del mercado de los cinco países analizados, y se da énfasis a algunas de las similaridades entre las tendencias en el uso de agentes farmacológicos en el tratamiento de la insuficiencia cardíaca y la hipertensión. Se analiza la actividad de prescripción de dos inhibidores de la ACE, enalapril y captopril, y se discute la actual tendencia hacia el incremento de una terapia antihipertensiva "individualizada" mediante la adición de un inhibidor de la ACE o un bloqueador de los canales del calcio a las formas tradicionales de terapia. También se analiza la percepción del médico en cuanto a la terapia antihipertensiva actual.

要約

本論文では，米国，英国，フランス，ドイツおよびイタリアにおける高血圧および心不全に対する薬剤使用の現状について総説する。ここでのデータは，以下のいくつかの資料源からとったものである。IMS 病院・薬局調査や MSDI 市場調査，英国，ドイツおよびフランスでの一般医の日誌調査，またこれらの国で行われた医師のインタビューや抽出群調査など。

従来の治療薬（高血圧における合成降圧薬，利尿薬および β 遮断薬，うっ血性心不全における利尿薬および心療法薬）の処方量は大量であるが，アンジオテンシン変換酵素（ACE）阻害薬と Ca 拮抗薬は少量ながらも両疾患領域での処方市場に著しい浸透を示している。総覧した 5 カ国の市場動向を比較対照し，心不全および高血圧における薬剤使用傾向の共通点についてのハイライトを示す。また，エナラプリルとカプトプリルの 2 つの ACE 阻害薬の処方状況についてまとめ，ACE 阻害薬および Ca 拮抗薬を従来の治療法に加えることによって，「個々の患者に対応した」降圧療法が増加する傾向にある点ついても考察した。最近の降圧療法に対する医師の認識についても概説する。

Cardiac and Renal Failure: An Expanding Role for ACE Inhibitors, edited by C. T. Dollery and L. M. Sherwood, Hanley & Belfus, Inc., Philadelphia.

DISCUSSION

HUGENHOLTZ: Referring to your data on physicians' perception of antihypertensive therapy, was the sample chosen from people who were friendly to the products?

McKINNEY: Market research samples are chosen at random, with a sample size that gives us a 95% confidence level that the data are projectable to that geographic region. Remember these data are from primary care physicians. If we looked at specialists or hospital-based physicians we might see a slightly different trend. In the congestive heart failure data, we did include specialists as they are the ones who most often treat this disease.

LANGMAN: How does the number of prescriptions relate to people with disease and therefore to the actual burden of disease?

McKINNEY: We generally use prescription data to show trends within a country. However we cannot add prescription data together from France, U.K., Germany, Italy, and U.S., because the prescription sizes are different in each country. The length of time that each prescription runs may vary considerably between countries. However, we do look at patient-days of therapy, and prescription data and patient-days of therapy data generally follow the same trends.

POOLE-WILSON: One has to be careful in looking at this set of data, particularly the data on heart failure. We have found large differences between hospital and community practice. The key problem is the reason for the diagnosis of heart failure in the community. The opinion of the general practitioner greatly affects the figures.

McKINNEY: Yes, that is an excellent point. Definitions of heart failure are different in different countries. For example it is difficult to say whether there are more patients with CHF in Germany or if they simply have a much broader definition of heart failure.

BAYLISS: I am puzzled by all this. First it seems to me that "heart failure" is a term for a variety of pathophysiologic abnormalities which have a large number of different causes. It seems sensible to treat the cause as much as the actual heart failure. Secondly we are faced with the old problem of the cart and the horse: I feel that you are telling us what the physicians are doing as if it were a perception of their independent scientific thinking. This is probably untrue. I believe you are showing us the outcome of the promotional expertise of representatives of all the pharmaceutical companies and the success and influence of this on clinical practice. I think we should be quite clear that this is what we are really learning about.

McKINNEY: It is important to remember that these data are based on what primary care physicians are doing or what they perceive that they are doing. It has been our experience over the years that the approach taken by academic physicians in the treatment of a disease is often significantly different from that taken by an average general practitioner.

Cardiac and Renal Failure: An Expanding Role for ACE Inhibitors, edited by C. T. Dollery and L. M. Sherwood, Hanley & Belfus, Inc., Philadelphia.

Roundtable 1: *Comparison of ACE Inhibitors with Other Agents*

Chairman: Colin I. Johnston
Panelists: Hans R, Brunner, Pierre Corvol,
Prof. Sir Colin Dollery, Trefor O. Morgan

Treatment of patients with hypertension can halve the incidence of stroke and reduce the incidence of heart failure, renal failure and cerebral hemorrhage. On the other hand, there is still an increased morbidity and mortality in treated hypertensives, even when their blood pressure has been reduced to normotensive levels.[1,2] None of the currently available antihypertensive drugs has had a significant impact on ischemic heart disease or the outcome of acute myocardial infarction,[3] and about 1 in 4 patients have to stop antihypertensive medication because of adverse effects.[4] There is a continuing need, therefore, to develop new antihypertensive drugs. But how should we manage our hypertensive patients today?

The main part of the discussion in this roundtable centered on which antihypertensive agent to use and when.

HOW TO CHOOSE THE RIGHT DRUG

The four most commonly used classes of antihypertensive drug are the beta-blockers, diuretics, calcium antagonists and ACE inhibitors. "The problem is," said Dr. Brunner, "to decide which of these drugs to use first." What are the factors involved in making the choice? Age of the patient may influence response to a particular type of drug, and cost, effectiveness, and side-effect profile also need to be taken into account. On this point, Dr. Dollery felt that at the general practitioner level, the drugs that cause the fewest adverse effects are most likely to be used. However, cost may affect prescribing of some drugs such as ACE inhibitors.

In an attempt to determine whether the response of a given patient to a particular drug can be predicted, a randomized cross-over study of the response to diltiazem (120 mg b.i.d.) or enalapril (20 mg q.d.) over a 6-week period was performed. Both treatments caused significant decreases in blood pressure. Although systolic blood pressure appeared to be better controlled with the ACE inhibitor, the difference observed did not reach statistical significance. However, Dr. Brunner stressed that only 16 patients completed the study. When individual responses to the drugs were analyzed, there was no relationship between age of the patient and response to either of the drugs. In addition, the hypothesis that there would be an inverse relationship between the response to the two drugs after 6 weeks of treatment was not upheld. Both classes of drug were equally active. "We are still reduced to the trial and error method of choosing the right drug for the right patient," said Dr. Brunner.

As Dr. Sonnenblick pointed out, hypertension is a heterogeneous disease, and it is unlikely that a single treatment will suit every patient. Dr. Brunner, in response described "his dream" as being "in an individual patient we will be able to predict what treatment is required."

NONPHARMACOLOGICAL TREATMENT

In a trial described by Dr. Morgan, dietary salt restriction (70 mmol/day) was shown to cause a significant but small fall in blood pressure, of about 5 mm Hg. This was accompanied by a rise in plasma renin. Initial plasma renin activity was not predictive of response to sodium restriction. The response to enalapril treatment was better in patients who were also on a sodium-restricted diet. However, there was no positive interaction between the two treatments. Further comparisons of the response to another ACE inhibitor, perindopril, in patients on low or high sodium diets confirmed the results obtained with enalapril. Thus, said Dr. Morgan, "sodium restriction and the other non-pharmacological methods do reduce blood pressure." He concluded that these treatments increase responsiveness to the ACE inhibitors, although only by a small amount. Extra response can be obtained by increasing the drug dose.

PHARMACOLOGICAL TREATMENT

Diuretics

According to Dr. Corvol, France has seen a continuing increase in sales of diuretics. A thiazide is usually prescribed in combination with a potassium-sparing agent such as amiloride or triamterene. Treatment with spironolactone is common. Dr. Corvol's group showed the same fall in blood pressure in three groups of hypertensive patients, treated with spironolactone alone, hydrochlorothiazide plus amiloride, or chlorothiazide plus triamterene. There were no adverse effects with thiazides, and no changes in cholesterol or triglyceride levels during long-term follow-up.

Beta-blockers

Dr. Dollery pointed out that there is some evidence to suggest that beta-blockers may have a more favorable effect on ischemic heart disease than the other antihypertensive drugs. His policy is to include beta-blockers in the treatment regimen of male hypertensives, since their main problem is mortality from ischemic heart disease. He cited a study that found a 6-fold increase in the relative risk of death from ischemic heart disease in both male and female hypertensives within the first 2 years of stopping beta-blockers. However, Dr. Mezey declared that "the biological price you pay with beta-blockers to get a decent antihypertensive effect is much too high." He went on to outline their possibly detrimental cardiac effects, including decreased cardiac output and increased peripheral resistance. There is also the possibility of respiratory problems arising during monotherapy with these agents.

HOW DO ACE INHIBITORS COMPARE WITH OTHER DRUGS?

As already described, sodium restriction lowers blood pressure in many patients, and enhances the effects of ACE inhibitors.

Dr. Brunner described a study in which he had participated. Nifedipine (10 mg p.o.) or enalaprilat (5 mg i.v.) were administered in a random order over 48 hours. Both produced a similar marked blood pressure reduction. However, nifedipine induced an increase in heart rate, and several patients complained of feeling ill after nifedipine administration. A longer-term comparison of enalapril with diltiazem also showed both drugs to be equally effective.

There was discussion over whether beta-blockers could be directly compared with ACE inhibitors in terms of their effectiveness as antihypertensive agents. "There is also the question of cost," said Dr. Sonnenblick. He wanted to know why the cheaper beta-blockers should be ignored when, he said, "there are a number of parallels between beta-blockers and ACE inhibitors." Although Dr. Corvol agreed that there is a definite price difference, he emphasized that the two types of drug are not directly comparable in their effects. "You can never suppress angiotensin II with beta-blockers like you can with an ACE inhibitor," he said.

DOES MILD TO MODERATE HYPERTENSION RELATE TO THE DEVELOPMENT OF CORONARY HEART DISEASE?

Dr. Dollery and Dr. Morgan both felt hypertension to be a risk factor for CHD. Dr. Morgan qualified this by saying that "cholesterol elevation and smoking are more potent risk factors," and was supported by Dr. Dollery, who thought smoking the most important factor, with cholesterol level second and hypertension third. In the MRC trial, patients who smoked had twice the chance of dying compared to nonsmokers with the same blood pressure.[5]

Among the other risk factors for CHD are lipids, obesity, physical inactivity, and genetics. Dr. Cohn referred to a recently reported American study of familial CHD and hypertension. Dr. Johnston, on the other hand, was of the opinion that mild to moderate hypertension and CHD are probably not causally related, although hypertension is a weak risk factor for IHD. However, according to Dr. Cohn, "the only reason for treating mild hypertension is to prevent the cardiovascular complications." He continued, "Our emphasis has always been on treating the blood pressure rather than identifying that subset of the mild hypertensive population who are at risk of developing cardiovascular complications."

WHICH DRUG TO REDUCE THE RISK OF CHD?

The speakers agreed that in order to determine whether ACE inhibitors are better than any other antihypertensive agent in preventing CHD, extensive analysis of large sets of data is required. Dr. Dollery emphasized that large numbers of patients will be required to participate in randomized trials, and that results should be based on an analysis of cause of death.

MATCHING THE TREATMENT TO THE PATIENT

All of the speakers agreed that the choice of drug can be difficult. Some patients have definite contraindications to the use of a particular type of drug. For instance, beta-blockers should not be given to patients with wheezy dyspnea, and diuretics are contraindicated in those with gout. Which ever drug you choose, there is always the problem of compliance, which appears to differ between different groups of patients. In addition, cost may be involved in the choice of drug. However, all other things being equal, Dr. Brunner summed up the problem when he said "in broad terms all the drugs we are discussing will lower the blood pressure in mild hypertension, so how do we choose between them?" The possible answer to this was given by Dr. Morgan who suggested that "you give all the drugs in turn for about a month, decide on which drug worked best with fewest side effects in the lowest doses, and in this way you would, in theory, have many patients on monotherapy."

SUMMARY

There is little doubt that hypertension should be treated. The main question appears to be which drug or drugs to use in individual patients. The general consensus at the workshop was that, in patients with mild hypertension, most antihypertensive agents are effective. The drug which is effective at the lowest dose and with the fewest side effects should therefore be employed.

The decision is more difficult in the severely hypertensive patient. Some patients may have contraindications to particular types of drug. Other than that, it is often a case of "trial and error," since there is no reliable method of predicting which patients will respond to any given drug or drug type. Combination therapy is often the most acceptable.

The role of hypertension as a risk factor for heart disease appears to be accepted. However, this needs to be put in perspective alongside the other factors, such as smoking and cholesterol levels, which represent more significant risks. If and when an antihypertensive agent is shown to be equally efficacious with a low adverse profile, but provides cardioprotection, it will obviously be a significant advance.

REFERENCES

1. Lindholm L, Ejlertsson G, Schersten B. High risk of cerebrocardiovascular morbidity in well treated male hypertensives. A retrospective study of 40–59 year old hypertensives in a Swedish primary care district. *Acta Med Scan* 1984; **216**:251–259.
2. Isles C, Walker LM, Beevers DG, Brown I, Cameron HL, Clarke J, Hawthorne V, Hole D, Lever AF, Robertson JIS, Wapshaw JA. Mortality in patients of the Glastow Blood Pressure Clinic. *J Hypertens* 1986; **4**:141–156.
3. MacMahon SW, Cutler JW, Furberg CD, Payne GH. The effects of drug treatment for hypertension on morbidity from cardiovascular disease: a review of randomized controlled trials. *Prog Cardiovasc Dis* 1986; **29(suppl 3)**:99–118.
4. Medical Research Council Working Party. Report of MRC Working party on mild to moderate hypertension: Adverse reactions to bendrofluazide and propranolol for the treatment of hypertension. *Lancet* 1981; **ii**:539–542.
5. Medical Research Council Working Party. MRC trial of treatment of mild hypertension and principal results. *Br Med J* 1985; **291**:97–104.

Cardiac and Renal Failure: An Expanding Role for ACE Inhibitors, edited by C. T. Dollery and L. M. Sherwood, Hanley & Belfus, Inc., Philadelphia.

The Primary Etiology of Heart Failure: Myocyte Loss, Reactive Hypertrophy, Dynamic Ischemia, and Ventricular Wall Remodeling

Edmund H. Sonnenblick, Stephen M. Factor, Calvin Eng, Thierry Le Jemtel, Pierro Anversa

Heart failure leading ultimately to congestive heart failure (CHF) and death presents a growing clinical problem. The mortality rates in late heart failure remain high, despite recent therapeutic advances to halt or modify adaptive and compensatory mechanisms that occur in response to heart failure. Apart from control of hypertension, correction of an uncompensated valve abnormality or amelioration of recurrent ischemia, little effort has been made to alter the primary events (sustained work or pressure overload causing myocardial hypertrophy) that lead to heart failure. This is not surprising since many of the primary events are poorly understood and heart failure may not be recognized clinically until it is far advanced. By this time the compensatory events, rather than the initiating events, have become the central problem.

This presentation is directed towards defining the initiating events which lead to heart failure, examining the adaptive responses to those events, and consideration of how these compensatory mechanisms may in turn become factors that advance the primary process itself.[1]

PRIMARY EVENTS LEADING TO HEART FAILURE

Heart failure most commonly develops as a result of severe myocardial hypertrophy[2] (Figure 1), usually caused by sustained work or pressure overload, but also as a response to loss of myocardium.[3] In a sense, the latter creates a "normotensive" work overload with "reactive" hypertrophy.[2] Myocyte loss occurs segmentally due to large-vessel coronary disease with myo-

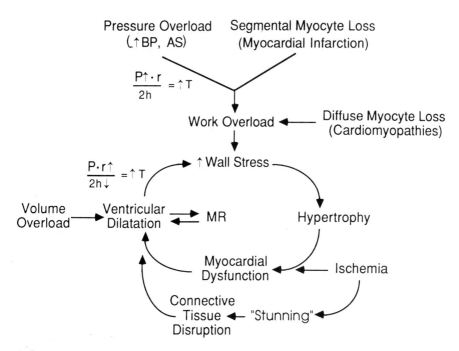

FIG. 1. The multiple factors that augment ventricular work load and result in hypertrophy. Secondary loads are created by augmented intraventricular volume that creates further stress via the LaPlace relation $t = \dfrac{PV}{2h}$ where T = tension in the ventricular wall, P = pressure, V = ventricular radius and h = thickness. Ventricular dilatation may be further increased by ventricular wall remodeling and create mitral regurgitation which is volume dependent.

cardial infarction, or diffusely perhaps as a result of small vessel disease in the form of microvascular spasm.[4]

"Reactive" or "normotensive" hypertrophy occurs after an acute myocardial infarction in direct proportion to the amount of myocyte loss.[3] This hypertrophy sets in motion a number of other compensatory mechanisms that may ultimately produce ventricular pump dysfunction. Thus, the extent of myocyte hypertrophy depends not only on the loading of the cell from pressure and volume but more subtly by the extent of myocyte cell loss. As will be discussed later, transient ischemia may lead to loss of intercellular myocyte connections[6] and this, together with compensatory ventricular volume changes, may lead to alterations in ventricular wall shape (remodeling), which, due to the LaPlace relation,[2] can place additional loads on an already compromised ventricle.

The primary events in heart failure may occur independently of symptoms of CHF, which only become manifest when cardiac output becomes limited or congestion occurs as compensatory mechanisms related to the peripheral circulation develop.[2] Peripheral compensations generally occur later, are more readily recognized, and are thus amenable to a therapeutic approach. If deaths from heart failure are to be prevented the primary events in the process will need to be addressed.

In order to examine therapeutic and prophylactic approaches to heart failure, a clear and comprehensive model of the disease is necessary (Figure 2). What is missing is the time base; the process commonly begins insidiously, is unrecognized, and progresses until the limitations of pump function become manifest and the peripheral circulation becomes disordered. (Figure 3).

Returning to the initial events in more detail, an increased systolic intraventricular pressure is the most commonly recognized form of work overload

HEART FAILURE: A two component problem

1. CARDIAC FAILURE

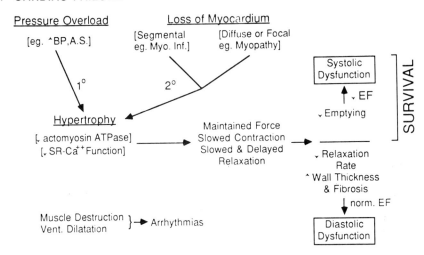

2. CONGESTIVE FAILURE

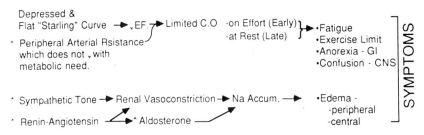

FIG. 2. Heart failure in terms of central (cardiac) and peripheral problems.

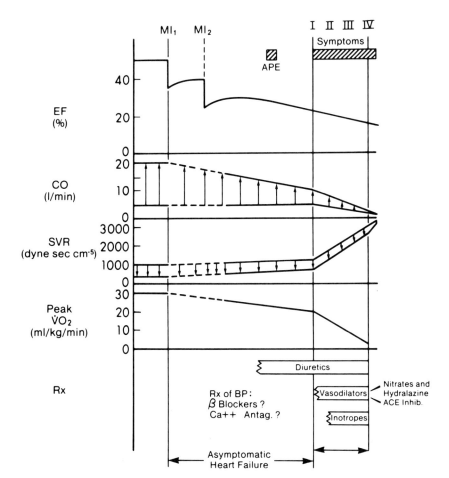

FIG. 3.   Hypothetical course of heart failure developing after two acute myocardial infarctions (MI). The period of asymptomatic heart failure may last months to years. APE = acute pulmonary edema. I–IV are clinical classes (NYHA).

leading to hypertrophy. In general, the ventricular wall thickens so as to normalize intraventricular wall tension, as expressed by the LaPlace relation.[2] With the development of hypertrophied myocardium, the workload can commonly be sustained with the systolic tension per unit myocardium being normalized, but certain biochemical adaptive mechanisms come into play that produce functional changes in myocardial contraction. Accordingly, when the mechanical behavior of left ventricular papillary muscle removed from the left ventricles of rats with experimental renal hypertension has been studied, total systolic force development is normal.[7] Nevertheless, the rate of force development is reduced and the time required to develop this force is delayed.[8] In addition, relaxation is slowed so that the total duration of contraction is prolonged. These mechanical alterations have electrophysiological and biochemical consequences. As hypertrophy occurs, there is a prolongation of the action potential[8] and a shift from the synthesis of the fast V_1 form of myosin ATPase to the relatively slower V_3 form.[8] The shift from the V_1 to the V_3 form of myosin correlates with a decrease in the unloaded velocity of shortening of the myocardium, presumably reflecting the rate of contractile bridge formation. It is likely that other slower isoenzymes may also be synthesized during this hypertrophic response, but this has not been studied critically.

With aging, mechanical and biochemical changes take place that parallel those caused by hypertrophy.[9] Moreover, the effects of hypertrophy and aging appear additive. In the renal hypertensive rat, when the arterial systolic load is normalized by removing the kidney, the mechanical,[10] electrophysiological,[8] and biochemical changes in the myocardium[10] are largely reversible as the hypertrophy resolves. A major question is whether other qualitative changes occur in heart failure or whether only a quantitative extension of these adaptive changes takes place. We would support the latter view, although ischemia and continued myocyte loss may complicate the matter. If the hypertrophic reaction occurs in response to loss of myocardium, for example after an acute myocardial infarction, an increase in intraventricular volume raises the systolic wall tension, encouraging further cellular hypertrophy.[2] In this situation the amount of reactive hypertrophy appears to be in direct proportion to the amount of myocardium that is lost.[11,12]

In terms of ventricular pump function, the consequence of severe hypertrophy alone may result in so-called "diastolic dysfunction." With the thickening of the myocardial wall and the delay in myocardial relaxation, relatively more time is spent in systole and diastole may be impinged upon. Thus ventricular filling would be impaired, resulting in a delay in ventricular diastolic filling and elevated end-diastolic pressures despite retained normal systolic emptying, producing some aspects of diastolic dysfunction of the ventricle.

VENTRICULAR WALL REMODELING

Myocellular hypertrophy continues over time, amplified by any further loss of myocytes. This will be discussed subsequently in terms of the effects of normal aging. The extent of hypertrophy can also be increased by alterations in the structure of the ventricular wall. With enlargement of ventricular end-diastolic volume and persistent elevated diastolic pressures, the ventricular diastolic volume progressively becomes larger to a greater degree than would be anticipated, i.e., the diastolic pressure volume curve is displaced to the right.[13] Although the pressure-volume is moved to the right, the compliance may actually be *reduced*, since the curve becomes very steep. This is also the case with primary volume overloads. In dogs in which a volume overload has been produced using an aortocaval shunt, sarcomeres in the left ventricular wall are not as long as one would anticipate from a simple increase in volume.[13] This suggests that myocellular slippage has occurred that would produce a decrease in the number of myocytes across the ventricular wall. Such a phenomenon has been termed *ventricular wall remodeling*.[3] An additional implication of these findings is that myocyte hypertrophy is greater than the increase in wall thickness would predict.

A reduction in the number of myocytes across the wall of the heart creates a generally unrecognized increase in load per myocyte. Thus, the extent of hypertrophy cannot be judged merely by measuring wall thickness. Ultimately the interaction between myocyte loss and ventricular wall remodeling leads to imbalances in the La Place relation that can lead to progressive ventricular dilatation and failure. Myocyte loss remains a central issue. In the Syrian hamster that develops an inherited *cardiomyopathy*, focal myocyte loss has been clearly demonstrated and this has been shown to be associated with microvascular spasm in the regions where myocyte loss occurs.[14,15] With the microvascular spasm and focal ischemia, cells that may be unable to tolerate an ischemic insult go on to necrosis, which heals with focal scarring.[16] This localized loss of cells is then compensated for by reactive hypertrophy. Ultimately, this process can lead to ventricular wall remodeling and the development of heart failure. It is of interest that verapamil has been shown to prevent the microvascular spasm and the development of the cardiomyopathy during the periods of therapy.[15,17] However, verapamil may also protect myocytes from calcium overloads that may lead to cardiac damage as well. It is also of interest that verapamil has an alpha-blocking effect that may relate to some of its protective action.[15]

We have also shown that streptozotocin-induced *diabetes* in rats may lead to the same contractile and biochemical alterations in the rat myocardium that occur in the presence of hypertrophy, but permanent damage, as occurs in the Syrian hamster, does not take place.[19] Insulin reverses these changes totally.[20] Nevertheless, if *renal hypertension* is induced in these diabetic animals, microvascular spasm occurs with resultant focal ischemia, focal necrosis, and scarring, with an end-stage cardiomyopathy that leads to heart failure and death of the animal.[21,23]

MYOCARDIAL INFARCTION, ACUTE ISCHEMIA AND HEART FAILURE

Recent observations suggest a link between acute myocardial infarction and reversible forms of acute ischemia that can contribute to heart failure. In the dog, transient and intermittent ischemia leads to loss of contractile activity in the affected region of the ventricular wall, and this may persist for hours and even days following the acute ischemic event, even though coronary blood flow is fully restored. This process has been termed "stunning" and has been generally thought to be benign. Nevertheless, after a period of "stunning" in the dog ventricle, although leading to no intracellular structural damage, we have observed significant damage to the *intercellular connective tissue*; this may contribute to unmooring of myocytes, which may then contribute to ventricular wall remodeling even though necrosis has not occurred.[6] Activation of collagenases that could produce these changes is poorly characterized. Superoxides, which are produced during reperfusion, may be involved.[24] Collagen breakdown is an intriguing mechanism, since it could lead to an increase in diastolic ventricular volume, which would augment systolic wall loads with resultant reactive hypertrophy. In the presence of diffuse coronary disease this might contribute to progressive ventricular dilatation and ultimately to a dilated ischemic cardiomyopathy. This possibility is being actively explored in our laboratories.

The extent of hypertrophy in the nonischemic portion of the ventricle remaining after an acute myocardial infarction is such as to restore the ventricular mass.[3,12] Whether this "reactive" hypertrophic tissue demonstrates the same alterations that occur in pressure overloads is only now being explored. We have preliminary evidence to indicate that this is indeed the case. Certainly, ventricular wall remodeling occurs in these circumstances and may further increase wall stress.

Whether the *extent* of myocellular hypertrophy is always adequate to normalize the tension in the ventricular wall, or may be limited by factors such as age or intercurrent disease, is unclear. This would also tend to increase ventricular dilatation and wall remodeling, since the myocardial wall tension would not be normalized.

Changes in systolic contraction occur while ventricular wall remodeling continues. This is characterized by a fall in ventricular ejection fraction, resulting in systolic dysfunction or heart failure. There may be few clinical symptoms of congestive heart failure, but the patient remains at risk while his ejection fraction becomes reduced.[25]

Signs and symptoms of CHF failure develop only as the peripheral circulation becomes disordered in response to a poorly functioning pump.[1] Accordingly, salt accumulation occurs with peripheral and central edema as the renin-angiotensin system is activated and aldosterone secretion by the adrenal cortex is increased. These changes in the peripheral circulation occur initially as adaptive mechanisms, but ultimately they become detrimental with progressive changes in the peripheral circulation and are associated with severe end stage symptoms of CHF. As shown in Figure 3, symptoms tend to occur a considerable time after the acute myocardial event. For example, the ejection fraction is reduced when the acute myocardial infarction occurs and remains reduced, although symptoms of CHF may not occur concomitantly. In the period between the acute infarction and congestive failure, ventricular wall remodeling may also occur, which could further reduce the ejection fraction.

Initially, cardiac output tends to remain normal at rest but may be somewhat limited during exercise. Later on, due to mechanisms that are still to be defined, the peripheral arterial resistance tends to rise so that the resting cardiac output is moderately reduced and the maximum increase in cardiac output during exercise decreases progressively. This reduction in peak cardiac output tends to correlate with a reduction of the maximum exercise response and reduced maximum VO^2. It should be noted that this late reduction in cardiac output both at rest and during exercise does not require a further reduction in the ejection fraction, and indeed treatment to improve the peripheral circulation leads to an increase in ejection fraction despite an improvement in VO^2 max.[1,26]

From the above it is clear that treatment affecting the periphery may not alter the course of the disease. The experimental cardiomyopathy in the *hypertensive diabetic* as well as the hereditary cardiomyopathy in the *Syrian hamster* will not be altered by either controlling salt metabolism or unloading the peripheral circulation, except to the limited theoretical extent that it may reduce or retard further reactive hypertrophy and dilatation. Similarly, in man, affecting the peripheral circulation and/or stimulating the failed myocardium does not alter the initial or primary etiology.[27] In such a circumstance, therapy would need to be directed toward protecting the myocardium itself and prevention of abnormal microvascular responses. A similar challenge is presented in human therapy, where the primary events may have nothing to do with the peripheral circulatory alterations that are readily amenable to therapeutic approach. This may help to explain why in the longer term mortality is not significantly altered by current forms of therapy. This does not reduce the importance of such forms of therapy on *immediate* (6-month) mortality,[28] which may relate to restoring circulatory competence and improving electrolyte balance so that circulatory failure may not occur acutely and electrolyte imbalance may not lead to life-threatening arrhythmias. However, this would not affect the long-term alterations in the myocardium.

Treatment of heart failure that alters the ultimate course of the disease involves limiting the initial damage to the myocardium or prevention of further damage to the ventricle, i.e., reduction in wall remodeling and prevention of further myocellular loss. On the other hand, symptoms related to CHF occur later and may be independent of the primary events that have damaged the myocardium. The peripheral adaptive alterations such as sodium accumulation and activation of the renin-angiotensin system may secondarily bring about these alterations in the myocardium. Thus, as a peripheral impedance rises there is a secondary increase in the load on the myocardium; further reactive hypertrophy may result with further augmentation of diastolic volume, causing ventricular wall remodeling of a progressive nature.[29] In this way, what are initially peripheral compensations serve to produce vicious cycles both peripherally and centrally.

EFFECTS OF AGING

Lastly, there is a major alteration in the ventricular wall that may be inexorable; this is due to the process of *aging*. We have clearly demonstrated that in the process of aging significant myocyte loss occurs that may result in reactive hypertrophy of the remaining myocardium.[30] The systolic hypertension of the elderly may further amplify this reactive hypertrophy. During the process of aging, there is also a decrease in the speed of actomyosin ATPase associated with a progressive V1 to V3 isoenzyme shift of myosin.[9] Contractile alterations that mimic those seen with hypertrophy occur,[9,31] namely a slowing of the rate of contraction, a prolongation of electrical activation, and a significant delay in relaxation, despite the fact that systolic force is well-maintained. Thus aging is a hypertrophic disease that adds to what other damage may be occurring. Exercise may improve some of these alterations, and this may be one of the benefits to be derived from an active life. Nevertheless, the process of myocyte loss needs further exploration; it may be an additional factor contributing to heart failure, especially in those who have other forms of cardiac damage such as coronary artery disease and hypertension.

CONCLUSIONS

In summary, heart failure ensues from hypertrophy that results either from a work overload or, equally importantly, myocyte loss. This myocyte loss may occur as a function merely of aging but can also occur during acute myocardial infarction or diffusely in the presence of cardiomyopathies, perhaps secondary to microvascular spasm. Therapy should be directed towards preserving the myocardium during the initial stages of heart failure. Later adaptive alterations in the peripheral circulation may secondarily produce CHF and limit cardiac output so that exercise performance is limited. These alterations in the periphery may well be structural as well as hormonally induced. Therapeutic approaches to deal with unwanted compensatory events will help to improve symptoms and to some extent prolong life, but the ultimate therapy of heart failure is in the preservation of the myocardium.

REFERENCES

1. Mancini DM, LeJemtel TH, Factor S, Sonnenblick EH. Central and peripheral components of cardiac failure. 1986; **80(suppl. 2B)**:2–13.
2. Sonnenblick EH, Strobeck JE, Capasso JM, Factor SM. Ventricular hypertrophy: models and methods. In Tarazi RC, Dunbar JB, eds. *Perspectives in Cardiovascular Research*, Vol. 8. New York, Raven Press 1983;13–20.
3. Anversa P, Ricci R, Olivetti G. Quantitative structural analysis of the myocardium during physiologic growth and induced cardiac hypertrophy: A review. *J Am Coll Cardiol* 1986; 7:1140–1149.
4. Sonnenblick EH, Factor S, Strobeck J, Capasso JM, Fein F. The pathophysiology of heart failure: The primary role of microvascular hyper-reactivity and spasm in the development of congestive cardiomyopathies. In Braunwald E, Mock MB, Watson J, eds. *Congestive Heart*

Failure: Current Research and Clinic. Applications. New York, Grune & Stratton, 1982;87–97.

5. Anversa P, Hiler B, Ricci R, Guideri G, Olivetti G: Myocyte cell loss and myocyte hypertrophy in the aging rat heart. *J Am Coll Cardiol* 1986; **8**:1441–1448.

6. Zhao M, Zang H, Robinson TF, Factor SM, Sonnenblick EH, Eng C. Profound structural alterations of the estracellular collagen matrix in post-ischemic dysfunctional but viable myocardium. *J Am Coll Cardiol* 1987; **10**:1322–1334.

7. Capasso JM, Strobeck JE, Sonnenblick EH. Myocardial mechanical alterations during gradual onset, long-term hypertension in rats. *Am J Phyisol* 1981; **241**:435–441.

8. Capasso JM, Aronson RS, Sonnenblick EH. Reversible alterations in excitation contraction coupling during myocardial hypertrophy in rat papillary muscle. *Circ Res* 1982; **51**:189–195.

9. Capasso JM, Malhotra A, Scheuer J, Sonnenblick EH. Myocardial biochemical, contractile, and electrical performance after imposition of hypertension in young and old rats. *Circ Res* 1986; **58**:445–460.

10. Capasso JM, Strobeck JE, Malhotra A, Scheuer J, Sonnenblick EH. Contractile behavior of rat myocardium after reversal of hypertensive hypertrophy. *Am J Physiol* 1982; **242**:(Heart Circ. Physiol. 11):H882–H889.

11. Anversa P, Beghi C, Kikkawa Y, Olivetti G. Myocardial response to infarction in the rat. Morphometric measurement of infarct size and myocyte cellular hypertrophy. *Am J Pathol* 1985; **118**:484–492.

12. Anversa P, Loud AV, Levicky V, Guideri G. Left ventricular failure induced by myocardial infarction. I. Myocyte hypertrophy. *Am J Physiol* 1985; **248**:H876–882.

13. Ross J Jr, Sonnenblick EH, Taylor RR, Spotnitz HM, Covell JW. Diastolic geometry and sarcomere lengths in the chronically dilated canine left ventricle. *Circ Res* 1971; **28**:49–61.

14. Sonnenblick EH, Factor S, Strobeck J, Capasso J, Fein F. The pathophysiology of heart failure: The primary role of microvascular hyper-reactivity and spasm in the development of congestive cardiomyopathies. In *Congestive Heart Failure: Current Research and Clinic. Applications.* Braunwald E, Mock MB, and Watson J, eds. New York, Grune & Stratton, 1982; 87–97.

15. Factor SM, Minase T, Cho S, Dominitz R, Sonnenblick EH. Microvascular spasm in the cardiomyopathic Syrian hamster: A preventable cause of focal myocardial necrosis. *Circulation* 1982; **66**:342–354.

16. Factor SM, Sonnenblick EH. Hypothesis: Is congestive cardiomyopathy caused by a hyper-reactive myocardial microcirculation (microvascular spasm)? *Am J Cardiol* 1982; **50**:1149–1152.

17. Factor S, Cho S, Scheuer J, Sonnenblick EH, Malhotra A. Prevention of hereditary cardiomyopathy in the Syrian hamster with chronic verapamil therapy. *J Am Coll Cardiol* (in press).

18. Sonnenblick EH, Fein F, Capasso JM, Factor SM. Microvascular spasm as a cause of cardiomyopathies and the calcium blocking agent (verapamil) as potential primary therapy. *Am J Cardiol* 1985; **55**:179B.

19. Fein FS, Kornstein LB, Strobeck JE, Capasso JM, Sonnenblick EH. Altered myocardial mechanics in diabetic rats. *Circ Res* 1980; **47**:922–933.

20. Fein FS, Strobeck JE, Malhotra A, Scheuer J, Sonnenblick EH. Reversibility of diabetic cardiomyopathy with insulin in rats. *Circ Res* 1981; **49**:1251–1261.

21. Factor SM, Minase T, Bhan R, Wolinsky H, Sonnenblick EH. Hypertensive diabetic cardiomyopathy in the rat: Ultrastructural features. *Virchows Archives (Pathol Anat).* 1983; **398**:305–317.

22. Factor SM, Minase T, Cho S, Fein F, Capasso JM, Sonnenblick EH. Coronary microvascular abnormalities in the hypertensive-diabetic rat: A primary cause of cardiomyopathy? *Am J Pathol* 1984; **116**:9–20.

23. Fein FS, Capasso JM, Aronson RS, Cho S, Nordin C, Miller-Green B, Sonnenblick EH, Factor SM. Combined renovascular hypertension and diabetes in rats: A new preparation of congestive cardiomyopathy. *Circulation* 1984; **70**:318–330.

24. Bolli R. Oxygen-derived free radicals and post-ischemic myocardial dysfunction "stunned" myocardium. *J Am Coll Cardiol* 1988; **12**:239–249.

25. Multicenter Postinfarction Research Group. Risk stratification and survival after myocardial infarction. *N Engl J Med* 1983; **309**:331–336,

26. LeJemtel TH, Gumbardo D, Chadwick B, Rutman HI, Sonnenblick EH. Milrinone for

long-term survival of severe heart failure: Clinical experience with special reference to maximal exercise tolerance. Circulation 1986; **73(suppl. III)**:111–213.

27. LeJemtel TH, Sonnenblick EH. Should the failing heart be stimulated? *N Engl J Med* 1984; **310**:1384–1385.

28. The CONSENSUS Trial Study Group. Effects of enalapril on mortality in severe congestive heart failure. *N Engl J Med* 1987; **316**:1429–1435.

29. Pfeffer MA, Lamas GA, Vaughn DE, Parisi AF, Braunwald E. Effect of captopril on progressive ventricular dilatation after anterior myocardial infarction. *N Engl J Med* 1988; **319**:80–86.

30. Hachamovich R, Wicker P, Capasso JM, Anversa P. Alterations of coronary blood flow and reverse with aging in Fischer 344 rats. *Am J Physiol* (in press).

31. Capasso JM, Malhotra A, Remily RM, Scheur J, Sonnenblick EH. Effects of age on mechanical and electrical performance of rat myocardium. *Am J Physiol* 1983; **243(Heart Circ. Physiol. 14)**:H72–H81.

SUMMARY

Heart failure, which leads ultimately to congestive heart failure and death, is a growing clinical problem. Heart failure is most commonly caused by myocardial hypertrophy either as a result of sustained work overload or myocyte loss. In recent years, dramatic clinical advances have been made to deal with the adaptive and compensatory mechanisms that occur in response to heart failure, but the events leading to heart failure remain poorly understood. This paper sets out to define the initiating events that lead to heart failure, examines the adaptive responses to these events and considers how, in turn, these adaptive and compensatory mechanisms advance the primary process. It is suggested that main therapy in heart failure should be directed toward preserving the myocardium in the initial stages, and prevention of further damage to the ventricle.

RÉSUMÉ

L'insuffisance cardiaque qui mène éventuellement à l'insuffisance cardiaque congestive et à la mort est un problème clinique d'actualité. La cause la plus courante de l'insuffisance cardiaque est l'hypertrophie du myocarde, à la suite soit d'un surcroît de travail soutenu soit d'une perte de myocytes. Ces dernières années on a fait des progès cliniques considérables concernant les mécanismes d'adaptation et de compensation qui se produisent face aux insuffisances cardiaques, mais les événements menant à l'insuffisance cardiaque ne sont toujours pas clairs. Cette étude a pour but de définir les facteurs qui favorisent l'insuffisance cardiaque. On examine les phénomènes d'adaptation et on essaie de déterminer comment, à leur tour, ces mécanismes d'adaptation et de compensation précipitent le processus initial. On suggère que le traitement de première intention de l'insuffisance cardiaque vise à préserver le myocarde et empêcher une détérioration ultérieure du ventricule.

ZUSAMMENFASSUNG

Herzinsuffizienz führt in ihrem Verlauf schliesslich zu hyperhämischer Herzinsuffizienz und zum Tod und stellt damit ein wachsendes klinisches Problem dar. Gewöhnlich wird Herzinsuffizienz durch myocarditische Hypertrophie ausgelöst; entweder als Resultat dauernder Arbeitsüberlastung oder Myocytenverlust. In den letzten Jahren sind dramatische klinische Fortschritte gemacht worden in der Behandlung der Anpassungs- und Kompensationsmechanismen, die aus der Herzinsuffizienz resultieren; jedoch bleiben die Ursachen, die zu Herzinsuffizienz führen, weiterhin wenig verstanden. Die vorliegende Veröffentlichung definiert zunächst die Ereignisse, die die Herzinsuffizienz einleiten, betrachtet damn die Anpassungsmechanismen an diese Erscheinungen und analysiert schliesslich die Art und Weise, wie umgekehrt diese Adaptations- und Kompensationsmechanismen den Primärprozess beeinflussen. Die Vorschläge gehen dahin, dass sich Terapiebemühungen für Herzinsuffizienz hauptsächlich auf die Erhaltung des Herzmuskels in den Anfangsstadien und auf Vermeidung weiteren Schadens an der Herzkammer richten sollten.

RIASSUNTO

L'insufficienza cardiaca, che alla fine conduce all'insufficienza cardiaca congestizia ed alla morte, è un crescente problema clinico. L'insufficienza cardiaca viene piú comunemente causata da ipertrofia miocardica, sia in seguito a sovraccarico di lavora sia a causa di perdita di miociti. Negli ultimi anni sono stati fatti drammatici passi avanti nell'agire sui meccanismi adattivi e compensatori che si verificano in reazione ad un'insufficienza cardiaca ma gli eventi che portano all'insufficienza cardiaca non sono ancora ben compresi. Questo articolo intende definire gli eventi iniziali che portano all'insufficienza cardiaca, esamina le reazioni d'adattamento a tali eventi e prende in considerazione come, a loro volta, tali meccanismi adattivi e compensatori facciano progredire il processo primario. Viene proposto che la terapia principale per l'insufficienza cardiaca dovrebbe essere diretta a preservare il miocardio negli stadi iniziali e a impedire che avvengano ulteriori danni al ventricolo.

SUMÁRIO

A insuficiência cardíaca, que filamente conduz à insuficiência cardíaca congestiva e à morte, é um problema clínico crescente. A insuficiência cardíaca é ocasionada mais comumente pela hipertrofia do miocárdio, quer como resultado de uma sobrecarga sostenida, quer como resultado de uma perda miocitária. Nos últimos anos, têm-se conseguido avanços clínicos dramáticos para controlar os mecanismos adativos e compensatórios que ocorrem em resposta à insuficiência cardíaca, mas os eventos que conduzem à insuficiência cardíaca ainda não são bem entendidos. Este trabalho começa com a intenção de definir os eventos iniciais que conduzem à insuficiência cardíaca, examina as respostas adativas a tais eventos e considera como, por sua vez, estes mecanismos adativos e compensatórios fazem avançar o processo primário. Sugere-se que a terapia principal na insuficiência cardíaca deve dirigir-se para a preservação do miocárdio nas etapas iniciais e à prevenção de lesões posteriores do ventrículo.

RESUMEN

La insuficiencia cardíaca, que finalmente produce insuficiencia cardíaca congestiva y la muerte, es un problema clínico que está en aumento. La insuficiencia cardíaca muy a menudo es causada por hipertrofia del miocardio, sea como resultado de una sobrecarga sostenida o pérdida miocitaria. En años recientes se han logrado grandes avances clínicos para controlar los mecanismos adaptivos y compensatorios que occurren en respuesta a la insuficiencia cardíaca, pero los sucesos que llevan a la insuficiencia cardíaca todavía no son bien comprendidos. Este trabajo tiene como propósito definir los sucesos iniciales que llevan a la insuficiencia cardíaca, examinar las respuestas adaptivas a estos sucesos, y considera cómo, a su turno, estos mecanismos adaptivos y compensatorios hacen avanzar el proceso primario. Se sugiere que la terapia principal en la insuficiencia cardíaca debe dirigirse hacia la preservación del miocardio en las etapas iniciales y a la prevención de lesiones posteriores del ventrículo.

要約

最終的にはうっ血性心不全からさらに死に至るという心不全は、臨床上大きな問題になっている。心不全は、最も一般的には心肥大によって起こり、これは継続的な心仕事量の負荷や心筋細胞損傷の結果でもある。

近年、心不全に対する反応として起こる適応性および代償性の機構についての臨床的研究は劇的な進歩を遂げたが、心不全に至る過程についてはまだほとんどわかっていない。

本論文では、心不全の引き金となる要因を明らかにし、これらの要因に対する適応反応について検討し、さらに翻って適応・代償機構が初期過程をどのように進展させるかを考察してみたい。

心不全の主要な治療法は、まず初期段階で心筋を保護し、損傷がさらに心室全体に及ぶのを防ぐことであると考えられる。

Cardiac and Renal Failure: An Expanding Role for ACE Inhibitors, edited by C. T. Dollery and L. M. Sherwood, Hanley & Belfus, Inc., Philadelphia.

Mechanogenic Transduction in the Hypertrophied Heart

Ketty Schwartz, Anne-Marie Lompre,
Diane de la Bastie, and Jean-Jacques Mercadier

In response to increasing functional demands, both cardiac and skeletal muscles rapidly adapt using several known mechanisms, such as augmented oxygen consumption, vasodilatation of capillaries, and enhanced contractility with stretch (Starling's law), all of which are simple extensions of the physiological properties of the tissue. Chronically, adaptation occurs by modifications in cardiac gene expression. These modifications lead to an enlarged organ containing proteins better adapted to the altered functional demand.[1] All of these mechanisms are useful adaptations that enable the ventricular chambers to sustain chronic hyperfunction and allow the heart to develop a normal tension at a low energy cost.[2] In this context, heart failure is not so much a disease as a process in which the limits of myocardial adaptation have been overcome. Improving our understanding of the mechanisms responsible for myocardial adaptation will thus help to elucidate the basis for the altered performance and for the transition from compensated hypertrophy to failure.

This article will focus on recent work from our laboratory concerning two mechanisms that have been shown to modify gene expression in the hemodynamically overloaded heart (Figure 1): (1) differential expression of contractile protein multigene families (myosin heavy chain and actin) that leads to a slower contraction and (2) modulation of single genes, such as those coding for the atrial natriuretic factor (ANF) that tends to improve the loading conditions of the cardiac pump, and the Ca^{++}-dependent ATPase of the sarcoplasmic reticulum that modifies cardiac relaxation.

115

MECHANOGENIC TRANSDUCTION

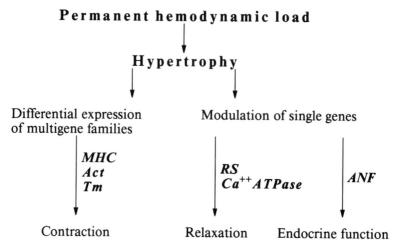

FIG. 1. Mechanisms that modify gene expression in the hemodynamically overloaded heart.

DIFFERENTIAL EXPRESSION OF MYOSIN HEAVY CHAIN AND ACTIN MULTIGENE FAMILIES

Myosin Heavy Chain

Because of the correlation observed between the maximum velocity of contraction of a given skeletal muscle with the specific activity of myosin adenosine triphosphatase (ATPase),[3] the early search for biochemical correlates of cardiac hypertrophy attempted to relate myosin ATPase activity to physiological function. In small mammals such as rat and rabbit, compensatory cardiac hypertrophy secondary to pressure overload has been associated with decreased maximum fiber-shortening velocity, myosin ATPase activity, and myocardial contractility.[4-6] We found that the shift in the different isoforms of myosin, the main contractile protein of the thick filament of the sarcomere, can account for the decrease in myosin ATPase activity.[7] This shift depends essentially on the potential of the tissue to regulate myosin isozymic composition (Table I). In the rat ventricle, almost all models of experimental systolic overload or of combined systolic and diastolic overload (including the spontaneously hypertensive strains) induce an isomyosin redistribution from V1 to V3, i.e., from myosin heavy chain α (αMHC) to βMHC.[8] In rats, due to the initial low level of V3 ($\sim 0 - 10\%$), the potential for increase is large: V3 can represent as much as 80% of myosin from hypertrophied rat ventricles, and its amount is correlated with the degree of hypertrophy. After treatment, the

TABLE I.   *Cardiac phenotypes of active and myosin heavy chain*

	Rat		Man	
	Atria	*Ventricles*	*Atria*	*Ventricles*
Myosin Heavy Chain				
Normal	α	$\alpha + \beta$	$\alpha + \beta$	$\beta + \alpha$
Mechanical Overload	?	$\alpha + \beta$	$\alpha + \beta$	β
Actin				
Normal	?	**card**	**card**	**card + skel**
Mechanical overload	?	**card** + skel	?	?

$\alpha = \alpha$ myosin heavy chain; $\beta = \beta$ myosin heavy chain
card = cardiac actin; skel = skeletal actin

shift is reversible in chronic hypertension.[9] Conversely, in pig and human hypertrophied ventricles, which contain mainly V3 (around 90%) no marked differences are found when compared to controls. However, human ventricles seem to lose the small amount of V1 that they normally contain, since this form is detected neither in autopsy material of patients suffering from hypertensive disease nor in perioperative biopsies of patients with valvular heart disease.[10,11] This isomyosin shift is too small to be enzymatically detectable.[10,12]

The situation is different in the human atria, since normal atrial myocardium essentially contains αMHC.[11] Chronic hemodynamic overload, whatever its type (mitral stenosis or mitral regurgitation), induces a transition from αMHC to βMHC, i.e., from an atrial to a ventricular MHC isoform.[11,13-15] The extent of change is correlated with the size of the atrium (left atrial area and left atrial diameter), suggesting that in the human atrium as in the rat ventricle, isomyosin transitions are related to the severity and/or the duration of the load whatever its type.[14]

With the availability of gene-specific DNA probes, it has been possible to ask at which level the α to βMHC transition is regulated. In collaboration with the team of Dr. V. Mahdavi, we performed S1 protection studies using a cDNA probe that contained 180 nucleotides of common coding sequence at the carboxyl end for α and βMHCs, in addition to the entire 3' untranslated sequence specific to the βMHC gene. In parallel experiments we determined the isomyosin pattern by pyrophosphate gel analysis. We found that aortic banding results in a rapid induction of the βMHC mRNA, followed by the appearance of comparable levels of the corresponding protein.[16] This indicates that the myosin heavy-chain transition induced by pressure overload is mainly regulated by pretranslational mechanisms.

A large body of evidence supports the idea that isomyosin shifts are functionally significant in the myocardium. A correlation has indeed been demonstrated between the initial speed of muscle shortening at zero load (V_{max}) and myosin isoenzyme pattern from both rat and rabbit hearts.[17,18,19] The V3 myosin isotype (or βMHC) is associated with a slower contraction together with a greater economy of force development. Conversely, the V1 myosin isotype is associated with a faster and less economic contraction.[2] Thus normal rats seem to sacrifice economy for the ability to develop tension rapidly. This enables the myocardium to beat at rapid rates to fulfill peripheral oxygen demands. Pressure-overloaded rat and rabbit hearts develop tension more economically than normal myocardium but at the expense of contraction speed.

Actin

The other main determinant of the *in vivo* ATPase activity of myosin is actin. It is the major structural component of the thin filament and *in vivo* it functions to activate myosin ATPase. Like myosin, actin is also encoded by a multigene family in mammals. Two sarcomeric actins exist, the α-skeletal and the α-cardiac isoforms. In small mammals α-cardiac actin mRNA and protein accumulate as the predominant actin type in adult hearts, whereas in larger mammals such as humans α-skeletal actin is also present.[20,21,22]

We found using mouse cDNA probes that, whereas α-skeletal actin mRNAs are hardly detectable in normal hearts ($0.6 \pm 0.16\%$), they accumulate significantly in the first days after aortic stenosis ($4.6 \pm 3.1\%$, $p < 0.001$ vs. controls) and then slowly decline (8–15 days, $3.2 \pm 1.7\%$ and 30–40 days, $1.6 \pm 0.6\%$, $p < 0.05$ and NS vs. controls).[23] The same observations were made in a similar experimental model with DNA probes corresponding to rat mRNAs.[24] Thus, in rat myocardium, the expression of mRNAs encoding the sarcomeric actins is altered at the onset of a pressure-overload hypertrophy. The functional significance of the different actin isoforms is not known. It is possible that the modifications between skeletal and cardiac actins may result in a fine-tuning of the actomyosin complex to respond transiently to altered physiological conditions. Our results, as well as the transitory isoform changes found for tropomyosin,[24] show that the thin filament participates as well as the thick filament in the response of cardiac muscle to new functional requirements.

Nonsynchronous Regulation of Myosin Heavy Chain and Actin Multigene Families

Rather strikingly, the time course of up-regulation of βMHC and α-skeletal actin genes is not the same (Figure 2). Whereas the amount of βMHC mRNA increases in proportion to the degree of hypertrophy and persists as long as the overload is maintained,[16] α-skeletal actin mRNA returns rapidly to control values.[23] Very recent experiments indicate that the early time course of appearance and the distribution of α-skeletal actin and βMHC mRNAs in the

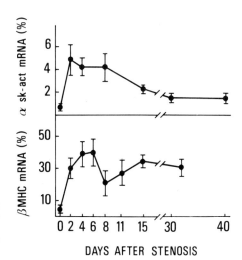

FIG. 2. Time course of the β myosin heavy-chain and α-skeletal actin mRNAs accumulation in the overloaded rat ventricle. Redrawn from Schwartz et al.[23] and Izumo et al.[16]

overloaded ventricle also differ. We have investigated, by *in situ* hybridization procedures, the distribution of βMHC and α-skeletal actin mRNAs during the early stages of cardiac hypertrophy, secondary to pressure overload (Schiaffino *et al.*, submitted). The α-skeletal actin gene was activated earlier than the βMHC gene. Moreover, whereas α-skeletal actin mRNA accumulation was seen throughout the entire left ventricle, that of βMHC mRNA was mainly observed around large coronary arteries and in the inner half of the left ventricular wall. This difference in the timing and the distribution of mRNA accumulation of the two contractile isogenes argues in favor of two different triggers. Increase in wall stress is known to be induced by pressure overload, which suggests that wall stress might be directly involved in the up-regulation of one of the two genes. Stimulation of the α1-adrenergic receptor could also contribute to the phenomena that we have observed.

MODULATION OF SINGLE GENES

Atrial Natriuretic Factor (ANF)

The fact that mammalian atrium is an endocrine gland that secretes ANF, a 28-amino acid peptide, which is diuretic, natriuretic, vasodilatory, and inhibitory of renin, arginine vasopressin, cortisol, and aldosterone has been known for several years. ANF and its precursors are stored in atrial granules and can be released in response to passive stretch of the atrial muscle.[25,26,27] The knowledge that ventricular myocytes also secrete ANF in various pathophysiological conditions is very recent, and most of the studies have been con-

ducted in rodents. Ventricular ANF peptides and mRNA have been identified
in the ventricles of fetal and neonatal rats, and after birth these levels decline
rapidly.[28,29] Although ANF mRNA is barely detectable in adult ventricles, it is
re-induced in congestive heart failure (cardiomyopathic hamster),[30,31] myocardial infarction,[32] spontaneously hypertensive rats,[33] and during acute and
chronic pressure and volume overload.[34-36] Recent results from our laboratory indicate that ANF mRNA accumulation in the overloaded ventricle in
response to coarctation is biphasic, which suggests that ventricular production
of ANF might be responsible for the temporal fluctuations in the ANF
circulating pool that occur in this model. At the stage of compensatory
hypertrophy, ANF mRNA in the ventricle is correlated with the degree of
hypertrophy. Although the mechanisms of ventricular release of the peptide
are not yet fully understood, one might hypothesize that in the overloaded
ventricle, the release of the hypotensive peptide is a compensatory mechanism that might help to normalize the loading conditions of the cardiac
pump.

Ca^{++} Dependent ATPase of the Sarcoplasmic Reticulum

Because the Ca^{++} ion plays a central role in the process of excitation-con-
traction coupling in the heart, alterations from normal in the subcellular
handling of Ca^{++} may provide a basis for cardiac contractile failure. Abnormal intracellular calcium handling was indeed found in experimental pressure overload as well as in myocardium from patients with end-stage heart
failure.[37,38] On the other hand, major alterations in relaxation occur during
cardiac hypertrophy induced by aortic stenosis in guinea pig,[39] and studies
conducted *in vitro* on microsomal vesicles demonstrated a reduction in calcium pump activity in failing hearts.[40,41] Taken together, these data strongly
suggested alterations of the sarcoplasmic reticulum (SR), the main intracellular organelle devoted to sequestration of cytosolic Ca^{++}, which could partially
account for the changes seen in relaxation with hypertrophy. Ca^{++} uptake by
SR is an ATP-supported process mediated by a (Ca^{++}, Mg^{++}) dependent
ATPase (Ca^{++}ATPase). Three isoforms of Ca^{++}ATPase have been described
in striated muscles, coded by two genes.[42,43] One gene, expressed exclusively
in fast skeletal muscle, generates by alternative splicing of the penultimate
exon two isoforms expressed sequentially during ontogenic development, one
in neonates and the other in adults.[44] The other gene codes for the protein
present in adult slow-twitch and cardiac muscles.

We have very recently studied the Ca^{++}ATPase gene expression in the
overloaded rat ventricle. Coarctation of the abdominal aorta was performed
in 8-week-old male Wistar rats (body weight 180–200g) by placing a partially
occluded Weck hemoclip (internal section 0.6 mm) around the abdominal
aorta between the renal and superior mesenteric arteries, as described pre-

viously.[8] This produces an aortic occlusion of about 75%. Sham-operated controls underwent anesthesia without placement of the clip. Six sham-operated rats and eight coarcted rats were killed 1 month after surgery, at the time of compensatory hypertrophy. As shown on Table II, the ratio left-ventricular weight/body weight (LVW/BW) was markedly increased in the coarcted animals, indicating severe hypertrophy of the cardiac tissue. The amount of mRNA coding for the Ca^{++}ATPase of the sarcoplasmic reticulum was determined by dot blot analysis with a 1.5 kb DNA probe complementary to the rat cardiac Ca^{++}ATPase mRNA (nucleotides -50 to $+1446$) (Lompré *et al.*, manuscript in preparation). The probe was labelled by random-priming (Amersham kit) to a specific activity of $1-3 \times 10^9$ dpm/μg. The same blot was dehybridized and rehybridized to a 24 mer-oligonucleotide specific to rat ribosomal 18S RNA (nucleotides $1046-1070$)[45] in order to normalize all results to the true amount of RNA spotted on the membrane. The relative amount of Ca^{++}ATPase message in each sample was then calculated as a percentage of the mean value obtained for the sham-operated animals. As shown in Table II, a 30% decrease in the Ca^{++}ATPase mRNA level was observed in severe hypertrophy. It remains to be determined whether this decrease corresponds to a parallel decrease of the protein. One might hypothesize that it is indeed the case, because regulation at the translational level has not been demonstrated to be frequently used as an adaptational mechanism in cardiac tissue. Our results would thus predict a decrease in the density of the Ca^{++}ATPase pumps per unit of contractile myocardium, which could be the molecular basis for the decreased function of the SR and for the altered intracellular Ca^{++} handling previously reported in the hypertrophied heart.

CONCLUSIONS

When the working conditions are changed, the intrinsic physiological properties of cardiac muscles are modified, allowing the muscle to adapt to the new environmental conditions. Two different mechanisms available to the cardiac genome have until now been described that can account, at least partly, for the alterations in contraction and relaxation. It should be emphasized that it is normal genes that are activated or deactivated and that the proteins pro-

TABLE II.   *SR Ca^{++} ATPase mRNA in severe cardiac hypertrophy*

	LVW/BW	SR Ca^{++} ATPase mRNA
Sham-operated rats ($n = 6$)	1.76 ± 0.07	99.9 ± 14.3
Coarcted rats ($n = 8$)	2.69 ± 0.14	$68.7 \pm 13^*$

*p < 0.001 by one-way analysis of variance

duced have a normal structure. Neither the multiple factors involved in this gene reprogramming, nor the sequence leading from the mechanical and perhaps also the hormonal triggers to this multifactorial gene modulation are known. Further work is now needed to clarify the question of how hemodynamic stimuli can lead to a myocardial phenotype better adapted to the new functional demands.

ACKNOWLEDGMENTS

We thank B. Swynghedauw and L. Rappaport for very constructive discussions, K. Boheler for reading the manuscript, T. Tarameli and P. Cagnac for their expert secretarial work.

REFERENCES

1. Swynghedauw B, Moalic JM, Lecarpentier Y, Ray A, Mercadier JJ, Aumont MC, Schwartz K. Adaptational changes of contractile proteins in chronic cardiac overloading: structure and rate of synthesis. In Alpert NR , ed. *Perspectives in Cardiovascular Research. Vol 7, Myocardial Hypertrophy and Failure.* New York, Raven Press, 1983;465–476.
2. Alpert NR, Mulieri LA. Increased myothermal economy of isometric force generation in compensated cardiac hypertrophy induced by pulmonary artery constriction in the rabbit. *Circ Res* 1982; **50**:491–500.
3. Barany M. ATPase activity of myosin correlated with speed of muscle shortening. *J Gen Physiol* 1967; **50**:197–216.
4. Bing OHL, Matsushita S, Fanburg BL, Levine HJ. Mechanical properties of rat cardiac muscle during experimental hypertrophy. *Circ Res* 1971; **28**:234–245.
5. Hamrell BB, Alpert NR. The mechanical characteristics of hypertrophied rabbit cardiac muscle in the absence of congestive heart failure. *Circ Res* 1977; **40**:20–25.
6. Spann JF, Buccino RA, Sonnenblick EH, Braunwald E. Contractile state of cardiac muscle obtained from cats with experimentally produced ventricular hypertrophy and heart failure. *Circ Res* 1967; **21**:341–354.
7. Lompré AM, Schwartz K, d'Albis A, Lacombe G, Thiem NV, Swynghedauw B. Myosin isoenzyme redistribution in chronic heart overload. *Nature* 1979; **282**:105–107.
8. Mercadier JJ, Lompré AM, Wisnewsky C, Samuel JL, Bercovici J, Swynghedauw B, Schwartz K. Myosin isoenzymic changes in several models of rat cardiac hypertrophy. *Circ Res* 1981; **49**:525–532.
9. Dussaule JC, Michel JB, Auzan C, Schwartz K, Corvol P, Menard JM. Effect of antihypertensive treatment on the left ventricular isomyosin profile in one-clip, two kidney hypertensive rats. *J Pharm Exp Ther* 1986; **236**:512–518.
10. Mercadier JJ, Bouveret P, Gorza L, Schiaffino S, Clark WA, Zak R, Swynghedauw B, Schwartz K. Myosin isoenzymes in normal and hypertrophied human ventricular myocardium. *Circ Res* 1983; **53**:52–62.
11. Gorza L, Mercadier JJ, Schwartz K, Thornell LE, Sartore S, Schiaffino S. Myosin types in the human heart. An immunofluorescence study of normal and hypertrophied atrial and ventricular myocardium. *Circ Res* 1984; **54**:694–702.
12. Schier JJ, Adelstein RS. Structural and enzymatic comparison of human cardiac muscle myosins isolated from infants, adults and patients with hypertrophic cardiomyopathy. *J Clin Invest* 1982; **69**:816–825.
13. Bouvagnet P, Léger J, Dechesne CA, Dureau G, Anoal M, Léger JJ. Local changes in myosin types in diseased human atrial myocardium: a quantitative immunofluorescence study. *Circulation* 1985; **72**:272–279.
14. Mercadier JJ, De la Bastie D, Ménasché P, N'Guyen Van Cao A, Bouveret P, Lorente P,

Piwnica A, Slama R, Schwartz K. Alpha-myosin heavy chain isoform and atrial size in patients with various types of mitral valve dysfunction: a quantitative study. *J Am Coll Cardiol* 1987; **9**:1024–1030.

15. Tsuchimochi H, Sugi M, Kuro-o M, Ueda S, Takaku F, Furuta SI, Shirai T, Yasaki Y. Isozymic changes in myosin of human atrial myocardium induced by overload; immunohistochemical study using monoclonal antibodies. *J Clin Invest* 1984; **74**:662–665.

16. Izumo S, Lompré AM, Matsuoka R, Koren G, Schwartz K, Nadal-Ginard B, Mahdavi V. Myosin heavy chain messenger RNA and protein isoform transitions during cardiac hypertrophy. *J Clin Invest* 1987; **79**:970–977.

17. Schwartz K, Lecarpentier Y, Martin JL, Lompré AM, Mercadier JJ, Swynghedauw B. Myosin isoenzymic distribution correlates with speed of myocardial contraction. *J Mol Cell Cardiol* 1981; **13**:1071–1075.

18. Ebrecht G, Rupp H, Jacob R. Alterations of mechanical parameters in chemically skinned preparations of rat myocardium as a function of isoenzyme pattern of myosin. *Basic Res Cardiol* 1982; **77**:220–234.

19. Pagani ED, Julian FJ. Rabbit papillary muscle myosin isozymes and the velocity of muscle shortening. *Circ Res* 1984; **54**:586–594.

20. Vandekerckhove J, Weber K. The complete amino acid sequence of actins from bovine aorta, bovine heart, bovine fast skeletal muscle, and rabbit slow skeletal muscle. *Differentiation* 1979; **14**:123–133.

21. Mayer Y, Czosnek H, Zeelon PE, Yaffe D, Nudel U. Expression of the genes coding for the skeletal muscle and cardiac actins in the heart. *Nucleic Acids Res* 1984; **12**:1087–2000.

22. Gunning P, Ponte P, Blau H, Kedes L. α-skeletal and α-cardiac actin genes are coexpressed in adult human skeletal muscle and heart. *Molec Cell Biol* 1983; **3**:1985–1995.

23. Schwartz K, De La Bastie D, Bouveret P, Oliviero P, Alonso S, Buckingham M. α skeletal muscle actin mRNA's accumulate in hypertrophied adult rat hearts. *Circ Res* 1986; **59**:551–555.

24. Izumo S, Nadal-Ginard B, Mahdavi V: Protooncogene induction and reprogramming of cardiac gene expression produced by pressure overload. *Proc Natl Acad Sci USA* 1988; **85**:339–343.

25. Bodak A, Cluzeaud F, Gastineau P, Hatt PY. Degree of granulation of atrial cardiocytes: its decrease after aorto-caval fistula in the rat. *Basic Res Cardiol* 1979; **74**:509–517.

26. Cantin M, Genest J. The heart as an endocrine gland. *Hypertension* 1987; **10**:I118–I121.

27. Goetz KL. Physiology and pathophysiology of atrial peptides. *Am J Physiol* 1988; **254**:E1–E15.

28. Bloch JD, Seidman JG, Naftilan JD, Fallon JT, Seidman CE. Neonatal atria and ventricles secrete atrial natriuretic factor via tissue-specific secretory pathways. *Cell* 1986; **47**:695–702.

29. Wei Y, Rody CP, Day ML, Wiegand RC, Needleman LD, Cole BR, Needleman P. Developmental changes in the rat atriopeptin hormonal system. *J Clin Invest* 1987; **79**:1325–1329.

30. Ding J, Thibault G, Gutkowska J, Garcia R, Karabatsos T, Jasmin G, Genest J, Cantin M. Cardiac and plasma atrial natriuretic factor in experimental congestive heart failure. *Endocrinology* 1987; **12**:248–257.

31. Franch HA, Dixon RAF, Blaine EH, Siegel PKS. Ventricular atrial natriuretic factor in the cardiomyopathic hamster model of congestive heart failure. *Circ Res* 1988; **62**:31–36.

32. Michel JB, Lattion AL, Salzmann JL, De Lourdes Cerol M, Philippe M, Camilleri JP, Corvol P. Hormonal and cardiac effects of converting enzyme inhibition in rat myocardial infarction. *Circ Res* 1988; **62**:641–650.

33. Arai H, Nakao K, Saito Y, Morij N, Sugawara A, Yamada T, Itoh H, Shiono S, Mukoyama M, Ohkubo H, Nakanishi S, Imura H. Augmented expression of atrial natriuretic polypeptide gene in ventricles of spontaneously hypertensive rats (SHR) and SHR-stroke prone. *Circ Res* 1988; **62**:926–930.

34. Lattion AL, Michel JB, Arnauld E, Corvol P, Soubrier F. Myocardial recruitment during ANF mRNA increase with volume overload in the rat. *Am J Physiol* 1986; **251**:H890–H896.

35. Mercadier JJ, Lompré AM, De La Bastie D, Wisnewsky C, Schwartz K. Left ventricular accumulation of messenger ribonucleic acid of atrial natriuretic factor in the rat at the compensated stage of pressure overload induced cardiac hypertrophy. *C.R. Acad Sci Ser III-Vie* 1987; **305**:79–82.

36. Day ML, Schwartz D, Wiegand RC, Stockman PT, Brunnert SR, Tolunay HE, Currie MG,

Standaert DG, Needleman P. Ventricular atriopeptin. Unmasking of messenger RNA and peptide synthesis by hypertrophy or dexamethasone. *Hypertension* 1987; **9**:485–491.

37. Gwathmey JK, Morgan JP. Altered calcium handling in experimental pressure-overload hypertrophy in the ferret. *Circ Res* 1985; **57**:836–843.
38. Gwathmey JK, Copelas L, MacKinnon R, Schoen FJ, Feldman MD, Grossman W, Morgan JP. Abnormal intracellular calcium handling in myocardium from patients with end-stage heart failure. *Circ Res* 1987; **61**:70–76.
39. Lecarpentier Y, Waldenstrom A, Clergue M, Chemla D, Oliviero P, Martin JL, Swynghedauw B. Major alterations in relaxation during cardiac hypertrophy induced by aortic stenosis in guinea pig. *Circ Res* 1987; **61**:107–116.
40. Lindenmayer GE, Sordahl LA, Harigaya S, Allen JC, Besch HR Jr, Schwartz A. Some biochemical studies on subcellular systems isolated from fresh recipient human cardiac tissue obtained during transplantation. *Am J Physiol* 1971; **27**:277–283.
41. Mead RJ, Peterson MB, Welty JD. Sarcolemmal and sarcoplasmic reticular ATPase activities in the failing canine heart. *Circ Res* 1971; **29**:14–20.
42. MacLennan DH, Brandl CJ, Korczak B, Green NM. Amino-acid sequence of a $Ca^{2+} + Mg^{2+}$-dependent ATPase from rabbit muscle sarcoplasmic reticulum, deduced from its complementary DNA sequence. *Nature* 1985; **316**:696–700.
43. Brandl CJ, Green NM, Korczak B, MacLennan DH. Two Ca^{2+} ATPase genes: homologies and mechanistic implications of deduced amino acid sequences. *Cell* 1986; **44**:597–607.
44. Brandl CJ, de Leon S, Martin DR, MacLennan DH. Adult forms of the Ca^{2+} ATPase of sarcoplasmic reticulum. *J Biol Chem* 1987; **262**:3768–3774.
45. Chan YL, Gutell R, Noller HF, Wool IG. The nucleotide sequence of a rat 18S ribosomal RNA gene. *J Biol Chem* 1984; **259**:224–230.

SUMMARY

Cardiac muscle is known to adapt to chronic changes in functional requirements. For example hemodynamic overload induces a cardiac hypertrophy accompanied by a reprogramming of some genes. Two mechanisms are involved: differential expression of contractile protein multigene families (myosin heavy chain and actin) and modulation of single genes, such as those coding for the atrial natriuretic factor and the Ca^{++}-dependent ATPase of the sarcoplasmic reticulum. These modifications lead to a new phenotype better adapted to the new functional demand, characterized by a slower and more efficient contraction, a slower relaxation, and a normalization of the loading conditions of the hypertrophied heart. The molecular mechanisms linking the mechanical event to cardiac gene reprogramming and the limits of this myocardial adaptation remain to be fully characterized.

RÉSUMÉ

On sait que le muscle cardiaque s'adapte aux changements chroniques des conditions fonctionnelles. La surcharge hémodynamique, par exemple, entraîne une hypertrophie cardiaque accompagnée d'une reprogrammation de quelques gènes. Deux mécanismes entrent en jeu: l'expression différentielle de familles multigènes de protéines contractiles (lourde chaîne myosine et actine) et la modulation de gènes uniques, tels que les codeurs du facteur natriurétique auriculaire et le Ca^{++}ATPase du reticulum sarcoplasmique.

Ces modifications mènent à un nouveau phénotype mieux adapté à la nouvelle demande fonctionnelle, caractérisée par une contraction plus lente et plus efficace, une relaxation plus lente, et une normalisation des conditions de remplissage du coeur hypertrophié. Il reste à caractériser les mécanismes moléculaires qui lient l'événement mécanique à la reprogrammation des gènes cardiaques, ainsi que les limitations de cette adaptation du myocarde.

ZUSAMMENFASSUNG

Es ist eine bekannte Tatsache, dass die Herzmuskulatur sich an chronische Veränderungen in den Funktionsbedingungen anpasst. Zum Beispiel verursacht hämodynamische Überlastung Herzmuskel-Hypertrophie, zusammen mit einer Neu-programmierung einiger Gene. Ausschlaggebend sind zwei Mechanismen: erstens der ausgleichende Ausdruck kontraktiler Multigen-Proteinfamilien (Myosin-Schwerketten und Aktin), und die Modulation einfacher Gene, so zum Beispiel solcher, die den atrialen natriuretischen Faktor kodieren und die Ca^{++} − abhängige ATPase des sarkoplastischen Retikulums. Diese Veränderungen führen zu einem neuen phänotyp, der besser an die neuen Funktionsbedingungen angepasst ist. Charakteristisch für diesen Phänotyp sind eine langsamere und wirkungsvollere Kontraktion, eine langsamere Relaxation und eine Normalisierung der Belastungsbedingungen für das von Hypertrophie betroffene Herz. Die molekularen Mechanismen, die die mechanische Auswirkung mit der Gen-Reprogrammierung verbinden, und die Grenzen dieser Herzmuskelanpassung sind noch nicht völlig geklärt.

RIASSUNTO

E' noto che il muscolo cardiaco si adatta ai cambiamenti cronici dei requisiti funzionali. Per esempio, il sovraccarico emodinamico induce un'ipertrofia cardiaca accompagnata da una riprogrammazione di alcuni geni. Due sono i meccanismi coinvolti: l'espressione differenziale di famiglie multigeniche di proteine contrattili (catena pesante di miosina e actina) e la modulazione di singoli geni, quali quelli che codificano il fattore natriuretico atriale l'ATPase CA^{++}−dipendente del reticolo sarcoplasmico. Queste modifiche portano ad un nuovo fenotipo più adatto alle nuove richieste sistemiche, caratterizzato da una contrazione più lenta e più efficiente, da un rilassamento più lento e da una normalizzazione delle condizioni di carico del cuore normalizzazione delle condizioni di carico del cuore normalizzazione delle condizioni di carico del cuore ipertrofizzato. I meccanismi molecolari che collegano l'evento meccanico alla riprogrammazione dei geni cardiaci ed i limiti di tale adattamento miocardico non sono ancora stati completamente caratterizzati.

SUMÁRIO

Sabe-se que o músculo cardíaco se adapta a mudanças crônicas nos requisitos funcionais. Por exemplo, a sobrecarga hemodinâmica induz a hipertrofia cardíaca acompanhada de uma reprogrammação de alguns genes. Dois mecanismos são envolvidos: a expressão diferencial de famílias multigênicas de proteína contrátil (cadeia forte de miosina e actina) e a modulação de genes individuais, tais como aqueles que codificam para o fator natriurético atrial e a ATPasa dependente de cálcio do retículo sarcoplasmático. Estas mudanças conduzem a um novo fenotipo melhor adatado à nova demanda funcional e caracterizado por uma contração mais lenta e eficiente, uma relaxação mais lenta e a normalização das condições de carga do coração hipertrofiado. Os mecanismos moleculares que associam o evento mecânico com a reprogramação do gene cardíaco e os limites desta adatação miocárdica ainda estão por serem plenamente caracterizados.

RESUMEN

Se sabe que el músculo cardíaco se adapta a cambios crónicos en los requisitos funcionales. Por ejemplo, la sobrecarga hemodinámica induce la hipertrofia cardíaca acompañada de una reprogramación de algunos genes. Dos mecanismos se hallan involucrados: expresión diferencial de familias multigénicas de proteína contráctil (cadena fuerte de miosina y actina) y modulación de genes unitarios, tales como aquellos que generan el código del factor natriurético atrial y la ATPasa dependiente del calcio++ del retículo sarcoplásmico. Estas modificaciones llevan a un nuevo fenotipo mejor adaptado a la nueva demanda funcional y caracterizado por una contracción más lenta y eficiente, una relajación más lenta, y la normalización de las condiciones de carga del corazón hipertrofiado. Todavía falta por explicar totalmente los mecanismos moleculares que asocian el evento mecánico con la reprogramación del gen cardíaceo, y los límites de esta adaptación miocárdica.

要約

心筋は、機能上の必要性から慢性的変化に適応することが知られている。たとえば血行動態の過負荷は、ある遺伝子の再プログラミングを伴う心肥大をひき起こす。これには2つの機序が関与する。収縮タンパクの多重遺伝子族（ミオシンH鎖およびアクチン）の異なった発現と、心房性ナトリウム利尿因子や筋小胞体のCa²⁺依存性ATPaseなどをコードする一重遺伝子の調節である。これらの修飾は新しい機能上の要求により適合した新しい表現型をつくりだし、これは緩徐なより強い収縮とか、ゆっくりとした弛緩、そして肥大心の負荷状態の正常化などのかたちをとる。心臓の機械的機能を遺伝子に関連させる分子レベルの機序と、この心筋の適応の限界についての詳細は、今後の検討課題である。

Cardiac and Renal Failure: An Expanding Role for ACE Inhibitors, edited by C. T. Dollery and L. M. Sherwood, Hanley & Belfus, Inc., Philadelphia.

Atrial Natriuretic Peptide in Heart Failure: Altered Gene Expression and Processing and Possible Pathophysiological Significance

H. Imura and K. Nakao

Atrial natriuretic peptide (ANP) was first isolated from human and rat atria as an agent with potent diuretic, natriuretic and vasorelaxant properties. Several different molecular forms of ANP were isolated, particularly from rat atria.[1] It is now generally agreed, however, that the major circulating form in man and rats is α-ANP (ANP 99–126), a 28–amino-acid peptide, whereas the major storage form in the atrium is γ-ANP (ANP 1–126), which is the precursor of α-ANP.[2,3] Another unique molecular form found only in human atria is β-ANP, which is an anti-parallel dimer of α-ANP.[4]

Secretion of ANP from the heart is enhanced by atrial stretch, which is usually caused by increased atrial pressure.[5] Any pathological state, therefore, associated with increased atrial pressure, such as congestive heart failure (CHF), hypertension and chronic renal failure, is known to accompany elevated plasma ANP levels.[6,7,8] Such elevation of plasma ANP concentrations in pathological states can be regarded as a compensatory mechanism because of its diuretic and vasorelaxant activities. It is still unclear, however, what is the role of ANP in these pathological states. In this article, we discuss the biosynthesis, secretion and possible action of ANP in pathological states, with special reference to CHF.

BIOSYNTHESIS AND SECRETION OF ANP IN PATHOLOGICAL STATES

In order to evaluate biosynthesis of ANP in human and rat heart, we measured the levels of messenger RNA (mRNA) for the ANP precursor by

Northern blot analysis and the content of the peptide by radioimmunoassay (RIA). We also studied secretion of ANP by using RIA for α-ANP.

Biosynthesis of ANP in the Atrium in Patients with CHF

Atrial tissues obtained at cardiac surgery were subjected to Northern blot analysis and RIA. Northern blot analysis using cDNA for the ANP precursor as a probe gave a single hybridization band of identical size in all atrial tissues studied. The amount of mRNA was significantly increased when right atrial pressure exceeded 10 mm Hg. There was a positive correlation between the amount of mRNA in the atrium and atrial pressure. These results suggest that atrial stretch due to increased atrial pressure is a determinant in regulating the expression of ANP gene in the atrium.

Immunoreactive ANP contents in atria measured by RIA for α-ANP were increased with the severity of heart failure as shown in Figure 1. We further

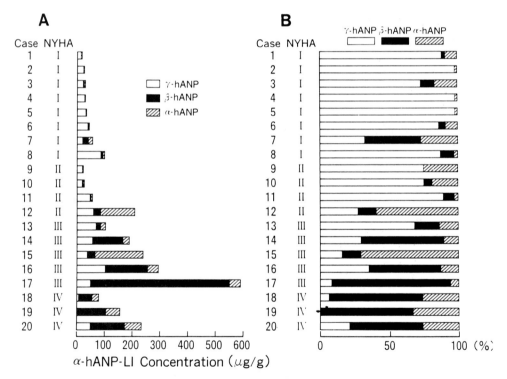

FIG. 1. Schematic illustrations of tissue concentrations of γ-, β- and α-ANP (A) and percentages of each fraction in the total ANP concentration (B) in right atria obtained from 20 patients. Cases are arranged in order of the severity of CHF classified by the criteria of NYHA. Reproduced from *J Clin Invest* 1988; **81**:1962, with permission.

analyzed molecular forms of ANP in these atria by using gel chromatography.[9] In patients with mild CHF, gel chromatography revealed that the predominant molecular form of ANP in atrial tissues was γ-ANP with minor peaks of α-ANP or β-ANP (an anti-parallel dimer of α-ANP). On the other hand, gel chromatography of atrial extracts from patients with severe CHF (grades III and IV according to the classification of the New York Heart Association) showed that γ-ANP was only a minor component, whereas β-ANP and/or α-ANP were predominant molecular forms.[9] Figure 1 illustrates absolute values and percentages of three peaks corresponding to γ-, β- and α-ANP in 20 atrial tissues. The percentage of γ-ANP fraction was decreased in patients with severe CHF, whereas β- and α-ANP fractions, especially β-ANP fraction, were significantly increased as shown in the right panel of Figure 1. The left panel of Figure 1 illustrates that an increase in total amounts of ANP in the atrium of severe CHF resulted from increases in the amounts of low molecular weight forms, α- and β-ANP.

The processing of γ-ANP, the precursor form in the heart, has not yet been fully elucidated. We have previously reported that the predominant molecular form of ANP in blood obtained at the coronary sinus during cardiac catheterization in man is α-ANP.[3] By using gel chromatography and high performance liquid chromatography,[3] we have also observed that peripheral blood of rats and perfusate of isolated beating rat heart contained predominantly α-ANP. These results suggest that the proteolytic processing of γ-ANP occurs immediately before, during or immediately after the secretion. In CHF, however, the processing seems to occur during storage, which gives rise to α-ANP and β-ANP. We have previously reported that β-ANP can be converted to α-ANP in blood and that the time course of its action is slower in onset but more prolonged than that of α-ANP.[10] It is concluded from these results that both the augmented expression of ANP gene and the accelerated processing of ANP precursor occur in the atrium in CHF.

Biosynthesis and Secretion of ANP in the Ventricle in Patients with CHF

It has been shown that fetal ventricles contain a significant amount of ANP, whereas only a trace of ANP could be detected from ventricles in human neonates and adults.[11] This suggests that the expression of ANP gene in the ventricle is markedly suppressed after birth. In fact only a trace of ANP could be detected from ventricular tissue of normal subjects. The amount of mRNA for the ANP precursor is also much less than that of the atrium. However, the ratios of tissue mRNA levels and tissue immunoreactive ANP contents in the ventricle were much greater than those in the atrium. It is likely that ANP synthesized in the ventricle is secreted more rapidly than that synthesized in the atrium.

In our previous study, we observed by RIA that the ventricle from a patient with dilated cardiomyopathy (DCM) contained a markedly increased amount of ANP, and we detected an increase of ANP mRNA by Northern blot analysis[12] (Figure 2). We further extended our studies and demonstrated that all ventricular tissues obtained from patients with DCM contained increased amounts of ANP (Table I).[13] Moreover, ventricular aneurysm tissues obtained from patients with heart failure due to old myocardial infarction also contained significantly increased amounts of ANP measured by RIA. The amount of ANP mRNA was also increased in both tissues.[13] All these data clearly indicate that the expression of ANP gene is augmented in the ventricle of the failing heart. A significant correlation was found between the ANP level in aneurysm tissues and pulmonary capillary wedge pressure (PCWP). This suggests that increased ventricular pressure is a determinant of altered expression of the ANP gene in the ventricle in CHF.

It is still unclear to what extent ventricular ANP secretion contributes to the elevated plasma ANP level in patients with CHF. In order to answer this question, we measured ANP concentration in blood at different levels during cardiac catheterization in patients with DCM who were assumed to produce an increased amount of ANP in the ventricle.[14] As shown in Table II, there was a significant step-up in ANP concentrations in blood obtained from the anterior interventricular vein in DCM patients but not in control patients. This suggests that ventricular ANP contributes to the elevated plasma ANP concentrations in CHF.

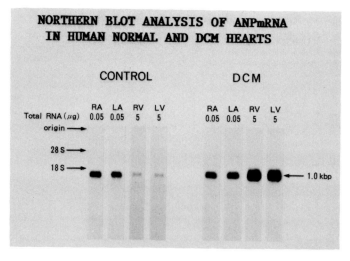

FIG. 2. Northern blot analysis of mRNA for the ANP precursor in control heart (left) and in DCM heart (right). Total RNA extracted from right and left atria and ventricles were fractionated on 2.0% agarose gel, transferred to a paper, and hybridized with ^{32}P-labeled cDNA for the ANP precursor. Reproduced from *Biochem Biophys Res Commun* 1988; **148**:211, with permission.

TABLE I. *Plasma and ventricular ANP concentrations and ventricular ANP mRNA levels in patients with dilated cardiomyopathy (DCM) and left ventricular aneurysm (LVA) due to old myocardial infarction*

	Plasma ANP level pg/ml	Tissue ANP level ng/g	Tissue ANP mRNA level arbitrary unit/μg RNA
Control	37 ± 5	18 ± 7	16 ± 8
DCM	1490 ± 459	986 ± 250	130 ± 10
LVA	517 ± 183	660 ± 122	140 ± 40

Biosynthesis and Secretion of ANP in the Heart of SHR-SP

We have previously observed an increase of ANP content in the ventricle of spontaneously hypertensive rats-stroke prone (SHR-SP) at the stage of established hypertension. Therefore, SHR-SP would be a suitable animal model to study ventricular biosynthesis and secretion of ANP. We studied biosynthesis of ANP by Northern blot analysis and RIA in SHR-SP, spontaneously hypertensive rats (SHR) and control Wistar Kyoto rats (WKY).[15] The RNA blot analysis revealed that atrial ANP mRNA levels were not significantly different among SHR-SP, SHR and WKY. On the other hand, ventricular ANP mRNA levels were moderately and markedly increased in SHR and SHR-SP, respectively. Taking the tissue weight into account, we could calculate that the total amount of ANP mRNA levels in the ventricle of SHR-SP was approximately twice as high as that of ANP mRNA in the atrium of control rats and SHR-SP. If the efficiency of translation is the same in the ventricle as in the atrium, 2 times more ANP can be released from the ventricle. Immunoreactive ANP content was also increased in the ventricle, although to a lesser extent than the increase in ANP mRNA. The ratio of mRNA level to immunoreactive ANP content was, therefore, smaller in the ventricle than in the atrium, suggesting more rapid secretion after biosynthesis in the ventricle.

In order to elucidate the secretory rate of ANP from the ventricle, we

TABLE II. *Plasma ANP levels from various sites during cardiac catheterization in control patients and dilated cardiomyopathy*

Sampling Point	Control n = 18 pg/ml	DCM n = 11 pg/ml
Aorta (Ao)	108 ± 42	454 ± 360
Anterior interventricular vein (AIV)	127 ± 55	915 ± 584
Great cardiac vein (GCV)	461 ± 224 ·	1310 ± 926
Coronary sinus (CS)	682 ± 341	1880 ± 1190

From Yasue, et al. *J Clin Invest* 1988 (in press), with permission.

performed perfusion of an isolated, beating rat heart on a Langendorff perfusion apparatus, as we previously reported.[16] After the period of 60 minutes of perfusion, both atria were quickly removed with scissors and the remaining heart was perfused for another 40 minutes. ANP concentrations in the perfusate were measured before and after atrial removal. ANP concentrations in the perfusate decreased after atrial removal to the level of less than 5% of the basal level in WKY or SHR rats. On the other hand, the ANP levels fell only to approximately 70% of the basal level in SHR-SP following atrial removal. These results indicate that the ventricle significantly contributes to an increased plasma level of ANP in SHR-SP. It is concluded from these results that the expression of ANP gene in the ventricle is augmented in rats with severe hypertension and with cardiac hypertrophy, much as in CHF.

These findings in man and rats suggest that the increased biosynthesis and secretion of ANP from the ventricle significantly contribute to the elevated plasma level of ANP in CHF or hypertension.

PATHOPHYSIOLOGICAL SIGNIFICANCE OF ANP AS A HORMONE

Since ANP has potent diuretic, natriuretic and vasorelaxant actions, the increased biosynthesis and secretion of ANP from the heart, especially from the ventricle in CHF and hypertension, can be interpreted as a compensatory mechanism to correct cardiovascular abnormalities. However, the biological actions of ANP can be observed only at pharmacological doses, and the physiological and pathophysiological significance have not yet been elucidated. We studied effects of chronic blockade of endogenous ANP by monoclonal antibody (MoAb) in rats with hypertension and also the effects of exogenous ANP in patients with CHF.

Effect of MoAb Against ANP on the Development of Hypertension in Rats

We raised two MoAbs against α-human ANP (α-hANP). MoAb (KY-ANP-II) recognizes the N-terminal portion of α-ANP[17] and, therefore, reacts equally with α-hANP and α-rat ANP (α-rANP). The other one recognizes the ring portion of α-hANP and reacts only with α-hANP.[18] The former was used for the experimental group, whereas the latter was for the control group. The ability of MoAb to neutralize ANP was tested by the following experiments. The decrease in blood pressure and the increase of plasma cyclic GMP induced by a single injection of 5 μg of α-hANP in SHR-SP were both reversed by the prior administration of 100 μl of MoAb (KY-ANP-II). To test whether the MoAb blocks the action of endogenous ANP, we studied the effect of immunoneutralization with MoAb on increases in plasma cyclic

GMP induced by the injection of vasopressin, and found a significant attenuation by the MoAb.[18]

Since the single injection of MoAb was shown to neutralize both exogenous and endogenous ANP, we next studied the effect of weekly, repeated injections of MoAb in SHR-SP, which were known to develop progressive hypertension, cardiomegaly and stroke. The increase in blood pressure observed in control SHR-SP was significantly augmented by the weekly injection of MoAb starting at the age of 6 weeks. After four injections ending at 10 weeks of age, the rats were followed for the next 4 weeks. The rats receiving the MoAb (KY-ANP-II) died significantly earlier than those receiving the MoAb (KY-ANP-I).[19]

We also studied the effect of the MoAb in DOCA salt-rats. The rats received weekly injections of 20 mg of deoxycorticosterone acetate (DOCA) and 1% NaCl as drinking fluid. As shown in Table III, the rats developed a gradual increase in blood pressure. This rise in blood pressure was significantly accelerated in rats receiving MoAb (KY-ANP-II) compared with those receiving MoAb (KY-ANP-I).[20] Plasma cyclic GMP levels were elevated in DOCA-salt rats compared with control untreated rats, but the elevation was more marked in those receiving KY-ANP-II. Both urine volume and urinary sodium excretion were also decreased in rats receiving the antibody compared with the control DOCA-salt rats, suggesting diuretic and natriuretic activities of endogenous ANP in these rats.

Use of Exogenous ANP in the Treatment of CHF

In order to elucidate whether ANP can be used in the treatment of heart failure, we studied the effect of intravenous infusion of α-ANP, 0.1 μg/kg body wt/min, over a period of 30 minutes on hemodynamic parameters measured by a Swan-Gantz catheter in patients with and without CHF.[20] Elevated PCWP in patients with CHF was markedly decreased by the infusion of α-ANP. A decrease was also observed, though less remarkably, in patients

TABLE III. *Changes of blood pressure in SHR-SP and DOCA-salt rats treated with monoclonal antibodies, KY-ANP-I and KY-ANP-II*

		MoAb KY-ANP-I	MoAb KY-ANP-II
SHR-SP	Before	148 ± 1	148 ± 2
	After 2 weekly injections	196 ± 3	216 ± 3*
DOCA-Salt Rats	Before	133 ± 6	139 ± 7
	After 9 weekly injections	175 ± 4	192 ± 6*

*Significantly different from rats treated with MoAb (KY-ANP-I): $p < 0.01$.

without CHF. The stroke volume index was decreased in patients without CHF but was slightly increased in patients with CHF. Total systemic resistance was decreased in both groups, especially in those with CHF. Urine volume was increased only in some patients by ANP infusion. These results suggest that the decrease in PCWP is caused by vasodilatation in patients with CHF. Both the decrease of PCWP and the increase of stroke volume index induced by ANP infusion suggest the potential usefulness of ANP for improving hemodynamic abnormalities in CHF. Similar results were obtained by other investigators.[21]

As mentioned above, plasma ANP levels are significantly elevated in patients with CHF, not infrequently reaching levels 100 times higher than normal values. Such an increase in ANP in blood may cause the down regulation of ANP receptors. Nevertheless, the infusion of ANP is effective in improving hemodynamics in CHF. This suggests that there is a dose-response relationship over a wide range of plasma ANP concentrations and that exogenous ANP given into patients with CHF is still effective despite increased plasma endogenous ANP levels.

REFERENCES

1. Cantin M, Genest J. The heart and the atrial natriuretic factor. *Endocr Rev* 1985; **6**: 107–127.
2. Bloch KD, Scott JA, Zisfein JB, Fallon JT, Margolis MN, Seidman CE, Matsueda GR, Homcy CJ, Graham RM, Seidman JG. Biosynthesis and secretion of proatrial natriuretic factor by cultured rat cardiocytes. *Science* 1985; **230**:1168–1171.
3. Nakao K, Sugawara A, Shiono S, Saito Y, Morii N, Yamada T, Itoh H, Mukoyama M, Arai H, Sakamoto M, Imura H. Secretory form of atrial natriuretic polypeptide as cardiac hormone in humans and rats. *Can J Physiol Pharmacol* 1987; **65**:1756–1761.
4. Kangawa K, Fukuda A, Matsuo H. Structural identification of β- and γ-human atrial natriuretic polypeptide. *Nature* 1985; **313**:397–400.
5. Dietz JR. Release of atrial natriuretic factor from rat heart-lung preparation by atrial distension. *Am J Physiol* 1984; **247**:R1093–R1096.
6. Sugawara A, Nakao K, Sakamoto M, Morii N, Yamada T, Itoh H, Shiono S, Imura H. Plasma concentration of atrial natriuretic polypeptide in essential hypertension. *Lancet* 1985; **2**:1426–1427.
7. Tikkanen I, Fyhrquist F, Metsarinne K, Leidenius R. Plasma atrial natriuretic peptide in cardiac disease and during infusion in healthy volunteers. *Lancet* 1985; **2**:66–69.
8. Cody RJ, Atlas SA, Laragh JH, Kubo SH, Covit AB, Ryman KS, Shakanovich A, Pondolfino K, Clark M, Camargo MJF, Scarborough RM, Lewicki JA. Atrial natriuretic factor in normal subjects and heart failure patients. *J Clin Invest* 1986; **78**:1362–1374.
9. Sugawara A, Nakao K, Morii N, Yamada T, Itoh H, Shiono S, Saito Y, Mukoyama M, Arai H, Nishimura K, Obata K, Yasue H, Ban T, Imura H. Synthesis of atrial natriuretic polypeptide (ANP) in human failing hearts—evidence for altered processing of ANP precursor and augmented synthesis of β-human ANP. *J Clin Invest* 1988; **81**:1962–1970.
10. Itoh H, Nakao K, Shiono S, Mukoyama M, Morii N, Sugawara A, Yamada T, Saito Y, Arai H, Kambayashi Y, Inouye K, Imura H. Conversion of β-human atrial natriuretic polypeptide into α-human atrial natriuretic polypeptide in human plasma in vitro. *Biochem Biophys Res Commun* 1987; **143**:560–569.
11. Kikuchi K, Nakao K, Hayashi R, Morii N, Sugawara A, Sakamoto M, Imura H, Mikawa H. Ontogeny of atrial natriuretic polypeptide in human heart. *Acta Endocr* 1987; **115**:211–217.

12. Saito Y, Nakao K, Arai H, Sugawara A, Morii N, Yamada T, Itoh H, Shiono S, Mukoyama M, Obata K, Yasue H, Ohkubo H, Nakanishi S, Imura H. Atrial natriuretic polypeptide (ANP) in human ventricle—increased gene expression of ANP in dilated cardiomyopathy. *Biochem Biophys Res Commun* 1987; **148**:211–217.

13. Saito Y, Nakao K, Arai H, Nishimura K, Okumura K, Obata K, Takemura G, Fujiwara H, Sugawara A, Yamada T, Itoh H, Mukoyama M, Hosoda K, Kawai C, Ban T, Yasue H, Imura H. Augmented expression of atrial natriuretic polypeptide gene in ventricle of human failing heart. *J Clin Invest* 1989; **83**:298–305.

14. Yasue H, Obata K, Okumura K, Kurose M, Ogawa H, Matsuyama K, Saito Y, Nakao K, Imura H. Increased secretion of atrial natriuretic polypeptide from the left ventricle in patients with dilated cardiomyopathy. *J Clin Invest* 1989; **83**:46–51.

15. Arai H, Nakao K, Saito Y, Morii N, Sugawara S, Yamada T, Itoh H, Shiono S, Mukoyama M, Ohkubo H, Nakanishi S, Imura H. Augmented expression of atrial natriuretic polypeptide (ANP) gene in ventricles of spontaneously hypertensive rats (SHR) and SHR-stroke prone. *Circ Res* 1988; **62**:926–930.

16. Saito Y, Nakao K, Morii N, Sugawara A, Shiono S, Yamada T, Itoh H, Sakamoto M, Kurahashi K, Fujiwara M, Imura H. Bay K 8644, a voltage-sensitive calcium channel agonist, facilitates secretion of atrial natriuretic polypeptide from isolated perfused rat heart. *Biochem Biophys Res Commun* 1985; **138**:1170–1176.

17. Mukoyama M, Nakao K, Yamada T, Itoh H, Sugawara A, Saito Y, Arai H, Hosoda K, Shirakami G, Morii N, Shiono S, Imura H. A monoclonal antibody against N-terminus of α-atrial natriuretic polypeptide (α-ANP): a useful tool for preferential detection of naturally circulating ANP. *Biochem Biophys Res Commun* 1988; **151**:1277–1284.

18. Mukoyama M, Nakao K, Sugawa H, Morii N, Sugawara A, Yamada T, Itoh H, Shiono S, Saito Y, Arai H, Morii T, Yamada H, Sano Y, Imura H. A monoclonal antibody to α-human atrial natriuretic polypeptide. *Hypertension* 1988; **12**:117–121.

19. Itoh H, Nakao K, Mukoyama M, Yamada T, Saito Y, Shiono S, Arai H, Hosoda K, Shirakami G, Morii N, Sugawara A, Imura H. Aggravation of hypertension in spontaneously hypertensive rats (SHR) and DOCA-salt rats by chronic blockade of endogenous atrial natriuretic polypeptide (ANP) with ANP monoclonal antibody. Abstracts of the Council for High Blood Pressure Research, 42nd Annual Fall Conference, ANA, Abstract No. 52, 1988.

20. Saito Y, Nakao K, Nishimura K, Sugawara A, Okumura K, Obata K, Sonoda R, Ban T, Yasue H, Imura H. Clinical application of atrial natriuretic polypeptide in patients with congestive heart failure: beneficial effects on left ventricular function. *Circulation* 1987; **76**:115–124.

21. Crozuer IG, Nicholls MG, Ikram H, Espiner EA, Gomez HJ, Warner NJ. Haemodynamic effects of atrial peptide infusion in heart failure. *Lancet* 1986; **2**:1242–1245.

SUMMARY

There are several compensatory mechanisms in the failing heart in order to correct functional abnormalities. Increased biosynthesis and secretion of ANP seem to be one of such compensatory mechanisms. Biosynthesis of ANP in the atrium is enhanced and the processing of the ANP precursor is accelerated in CHF. In addition, the expression of the ANP gene in the ventricle, which is usually suppressed under normal conditions after birth, is reactivated. Secretion of ANP from the ventricle in the failing heart significantly contributes to the elevated plasma ANP level in CHF. Circulating ANP seems to play a role in restoring hemodynamic abnormalities through its vasodilatory and diuretic actions.

RÉSUMÉ

Il y a plusieurs mécanismes de compensation dans les insuffisances cardiaques qui permettent de restaurer les anomalies fonctionnelles. Une augmentation de la biosynthèse et de la sécrétion de peptide natriurétique atriale semble être un de ces mécanismes de compensation. La biosynthèse du peptide natriurétique atrial est accrue dans l'oreillette et la transformation du précurseur de la peptide natriurétique atriale est accélérée dans les cas d'insuffisance cardiaque congestive. De plus, l'expression du gène peptide natriurétique atrial dans le ventricule, qui est généralement supprimé après la naissance dans des conditions normales, est réactivé. La sécrétion de peptide natriurétique atrial du ventricule contribue largement au taux plasmatique élevé du peptide natriurétique atrial chez les patients atteints d'insuffisance cardiaque congestive. Le peptide natriurétique atrial qui circule contribue, semble-t-il, à restaurer les anomalies hémodynamiques de par son action vasodilatatrice et diurétique.

ZUSAMMENFASSUNG

Verschiedene Anpassungsmechanismen erlauben es dem versagenden Herz, Abnormalitäten in der Funktion auszugleichen. Solche Kompensationsmechanismen sind wahrscheinlich die erhöhte Biosynthese und die Absonderung von atrialem natriuretischem Peptid (ANP). Bei hyperhämischer Herzinsuffizienz (CHF) tritt verstärkte Biosynthese des ANP im Atrium auf, und man beobachtet eine beschleunigte Weiterverarbeitung des ANP-Vorläufers. Ausserdem wird die Expression des ANP-Gens in der Herzkammer reaktiviert, die gewöhnlich nach der Geburt unter normalen Umständen desaktiviert wird. Der erhöhte Plasma-ANP-Gehalt bei hyperhämischer Herzinsuffizienz ist deutlich zurückzuführen auf die Absonderung des ANP in der Herzkammer des versagenden Herzens. Zirkulierendes ANP scheint durch seine gefässerweiternde und diuretische Wirkung eine wichtige Rolle in der Wiederherstellung hämodynamischer Abnormalitäten zu spielen.

RIASSUNTO

Esistono vari meccanismi compensatori nel cuore affetto da insufficienza per riparare le anormalita funzionali. L'aumento della biosintesi e della secrezione di peptide natriuretico atriale (PNA) sembrano essere uno di tali meccanismi compensatori. La biosintesi di PNA nell'atrio viene ottimizzata e l'elaborazione del precursore del PNA viene accelerata nell'insufficienza cardiaca congestizia. Inoltre, l'espressione del gene del PNA nel ventricolo, che di solito in condizioni normali viene soppressa dopo la nascita, viene riattivata. La secrezione di PNA dal ventricolo nel cuore insufficiente contribuisce significativamente all'elevato livello di PNA nel plasma riscontrato nell'insufficienza cardiaca congestizia. Il PNA circolante sembra svolgere un ruolo nel compensare le anormalita emodinamiche mediante le sue azioni vasodilatanti e diuretiche.

SUMÁRIO

Na insuficiência cardíaca, há vários mecanismos para restaurar as anormalidades funcionais. A biosíntese aumentada e a secreção do peptídio natriurético atrial (ANP) parecem ser um destos mecanismos compensatórios. Durante a insuficiência cardíaca congestiva (CHF), a biosíntese do ANP no átrio é aumentada e o processamento do precursor do ANP é acelerado. Além disso, a expressão do gene do ANP no ventrículo, que usualmente é suprimida sob condições normais após do nascimento, é reativada. A secreção do ANP desde o ventrículo na insuficiência cardíaca contribui significativamente ao elevado nível plasmático do ANP na CHF. O ANP circulante parece ter um papel na restauração de anormalidades hemodinâmicas através de suas ações vasodilatoras e diuréticas.

RESUMEN

En la insuficiencia cardíaca se presentan varios mecanismos que tienen como fin compensar las anormalidades funcionales. El incremento de la biosíntesis y la secreción del péptido natriurético atrial (ANP) parece ser uno de estos mecanismos compensatorios. Durante la insuficiencia cardíaca congestiva (CHF), la biosíntesis del ANP en el atrio es mejorada y el procesamiento del precursor del ANP es acelerado. Además, la expresión del gen del ANP en el ventrículo, que usualmente se ve suprimida bajo condiciones normales después del nacimiento, es reactivada. La secreción del ANP desde el ventrículo en la insuficiencia cardíaca contribuye significativamente al elevado nivel plasmático del ANP en la CHF. El ANP circulante parece tener un papel en la restauración de anormalidades hemodinámicas a través de sus acciones vasodilatadoras y diuréticas.

要約

心不全には機能異常を回復するためのいくつかの代償機構が存在する。心房性ナトリウム利尿ペプチド（ANP）の生合成と分泌の亢進は、この代償機構の1つであろう。うっ血性心不全（CHF）においては、心房でのANPの生合成が促進され、ANP前駆物質のプロセッシングが加速される。さらには、正常状態では生後抑えられている心室のANP遺伝子の発現が再び活性化される。CHFにおいては、心室からのANP分泌は血漿ANP濃度の上昇に明らかに寄与する。血中のANPは、その血管拡張作用と利尿作用によって、血行動態の異常を回復させる役割を果たすと考えられる。

Cardiac and Renal Failure: An Expanding Role for ACE Inhibitors, edited by C. T. Dollery and L. M. Sherwood, Hanley & Belfus, Inc., Philadelphia.

Discussion

LUTHY: There is obviously a dose response curve with atrial natriuretic peptide (ANP). What are the adverse effects of high doses?

IMURA: This is a problem. If we use a high dose of ANP, a sudden fall in blood pressure may occur both in CHF and also in normal subjects. We therefore choose a relatively low dose. The mechanism by which hypotension is induced by ANP is not clear.

CORVOL: The very interesting observation that there is an increase in the processing of the ANP precursor into ANP raises the question of which enzyme is responsible for it and which cell is involved. If it is not the cardiocytes, do you suppose there is another cell that could be turned on during chronic volume overload and could, therefore, increase the synthesis of the processing enzyme?

IMURA: That is a difficult question to answer. We do not know why the processing is enhanced in heart failure. There are probably some changes in the proteolytic enzymes, but we still do not know what type of enzymes are involved.

JOHNSTON: Dr. Schwartz, could you tell us how much you think turning on the gene is due to the mechanical stimulus or due to other secondary changes. Tying the aorta in a rat leads to a number of hormonal and hemodynamic changes.

SCHWARTZ: I have no direct answer to your question. This would need experimental models which might reproduce *in vitro* stretching or mechanical increases on isolation myocytes. This type of model is being developed for skeletal muscle and skeletal myocytes (Vandeburgh in the United States) and we are now succeeding in isolating adult myocytes. Dr. Jane-Lyse Samuel is going to the United States to try to make a model of stretching these cardiomyocytes. Dr. Cooper has tried to stretch isolated myocytes and has shown stretching induces increased protein synthesis. Other work done by Howard Morgan using isolated perfused heart in a Langerdorff preparation showed that when the pressure is raised for 1 or 2 hours there is increasing synthesis. Dr. B. Swynghedaav, using the same type of model, showed activation of two protooncogenes, myc and fos. Other factors may be involved; it is known that in neonate cells the alpha-1 adrenergic agonist induces an increase in protein synthesis, but whether this applies in adults is still very controversial.

LEDINGHAM: You had two models to induce left ventricular hypertrophy—aortic stenosis and aortic tie. I think you can also induce hypertrophy in animals such as rat by making them swim or exercise. Are there differences in that form of hypertrophy?

SCHWARTZ: We have no experience of that, but Dr. James Scheuer has done this work. Exercise induces hypertrophy, increases in protein synthesis, and enlargement of the heart. The changes that have been shown concerning the myosin heavy chain are opposite; it is the alpha type that is induced in this model. Professor Ganten's observation that a low dose of an ACE inhibitor can induce an increase in blood pressure without inducing cardiac hypertrophy might help us to find a way to answer this question.

GANTEN: Dr. Imura, have you given any thought to the possibility of an interaction between the two natriuretic factors, the one from the brain (the sodium-potassium ATPase inhibitor) and the cardiac one you discussed. The sodium potassium ATPase inhibitor will increase cellular sodium and calcium concentration, and as Dr. Lang has shown with ouabian, could subsequently increase ANP release. Have you looked at any possible interactions between these two factors? Secondly, in cardiac hypertrophy there appears to be a switch of ANP release from the atrium to the ventricles. As we have seen in Dr. Schwartz's presentation of the sodium-potassium ATPase, it may be different in hypertrophic hearts. Could there be a link between the effects of the hypothalamic natriuretic factor on sodium-potassium ATPase and could this be a molecular link between the atrial and the ventricular sodium-potassium ATPase?

IMURA: It is an interesting point, but we have not done such experiments yet.

SCHWARTZ: I have no experience with this, but I would like to add a comment concerning the sodium-potassium ATPase. It is true that the blinding affinity of the sodium-potassium ATPase has been shown to be modified in cardiac hypertrophy with kinetics of binding which strongly resemble those of the neonate heart. Again it seems to be a reactivation of the fetal phenotype. Dr. Charlemagne in our unit has just begun to do some experiments in collaboration with the team of J Lingrell from Cincinnati to determine which type of RNAs were expressed in cardiac hypertrophy but the preliminary results are not clearcut.

SONNENBLICK: I must emphasise that I do not think this is a disease. It is an adaptation that is totally reversible and only ends up as a disease state except when cells are lost.

SCHWARTZ: I fully agree with this idea that it is not a disease but an adaptation. It is not abnormal genes that are produced but normal genes which are activated at different times, either reactivated or repressed. This is a completely different mechanism in genetic disease. In cardiomyopathy we do not know what occurs and it could be something completely different but in this type of hypertrophy (hemodynamic overload) it is purely adaptation.

SHERWOOD: Dr. Sonnenblick, how early do you think the stimulus for ventricular remodeling occurs after ischemia and how early do you have to intervene in order to prevent it?

SONNENBLICK: Firstly, you are born with the stimulus for remodeling. You can see changes in heart weight within three days and I suspect that Dr. Schwartz sees RNA changes almost immediately. A delay of one week, 10 days or two weeks in preventing the remodeling is too long. It is an immediate response to the load and is manifest grossly within a few days and I am sure biochemically, immediately.

POOLE-WILSON: I would like to raise the question of models. I really wonder whether the rat is a good animal in which to study heart failure and hypertrophy. It is a species with V1 and V3 which humans don't have. Colin Johnston has reported heart failure without an increase in total blood sodium, so there seem to be many ways in which the rat differs from the human. We should be extremely cautious about jumping from one species to another and particularly this species.

SONNENBLICK: This is why we look at the rat, the cat, the dog and the guinea-pig. I think you are mixing up salt metabolism with what goes wrong with the heart. These are two separate issues. We are talking about what happens to the myocardium and its method of response. Once you have the mechanisms in hand you can apply them broadly across animal species. We could do the same with ischemic heart disease. We have learned a vast amount about the coronary circulation from the dog. You do your ultimate studies in man and change your concepts accordingly.

Cardiac and Renal Failure: An Expanding Role for ACE Inhibitors, edited by C. T. Dollery and L. M. Sherwood, Hanley & Belfus, Inc., Philadelphia.

Pharmacological Properties of Angiotensin-Converting Enzyme Inhibitors in Experimental Models of Congestive Heart Failure and Myocardial Ischemia

Charles S. Sweet

Human congestive heart failure (CHF) is a complex disease process with multiple etiologies in which the diseased heart can no longer provide adequate tissue perfusion for normal physical activities. In the pathophysiology of this disease, adaptive processes within the myocardium (hypertrophy, coronary collateral development) as well as the activation of multiple reflex compensatory mechanisms, such as the sympathetic nervous system, the renin-angiotensin-aldosterone system, and the atrial peptide system, hitherto provided the necessary hemodynamic support to maintain blood pressure despite a falling cardiac output.

One of the challenges in experimental biology is the development of animal models that mimic some of these varied changes. Lacking in most animal models is some degree of coronary atherosclerosis, a component of many forms of human CHF. Furthermore, in view of the slowly evolving multiple mechanisms in the human disease, the development of a single animal model with all the right features is probably unrealistic. Smith and Nuttall[1] have critically reviewed a number of experimental models and concluded that some of these can be used to address specific questions not easily answered in patients.

The purpose of this report is to review the existing animal data as they relate specifically to the therapeutic effects of converting enzyme inhibitors in animal models of myocardial ischemia and heart failure.

141

EFFECTS OF ACE INHIBITORS ON ISCHEMIC ISOLATED AND INTACT HEARTS

In Vitro Studies

Experimental myocardial ischemia and the mechanism of reperfusion arrhythmias have been the subject of a great deal of interest. vanGilst and colleagues[2,3] have evaluated the *in vitro* effects of the ACE inhibitors captopril, enalapril and HOE-498 in isolated rat hearts subjected to short periods of global ischemia followed by reperfusion. On the assumption that captopril may attenuate the synthesis and release of catecholamines induced by angiotensin II (ANG II) or may interfere with neurogenic transmission independently of ANG II, these authors found that captopril-treated hearts (80 μg/ml) fibrillated less and had better mechanical function during ischemia and reperfusion through a mechanism that may involve the preservation of high energy phosphates.[2] Consistent with their hypothesis, the norepinephrine overflow with reperfusion was blunted by these ACE inhibitors. An interaction with prostaglandins was suspected because indomethacin blocked the effects of captopril. Predictably, the pro-drug enalapril and the prodrug form of HOE-498 were not effective in this assay.[3] Although the concentrations of inhibitors in these studies (estimation: 50–300 μM) far exceeded their potency as converting-enzyme inhibitors (low nanomolar levels), a mechanism common to ACE inhibition is suspected because both captopril and the structurally diverse HOE-498 shared similar effects *in vitro.*

The possibility that ACE inhibitors may act in the heart through a local renin system[4,5] has support from studies demonstrating that hearts from rats pretreated (1 hour) with enalapril and ramipril displayed reduced tissue levels of ACE (measured biochemically) for 24 hours.[6] In addition, ramipril pretreatment significantly reduced the *in vitro* responses to sympathetic activation of the intact nerve supply to the heart.[6]

Some of the *in vitro* studies, which have examined coronary blood flow following direct administration of ACE inhibitors, have used substantial doses of these drugs. A recent study by vanGilst, however, has demonstrated that hearts from rats pretreated for 48 hours with ACE inhibitors had higher coronary flow compared to untreated controls by a mechanism that involves prostaglandin activation.[7] Other workers using a 1-hour pretreatment with enalapril[8] showed that coronary blood flow was significantly higher than controls following reperfusion.

It has been reported recently that the sulfhydryl (SH) moiety of captopril plays an important (and perhaps a unique) role in reperfusion-induced myocardial dysfunction.[9] Captopril (2–100 μM), but not teprotide or enalaprilat (>1000 μM), scavenged superoxide anion as assayed by two *in vitro* methods. Interestingly, however, ventricular fibrillation *in vivo* occurred in 37% of control dogs upon reperfusion, but only 9% in the enalaprilat group and 0% in the captopril group. Complex mechanisms are undoubtedly involved, because the isomer of captopril that lacks ACE inhibitory properties (but was a scavenger) was not antifibrillatory. As will be discussed later in this report, additional beneficial mechanisms of ACE inhibitors on reperfusion arrhythmias may be related to a hemodynamic profile that improves regional coronary blood flow and ameliorates ischemia.

In summary, isolated hearts treated *in vitro* or *ex vivo* with ACE inhibitors have been shown to perform better than untreated hearts during occlusion/reperfusion experiments. Several mechanisms have been advanced to explain this beneficial action, including preservation of high energy phosphates, release of vasodilator/antifibrillatory prostacyclin, attenuation of noradrenalin release, and scavenging toxic free radicals. As will be discussed later, some of these findings have been confirmed in whole animals given therapeutic doses of these drugs.

Coronary Blood Flow

ACE inhibitors given in therapeutic concentrations do not have a direct vascular action. In contrast, angiotensin I (ANG I) and particularly ANG II are potent coronary vasoconstrictors, the latter participating in modulating coronary tone in high renin states in animals and humans.[10] In the coronary circulation, ACE inhibitors have been shown to be antivasoconstrictor when assayed against the angiotensins, and high doses of some ACE inhibitors are claimed to vasodilate the coronary bed under certain circumstances (Langendorff preparations).[7] More relevant, perhaps, have been experiments demonstrating that baseline coronary flow in isolated hearts from rats pretreated with ACE inhibitors for several hours before setup have higher coronary flows than controls.[7,8] The direct relaxant effect of ACE inhibitors on isolated coronary arteries is unlikely and has not been reported, but one study has demonstrated that enalaprilat (0.5 to 1 μg/ml), but not captopril (250 μg/ml), behaved as if it were an ANG II antagonist on isolated cat coronary arteries.[11]

In analyzing the importance of either a local renin system or the effects of circulating angiotensin on coronary hemodynamics, it is important to recognize that coronary blood flow is mainly determined by local factors that are dependent on myocardial oxygen needs. However, when the renin system is turned on with a diuretic such as hydrochlorothiazide in rats,[10] or dogs under sodium deprivation,[12] important effects of ACE inhibitors can be demonstrated, such as epicardial artery dilation[12] with enalaprilat, and changes in coronary blood flow with captopril that were significantly correlated with control plasma renin activity (PRA) levels.[10] In normal renin states, it is difficult to demonstrate a direct coronary action of ACE inhibitors. For example, intracoronary artery infusions of captopril in anesthetized dogs administered at reasonable concentrations (0.01 mg/min) that inhibited ACE (unlike high doses given as an injection) produced no direct cardiac effects.[13] In summary, in high renin states the effect of converting-enzyme inhibitors can best be understood as a consequence of reduction in ANG II levels, although a possible contribution by increased bradykinin or particularly stimulated prostaglandins cannot be completely ruled out. Whether the site of action is in the plasma or a local tissue site remains to be elucidated.

In Vivo Studies in Myocardial Ischemia/Myocardial Infarction Anesthetized and Conscious Dogs

Myocardial ischemia in many animal models and certainly myocardial infarction (MI) causes hypotension. To maintain blood pressure, at least two neurohumoral adjustments participate early in this complex process. There is activation of the sympathetic nervous system, which, in concert with other mechanisms, causes a release of renin. The high circulating catecholamines and the ANG II formed from renin directly constrict the peripheral vasculature. ANG II, formed in the plasma or released locally near the nerve terminal, can increase the release of more catecholamines. The consequence of this interaction is an undesirable increase in oxygen demand and a reduction in oxygen supply. With the availability of long-lasting and orally active converting-enzyme inhibitors, it became possible to determine the value of interfering with the production of ANG II in these models.

Global left ventricular dysfunction/ischemia can be produced by selective coronary embolization with a variety of occlusive agents.[1] In a closed-chest dog model characterized by elevated ANG II levels, moderate left ventricular dysfunction occurs after selective coronary embolization with 50 micron plastic microspheres. Depending on the amount of microspheres given, ischemic failure with a 40% reduction in cardiac output and a moderate elevation in left ventricular end-diastolic pressure (LVEDP) can be achieved. Enalaprilat, given after heart failure had stabilized, reduced arterial pressure, total peripheral resistance, and double product, while maintaining coronary vascular resistance.[14] Enalapril has also been studied in another acute embolization model (mercury), and the drug given by infusion over 15 min did not significantly alter hemodynamics.[15] However, in a chronic variation of this model (glass beads), these workers were able to demonstrate a fall in total peripheral resistance and a rise in cardiac output with this agent.[15]

There have been several studies with ACE inhibitors in dogs with acute MI. In *anesthetized* dogs with acute MI, captopril has been studied to determine whether it can improve regional myocardial blood flow (tracer microspheres) in the ischemic region. Six hours after left anterior descending artery (LAD) occlusion, regional myocardial blood flow remained constant in control dogs in the ischemic zone, but increased in dogs treated acutely with captopril.[16]

This effect, combined with a lowering of blood pressure, was thought to be important in the limitation of infarct size found by Ertl et al.[16] Other studies have shown that enalapril significantly increased regional myocardial blood flow in dogs with acute left ventricular failure,[17] and in spontaneously hypertensive rats.[18]

In acute MI in *conscious* dogs, a favorable hemodynamic response to captopril (15-hour infusion begun 10 min post-MI) was confirmed by Daniell et al.;[19] however, these authors found no differences in MI size, creatinine kinase (CK) levels, or incidence of arrhythmias between treated and untreated groups. The favorable hemodynamic response to ACE inhibitors in MI is related to the acute activation of the renin system,[20] which explains the finding that teprotide plus oral captopril given for 24 hours reduced total peripheral resistance and improved cardiac output in dogs with MI. However, Daniell et al. did not find an increase in blood flow to the ischemic myocardium using somewhat different experimental preparations from those used by Ertl et al.[16]

Coronary Occlusion/Reperfusion Models

Coronary occlusion/reperfusion models have been widely studied to investigate the mechanisms of lethal arrhythmias that contribute to sudden death upon restoration of blood flow in a previously occluded vessel. One current theory holds that it is the severity of the arrhythmias during the occlusion period that influences the lethality of the arrhythmias in the subsequent reperfusion period.[21 and refs. therein] It is of interest, therefore, that enalapril (0.5 mg/kg i.v.), but surprisingly not captopril (0.5 mg/kg i.v.), given before LAD occlusion reduced the incidence of ventricular fibrillation (VF) during reperfusion.[21] Westlin and Mullane[9], however, showed that both captopril (5 mg/kg i.v.) and enalaprilat (1.6 mg/kg i.v.) were antifibrillatory in this model. Although different doses of captopril were used in each study, the drug concentrations were certainly sufficient in both studies to inhibit plasma ACE fully, since the ED_{50} of captopril is about 60 μg/kg i.v. in the dog. According to Elfellah and Ogilvie,[21] not all vasodilators that improve ischemia when given during the occlusion period, in fact, exert beneficial antiarrhythmic effects during the reperfusion period. Thus, captopril, felodipine, nifedipine or ketanserin did not significantly lower the incidence of VF.

Some preliminary electrophysiological studies have been undertaken with ACE inhibitors. In one such study in Yorkshire swine with a healed MI, programmed electrical stimulation induced ventricular tachycardia (VT). Five minutes after intravenous captopril (0.6–1.2 mg/kg i.v.), VT could not be induced.[22]

There are other confirmatory reports with ACE inhibitors that have demonstrated an improvement in left ventricular function in dogs with acute

LAD occlusion.[23] Confirming the work of Elfellah and Ogilvie,[21] beneficial hemodynamic and antifibrillatory effects of enalapril have been reported in dogs,[24] as well as improvements in contractile function of the postischemic stunned myocardium,[25] and in acute myocardial ischemia in cats.[27] In view of the conflicting data between laboratories, there is a need for carefully controlled comparative dose-response studies with several ACE inhibitors (as well as Class III antifibrillatory drugs) in these and other models.

EFFECTS OF ACE INHIBITORS IN LOW AND HIGH CARDIAC OUTPUT FAILURE MODELS

Several important hemodynamic and humoral adjustments occur during the development of heart failure in these interesting models. Low-output failure in dogs is produced by constriction of the inferior vena cava. These animals retain sodium and develop ascites[27,28] as part of a compensatory mechanism to maintain blood pressure. There is an early phase in which blood pressure is restored by activation of the renin system, whereas in the later stages restoration of arterial pressure is dependent upon an increase in plasma volume.[27] Long-term ascites and edema are common. The nonapeptide ACE inhibitor, teprotide, when given as an infusion early in the pathogenesis of the disease when renin is high, prevented the restoration of blood pressure.[27] Subacute administration of captopril has been studied in this model as well and, consistent with the important role of the renin-angiotensin-aldosterone system, the drug caused a fall in plasma aldosterone, a decrease in arterial pressure, and an improvement in sodium balance.[28]

High output heart failure in rats[29] and dogs[30] produced by an aortic-caval fistula also has a renin component. In this model, an elevation in cardiac output compensates almost entirely for shunt flow. However, the mechanisms that contribute to the increase and maintenance of cardiac output differ over time. There is a causative role for ANG II in the sodium retention in this model, based on the fact that captopril can reduce arterial pressure and increase sodium excretion over 3 days in dogs.[30] In rats, captopril elevates PRA and reduces blood pressure.[29] Severe edema accompanies the heart failure in these rats, a feature not found in rats with heart failure secondary to healed myocardial infarction. Because vasopressin and catecholamines are elevated in addition to ANG II in rats with high output failure, Riegger et al.[29] found a weak correlation between the pretreatment PRA and the subsequent fall in mean arterial pressure (MAP) with captopril.

HEART FAILURE MODELS IN DOGS WITH CHRONIC RAPID VENTRICULAR PACING

The model of CHF produced by rapid ventricular pacing has the advantage of being surgically simple, with a circulation that is anatomically intact. In addition, the hemodynamic derangements are slowly reversible upon termination of the pacemaker. Because rapid pacing in the dog interferes with ventricular emptying, the CHF develops over time and is characterized by elevated LVEDP and ascites.[31,32] In addition, there is a gradual increase in the plasma levels of renin, ANG II, aldosterone, noradrenaline and adrenaline.[32] In unanesthetized paced dogs, subacute administration of captopril blunted the expected increases in mean pulmonary arterial pressure (MPAP) and peripheral resistance compared with untreated control dogs.[33] In another preliminary study in this form of low output failure, enalapril given over 8 days was also effective.[34] Underperfusion of skeletal muscle and poor treadmill performance are also features of this model.[35] Recent experiments with more extended pacing lasting 2 months has revealed biventricular failure and chamber dilatation.[36] It would be interesting to examine whether ACE inhibitors might improve exercise performance and lessen cardiac enlargement under these conditions.

HEART FAILURE IN RATS WITH ACUTE AND CHRONIC MYOCARDIAL INFARCTION

Experimental MI in the rat was first described in 1946[37] and has been modified over the years[38-41] to the point where a major portion of the left ventricular muscle can be infarcted in a reproducible manner. With miniaturization of catheters and flow transducers to measure cardiovascular function *in vivo,* the rat with the healed MI has become an important model for the study of chronic heart failure.[41-43] There have been numerous studies published over the years in which the rat with acute MI has been used to examine hemodynamic change, arrhythmia production, and pharmacological reduction in infarct size. However, because the rat has little or no collateral coronary blood flow, Hearse *et al.*[44] have raised questions about infarct size measurements in pharmacological experiments (salvage) during the evolution of ischemia. With this in mind, it is interesting that enalaprilat (given after occlusion) has been shown to salvage tissue during sustained ischemia in the rat heart, based on reducing the fall in left ventricular free wall CK.[45]

ACE inhibitors have been studied more extensively in rats in which the infarction was allowed to heal. One important feature of this chronic preparation is that the enlargement of the ventricular chamber depends on the size of the infarct, and ventricular enlargement continues after healing. Interestingly, chronic captopril improved the pumping ability of the heart and lessened ventricular enlargement.[43] The precise mechanisms whereby ACE inhibitors alter this cardiac remodeling is not known, but they exert a favorable hemodynamic profile in this model. For example, enalaprilat given acutely to rats with CHF approximately 76 days post-infarction, reduced mean arterial pressure and preload without altering heart rate or cardiac contractility.[46] Drexler *et al.*[47] have studied the distribution of cardiac output in rats with healed MI at rest and during exercise. Captopril caused a preferential renal dilation with some increase in total myocardial blood flow. The ACE inhibitor, perindopril, given over 2 months to rats with healed MI and failure, lowered blood pressure, altered the cardiac isomyosin forms and reduced the volume density of collagen in these hearts.[48]

Three studies have addressed the important issue of whether ACE inhibitors will improve life expectancy when given over the lifespan of rats with heart failure.[49-51] In the first study of this kind,[49] captopril improved survival (48%) in rats with moderate infarct sizes compared to untreated controls (21%). In this study, the relative risk of death rose dramatically in rats with infarct sizes between 40-50%. In a second lifetime study performed in our laboratories, enalapril was shown to increase the median survival time from 104 days (controls) to 165 days in rats with an average MI size of about 40% of the left ventricle.[50] Rats with infarct sizes of this magnitude were shown to have overt heart failure with LV dilatation.[43] The prolongation of survival with enalapril was associated with lessened cardiac hypertrophy and presumably less ventricular dilatation.[50] A favorable therapeutic response was also confirmed in a second mortality study when enalapril was coadministered with milrinone for 365 days.[51] The expectations of these animal experiments with this class of vasodilator have been borne out in a large clinical trial.[52]

CONCLUSIONS

Several animal models that mimic some of the pathophysiological changes of human CHF have been used to examine the efficacy of both short-term and chronic administration of ACE inhibitors. These vasodilator drugs have been evaluated in a range of models spanning the isolated ischemic hearts to animals with various forms of high- and low-output failure, including survival studies in rats with healed MI and heart failure.

The principal mechanism most often cited in various *in vivo* studies is peripheral vasodilation, which by "unloading" the left ventricle permits more complete ejection of blood. It is not known with certainty exactly how ACE inhibitors improve the hemodynamic profile through vasodilation. Afterload reduction in association with such beneficial actions as an increase in regional myocardial blood flow to ischemic myocardium, lack of reflex tachycardia, improvement in renal perfusion, attenuation of the action of ANG II on the nerve terminal, preservation of high energy phosphates, and release of vasodilatory/antifibrillatory prostacyclin have been proposed to explain the beneficial actions of these drugs in some models of experimental ischemia and heart failure.

It is still not clear whether subtle differences amongst ACE inhibitors such as lipid solubility, tissue penetration, or other chemical characteristics provide unique profiles of activity in one model but not another. In the future, our knowledge of how these drugs act will be aided by molecular biochemical studies of the renin system in the circulation and at the cardiac and vascular level in models of ischemia/heart failure. From studies with ACE inhibitors, the weight of available evidence suggests that ANG II is a suitable mediator for ischemia-induced myocardial damage. Furthermore, in view of the reports that ACE inhibitors can prevent ventricular dilatation on long-term treatment in rats with heart failure, the possibility is raised that ANG II through a variety of mechanisms extends ischemic damage during permanent coronary occlusion.

The role of the renin-angiotensin system in myocardial ischemia and heart failure has been aided by the development of orally-acting inhibitors of converting enzyme. It is conceivable that in the future, new mechanisms to inhibit ANG II at its numerous effectors will be developed that will further clarify the role of the renin system in myocardial ischemia and heart failure.

REFERENCES

1. Smith HJ, Nuttall A. Experimental models of heart failure. *Cardiovasc Res* 1985; **19**:181–186.
2. vanGilst WH, deGraeff PA, Kingma JH, Wesseling H, deLangen CDJ. Captopril reduces purine loss and reperfusion arrhythmias in the rat heart after coronary artery occlusion. *Eur J Pharmacol* 1984; **100**:113–117.
3. vanGilst WH, deGraeff PA, Wesseling H, deLangen CDJ. Reduction of reperfusion arrhythmias in the ischemic isolated rat heart by angiotensin converting enzyme inhibitors: A comparison of captopril, enalapril and HOE-498. *J Cardiovasc Pharmacol* 1986; **8**: 722–728.
4. Lindpaintner K, Jin M, Wilhelm MJ, et al. Intracardiac generation of angiotensin and its physiologic role. *Circulation* 1988; **77**(suppl 1):I-18–I-23.
5. Dzau V. Circulating versus local renin-angiotensin system in cardiovascular homeostasis. *Circulation* 1988; **77**(suppl 1):I-4–I-13.
6. Xiang J, Linz W, Becker H, et al. Effects of converting enzyme inhibitors ramipril and enalapril on peptide action and sympathetic neurotransmission in the isolated heart. *Eur J Pharmacol* 1985; **113**:215–223.
7. vanGilst WH, Scholtens E, deGraeff PA, deLangen CDJ, Wesseling H. Differential influences of angiotensin converting enzyme inhibitors on the coronary circulation. *Circulation* 1988; **77**(suppl 1):I-24–I-29.
8. Li K, Chen X. Protective effects of captopril and enalapril on myocardial ischemia and reperfusion damage of rat. *J Moll Cell Cardiol* 1987; **19**:909–915.
9. Westlin W, Mullane K. Does captopril attenuate reperfusion-induced myocardial dysfunction by scavenging free radicals? *Circulation* 1988; **77**(suppl 1):I-30–I-39.
10. Magrini F, Shimizu M, Roberts N, Fouad FM, Tarazi RC, Zanchetti A. Converting-enzyme inhibition and coronary blood flow. *Circulation* 1988; **75**(suppl 1):I-168–I-174.
11. Lefer DJ, Lefer AM. Coronary vascular actions of the converting enzyme inhibitor enalapril. *Proc Soc Exp Biol Med* 1984; **175**:211–214.
12. Holtz J, Busse R, Sommer O, Bassenge E. Dilation of epicardial arteries in conscious dogs induced by angiotensin-converting enzyme inhibition with enalaprilat. *J Cardiovasc Pharmacol* 1987; **9**:348–355.
13. Noguchi K, Kato T, Ito H, Aniya Y, Sakanashi M. Effect of intracoronary captopril coronary blood flow and regional myocardial function in dogs. *Eur J Pharmacol* 1985; **110**:11–17.
14. Sweet CS, Ludden CT, Frederick CM, Bush LR, Ribeiro LGT. Comparative hemodynamic

effects of MK-422, a converting enzyme inhibitor, and a renin inhibitor in dogs with acute left ventricular failure. *J Cardiovasc Pharmacol* 1984; **6**:1067–1075.

15. Leddy CL, Wilen M, Franciosa JA. Effects of a new converting enzyme inhibitor, enalapril, in acute and chronic left ventricular failure in dogs. *J Clin Pharmacol* 1983; **23**:189–198.

16. Ertl G, Kloner RA, Alexander RW, Braunwald E. Limitation of experimental infarct size by an angiotensin-converting inhibitor. *Circulation* 1982; **65**:40–48.

17. Hall C, Morkrid I, Kjekshus J. Effects of ACE inhibition on regional blood flow during acute left ventricular failure in the dog—preliminary report. *Scand J Urol Nephrol* 1984; **79(suppl 1)**:I-21–I-24.

18. Richer C, Doussau MP, Giudicelli JF. Effects of captopril and enalapril on regional vascular resistance and reactivity in spontaneously hypertensive rats. *Hypertension* 1983; **5**:312–320.

19. Daniell HB, Carson RR, Ballard KD, Thomas GR, Privitera PJ. Effects of captopril on limiting infarct size in conscious dogs. *J Cardiovasc Pharmacol* 1984; **6**:1043–1047.

20. Liang C, Gavras H, Black J, Sherman LG, Hood WB Jr. Renin-angiotensin system inhibition in acute myocardial infarction in dogs. *Circulation* 1982; **66**:1249–1255.

21. Elfellah MS, Ogilvie RI. Effect of vasodilator drugs on coronary occlusion and reperfusion arrhythmias in anesthetized dogs. *J Cardiovasc Pharmacol* 1985; **7**:826–832.

22. Kingma JH, deGraeff PA, vanGilst WH, van Binsbergen E, deLangen CDJ, Wesseling H. Effects of intravenous captopril on inducible sustained ventricular tachycardia one week after experimental infarction in the anesthetized pig. *Postgrad Med J* 1986; **62(suppl 1)**:159–163.

23. Shionoiri H, Jinno Y, Kobayashi H, et al. Cardiovascular effects of the converting enzyme inhibitors captopril, enalaprilat or ramiprilat in anesthetized dogs with acute ischemic heart. *Curr Ther Res* 1987; **42**:988–994.

24. Li-Yang L, Xiu C, Kai L, Wen-Jian W. Beneficial effects of enalapril on reperfusion arrhythmia and segmental contraction in anesthetized dogs. *Acta Pharm Sin* 1987; **8**:434–438.

25. Przyklenk K, Kloner RA. Acute effects of hydralazine and enalapril on contractile function of the postischemic "stunned" myocardium. *Am J Cardiol* 1987; **60**:934–936.

26. Lefer A, Peck RC. Cardioprotective effects of enalapril in acute myocardial ischemia. *Pharmacology* 1984; **29**:61–69.

27. Watkins LJ, Burton JA, Hubeer TR, Cant F, Smith FW, Barger AC. The renin angiotensin system in congestive heart failure in conscious dogs. *J Clin Invest* 1976; **57**:1606–1617.

28. Freeman RH, Davis JO, Williams GM, deForrest JM, Seymour AA, Rowe BP. Effects of oral converting enzyme inhibitor, SQ 14,225, in a model of low output heart failure. *Circ Res* 1979; **5**:540–545.

29. Riegger GAJ, Liebau G, Bauer E, Kochsiek K. Vasopressin and renin in high output heart failure of rats: Hemodynamic effects of elevated plasma hormone levels. *J Cardiovasc Pharmacol* 1985; **7**:1–5.

30. Williams GM, Davis JO, Freeman RH, deForrest JM, Seymour AA, Rowe BP. Effects of the oral converting inhibitor, SQ 14,225, in experimental high output failure. *Am J Physiol* 1979; **236**:F541–F545.

31. Coleman HN, Taylor RR, Pool PE, et al. Congestive heart failure following chronic tachycardia. *Am Heart J* 1971; **81**:790–798.

32. Riegger AJG, Liebau G. The renin-angiotensin-aldosterone system, antidiuretic hormone and sympathetic nerve activity in experimental model of congestive heart failure in the dog. *Clin Sci* 1982; **62**:465–469.

33. Riegger GAJ, Liebau G, Holzschuh M, Witkowski D, Steilner H, Kochsiek K. Role of the renin-angiotensin system in the development of congestive heart failure in the dog as assessed by chronic converting enzyme blockade. *Am J Cardiol* 1984; **53**:614–618.

34. Bassenge E, Holtz J. Converting enzyme inhibition by enalapril in experimental heart failure; cardioprotection by mechanisms in addition to vasodilation? Proceedings of the 12th Scientific Meeting of the International Society of Hypertension, 1988.

35. Wilson JR, Falcone R, Ferraro N, Egler J. Mechanism of skeletal muscle underperfusion in a dog model of low output heart failure. *Am J Physiol* 1986; **251**:H227–H235.

36. Wilson JR, Douglas P, Hickey, et al. Experimental congestive heart failure produced by rapid ventricular pacing in the dog: cardiac effects. *Circulation* 1987; **75**:857–867.

37. Heimburger RF. Injection into pericardial sac and ligation of coronary artery of the rat. *Arch Surg* 1946; **52**:677–689.

38. Fabiani JN, Deloche A, Camilleri JP, *et al.* Etude experimentale de la microcirculation dans l'infarctus myocardique revascularise du rat. *Coeur Med Interne* 1976; **15**:543–555.
39. Johns TNP, Olson BJ. Experimental myocardial infarction 1. A method of coronary occlusion in small animals. *Ann Surg* 1954; **140**:675–682.
40. Selye H, Bajusz E, Grasso S, Mendell P. Simple technique for surgical occlusion of coronary vessels in the rat. *Angiology* 1960; **11**:398–407.
41. Pfeffer MA, Pfeffer JM, Fishbein C, *et al.* Myocardial infarct size and ventricular function in rats. *Circ Res* 1979; **44**:503–512.
42. Fletcher PJ, Pfeffer MT, Pfeffer JA, Braunwald E. Effects of hypertension on cardiac performance in rats with myocardial infarction. *Am J Cardiol* 1982; **50**:488–496.
43. Pfeffer JM, Pfeffer MA, Braunwald E. Influence of chronic captopril therapy on the infarcted left ventricle of the rat. *Circ Res* 1985; **57**:4–95.
44. Hearse DJ, Richard V, Yellon DM, Kingma JG Jr. Evolving myocardial infarction in the rat *in vivo*: An inappropriate model for the investigation of drug-induced infarct size limitation during sustained regional ischemia. *J Cardiovasc Pharmacol* 1988; **11**:701–710.
45. Hock CE, Ribeiro LGT, Lefer AM. Preservation of ischemic myocardium by a new converting enzyme inhibitor, enalaprilic acid, in acute myocardial infarction. *Am Heart J* 1985; **109**:222–228.
46. Emmert SE, Stabilito II, Sweet CS. Acute and subacute hemodynamic effects of enalaprilat, milrinone and combination therapy in rats with chronic left ventricular dysfunction. *Clin Exp Hypertens* 1987; **A9**:297–306.
47. Drexler H, Depenbusch JW, Truog AG, Zelis R, Flaim S. Acute regional vascular effects of intravenous captopril in a rat model of myocardial infarction and failure. *J Pharmacol Exp Ther* 1987; **241**:13–19.
48. Michel JP, Lattion AL, Salzmann JL, *et al.* Cardiac effects of converting enzyme inhibition in rat myocardial infarction. *Circ Res* 1988; **62**:641–650.
49. Pfeffer MA, Pfeffer JM, Steinberg C, Finn P. Survival after an experimental myocardial infarction: beneficial effects of long-term therapy with captopril. *Circulation* 1985; **72**:406–412.
50. Sweet CS, Emmert SE, Stabilito II, Ribeiro LGT. Increased survival in rats with congestive heart failure treated with enalapril. *J Cardiovasc Pharmacol* 1987; **10**:636–642.
51. Sweet CS, Ludden CT, Stabilito II, Emmert SC, Heyse JF. Beneficial effects of milrinone and enalapril on long-term survival of rats with healed myocardial infarction. *Eur J Pharmacol* 1988; **147**:29–37.
52. The Consensus Trial Study Group. Effects of enalapril on mortality in severe congestive heart failure. *N Engl J Med* 1987; **316**:1429–1435.

SUMMARY

The formation of angiotensin II (ANG II) is a physiologically important compensatory adjustment to the hypotension that accompanies some experimental models of heart failure and myocardial ischemia. As these diseases progress, this important vasoconstrictor and sodium-retaining mechanism, in concert with other vasoconstrictor mechanisms (e.g., catecholamines and vasopressin), are thought to aid cardiovascular hemostasis through a complex series of interactions. At some point, however, these vasoconstrictor mechanisms play an increasingly dominant and potentially deleterious role. Several *in vitro* and *in vivo* animal models of myocardial ischemia and heart failure have been used to elucidate the role of ANG II. Isolated ischemic rat hearts treated *in vitro* or *ex vivo* with high doses of ACE inhibitors have better mechanical/coronary flow properties and produce fewer arrhythmias. In models of acute heart failure (coronary embolization, myocardial infarction),

ACE inhibitors reduced the elevated peripheral resistance, lowered blood pressure, and improved the imbalance in oxygen supply/demand by increasing regional myocardial blood flow. In *in vivo* models of coronary occlusion/ reperfusion, the incidence of ventricular fibrillation during reperfusion was lessened with some ACE inhibitors. In models of low-output failure (rapid ventricular pacing, constriction of inferior vena cava) and high-output failure (aortic-caval fistula), various inhibitors of ACE have been reported to reduce blood pressure, improve sodium balance, and attenuate the expected rise in pulmonary artery pressure and total peripheral resistance. In the rats with healed myocardial infarction and heart failure, chronic treatment with ACE inhibitors resulted in better cardiac pumping ability, lessened ventricular enlargement, preferential renal and myocardial dilatation, and improved long-term survival.

The precise mechanisms that are ultimately responsible for the improved hemodynamic status of animals treated with ACE inhibitors are not known. However, based on the *in vivo* responses to ACE inhibitors in various models of experimental heart failure, it is now possible to conclude that the renin-angiotensin system plays an increasingly dominant role as the heart failure state progresses.

RÉSUMÉ

La formation de l'agiotensine II est un phénomène de compensation physiologiquement important relativement à l'hypotension qui accompagne plusieurs modèles expérimentaux d'insuffisance cardiaque et d'ischémie myocardique. Comme ces maladies progressent, on pense que cet important mécanisme vasoconstricteur et de rétention sodée. de concert avec d'autres mécanismes vasoconstricteurs (tels les catécholamines et la vassopressine) contribuent à l'hémostasie cardiovasculaire par une série complexe d'interactions. A un certain moment, cependant, ces mécanismes vasoconstricteurs jouent un rôle de plus en plus importants et peuvent avoir des effets délétères. On a utilisé plusieurs modèles animaux *in vitro* et *in vivo* d'ischémie myocardique et d'insuffisance cardiaque pour élucider le rôle de l'angiotensine II. Des coeurs de rats isolés ischémiques traités *in vitro* ou *ex vivo* à fortes doses d'inhibiteurs de l'enzyme de conversion de l'agiotensine ont de meilleures propriétés mécaniques et aussi de meilleures propriétés du flux coronarien et présentent moins d'arythmies. Parmi les modèles d'insuffisance cardiaque aigue (embolisme coronarien, infarctus du myocarde), les inhibiteurs de l'enzyme de conversion de l'angiotensine ont diminué la résistance périphérique élevée, ont fait baisser la pression artérielle, et ont amélioré le déséquilibre des apports d'oxygène en augmentant le flux sanguin du myocarde régional. Dans les modèles *in vivo* d'occlusion/reperfusion coronarienne, les inhibiteurs de l'enzyme de conversion de l'angiotensine ont minoré les incidences de fibrillation ventriculaire pendant la reperfusion. Dans les modèles d'insuffisance légère (rythme ventriculaire rapide, constriction de la veine cave inférieure) et sévère (fistule aortique-cave), on a constaté que différents inhibiteurs de l'enzyme de conversion de l'angiotensine réduisaient la pression artérielle, amélioraient l'équilibre de sodium et atténuaient l'augmentation prévue de la pression arterielle pulmonaire et de la résistance périphérique totale. Chez les rats guéris d'un infarctus dy myocarde et d'une insuffisance cardiaque, l'administration chronique d'inhibiteurs de l'enzyme de conversion de l'angiotensine a entraîné une meilleure performance cardiaque, a minoré l'hypertrophie ventriculaire, la dilatation rénale et myocardique préférentielle, et a amélioré la survie à long terme. On ignore les mécanismes précis qui ont éventue llement provoqué l'amélioration des paramètres hémodynamiques chez les animaux traités avec les inhibiteurs de l'enzyme de conversion de l'angiotensine. Cependant, si l'on se base sur les réponses *in vivo* aux inhibiteurs de l'enzyme de conversion de l'angiotensine parmi les différents modèles d'insuffisance cardiaque expérimentale, il est maintenant possible de conclure que le système rénine-angiotensine, face à la détérioration progressive de la performance cardiaque, joue un rôle de plus en plus important.

ZUSAMMENFASSUNG

Die Bildung von Angiotensin (ANG II) ist ein physiologisch wichtiger Kompensationsmechanismus zum Ausgleich von Hypotension, die in einigen experimentellen Modellen die Herzinsuffizienz und die Herzmuskelischämie begleitet. Es wird angenommen, dass im Verlauf dieser Krankheiten die Blutstillung in den Herzgefässen in einer komplexen Serie von Interaktionen durch diesen wichtigen gefässkontraktierenden und natriumhaltenden Mechanismus, zusammen mit anderen gefässverengenden Mechanismen (wie Brenzkatechinethanolamin und Vasopressin), unterstützt wird. Jedoch erreichen diese gefässverengenden Mechanismen einen Punkt, an dem sie eine immer dominantere und potentiell schädliche Rolle spielen. Verschiedene in vitro- und in vivo- Tier modelle für myocarditische Ischämie und Herzinsuffizienz sind zur Aufklärung der Rolle des ANG II herangezogen worden. Isolierte blutleere Rattenherzen, die in vitro oder ex vivo mit hohen Dosierungen an Inhibitoren des angiotensin-konvertierenden Enzyms ACE behandelt worden waren, zeigten bessere mechanische/koronare Durchblutungseigenschaften und produzierten weniger Herzschlagun regelmässigkeiten. In Modellen für akute Herzinsuffizienz (Koronarembolie, Myocardialinfarkt) reduzierten ACE-Inhibitoren den erhöhten peripheren Widerstand, erniedrigten den Blutdruck und verbesserten die Bilanz des Sauerstoffzufuhrs und -bedarfs durch verstärkte regionale Herzmuskeldurchblutung. Bei in vivo-Modellen für Koronarokklusion/Reperfusion wurde das Auftreten von Herzkammerflimmern während der Reperfusion durch einige ACE-Inhibitoren verringert. Bei Modellen für niedriges Leistungsversagen (schneller Herzkammerrhythmus, Zusammenziehen der unteren Hohlvene) und für hohes Leistungsversagen (Aortahöhlenfistel) reduzierten diverse ACE-Inhibitoren den niedrigen Blutdruck, verbesserten die Natriumbilanz und verringerten den erwarteten Anstieg des Arteriendrucks in der Lunge und den gesamten äusseren Widerstand. Untersuchungen an Ratten mit geheiltem Herzmuskelinfarkt und Herzinsuffizienz zeigten, dass chronische Behandlung mit ACE-Inhibitoren die Pumpfähigkeit des Herzens verbessert, die Vergrösserung der Herzkammer verringert, die Nieren- und Herzmuskelerweiterung unterstützt und die langzeitigen Überlebenschancen verbessert. Unbekannt sind die genauen Mechanismen, die schliesslich und endlich verantwortlich sind für den verbesserten hämodynamischen Zustand der mit ACE-Inhibitoren behandelten Tiere. Jedoch ist es möglich, auf der Basis der in vivo-Resultate mit ACE-Inhibitoren bei verschiedenen Modellen für experimentelles Herzversagen die Schlussfolgerung zu ziehen, dass das Renin-Angiotensin-System im Verlauf der Herzinsuffizienz eine zunehmend wichtigere Rolle spielt, wenn die Krankheit fortschreitet.

RIASSUNTO

La formazione di angiotensina II (ANG II) è un adattamento compensatorio fisiologicamente importante all'ipotensione che si verifica in alcuni modelli sperimentali d'insufficienza cardiaca e ischemia miocardica. Si pensa che, man mano che la malattia progredisce, questo importante meccanismo vasocostrittore e sodio-ritenente, assieme ad altri meccanismi vasocostrittori (p. es.: catecolamine e vasopressina), favorisca l'emostasia cardiovascolare mediante una complessa serie di interazioni. Ad un certo punto, però, questi meccanismi vasocostrittori svolgono un ruolo sempre più dominante e deleterio. Sono stati usati vari modelli animali in vitro ed in vivo di ischemia miocardica e d'insufficienza cardiaca per elucidare il ruolo dell'ANG II. Cuori di ratto ischemici isolati trattati in vitro o ex vivo con alte dosi di inibitori dell'EIA (enzima isomerizzante dell'angiotensina) possiedono migliori proprietà di flusso meccanico/coronario e producono meno aritmie. In modelli di acuta insufficienza cardiaca (embolizzazione coronaria, infarto miocardico), gli inibitori dell'EIA riducevano l'elevata resistenza periferica, abbassavano la pressione sanguigna e alleviavano lo squilibrio nella richiesta/alimentazione d'ossigeno facendo aumentare il flusso regionale di sangue miocardico. In modelli in vivo di occlusione/riperfusione coronaria, l'incidenza di fibrillazione ventricolare nel corso della riperfusione veniva diminuito con certi inibitori dell'EIA. E'stato documentato che in modelli con insufficienza dovuta a bassa gettata (ritmo ventricolare rapido, costrizione della vena cava inferiore) e ad alta gettata (fistula aortico-cavale), vari inibitori dell'EIA hanno ridotto la pressione sanguigna, migliorato l'equilibrio del sodio ed attenuato l'atteso aumento di pressione dell'arteria polmonare e della resistenza periferica totale. Nei ratti guariti da infarto miocardico e insufficienza cardiaca, il somministro cronico di inibitori dell'EIA ha avuto come risultato una maggiore capacità di pompaggio cardiaco, una diminuzione dell'ingrossamento ventricolare, una dilatazione preferenziale renale e miocardica nonché un aumento della sopravvivenza a lungo termine. Gli esatti meccanismi che in definitiva sono responsabili del migliore stato emodinamico degli animali trattati con inibitori dell'EIA non sono noti. Tuttavia, in base alle reazioni in vivo algi inibitori dell'EIA in vari modelli di insufficienza cardiaca sperimentale, adesso è possibile concludere che il sistema renina-angiotensina svolge un ruolo sempre maggior man mano che lo stato di insufficienza cardiaca progredisce.

SUMÁRIO

A formação da angiotensina II (ANG II) constitui um importante ajuste compensatório fisiológico em resposta à hipotensão que acompanha alguns modelos experimentais de insuficiência e isquemia miocárdica. À medida que as doenças progressam, este importante mecanismo vasoconstritor e de retenção de sódio, em conjunção com outros mecanismos vasoconstritores (por exemplo, catecoleminas e vasopresina), aparentemente ajudam a hemostase vascular através de uma complexa série de interações. Contudo, em algum momento estos mecanismos vasoconstritores jogam um papel cada vez mais dominante e potencialmente nocivo. Têm-se utilizado vários modelos animais *in vitro* e *in vivo* de isquemia miocárdica e insuficiência cardíaca para esclarecer o papel da ANG II. Corações isquémicos de rato islados e tratados *in vitro* ou *in vivo* com doses elevadas de inibidores da enzima convertidora da angiotensina (ACE) presentam melhores propriedades mecânicas e de fluxo cardíaco, e produzem menos arritmias. Em modelos de insuficiência cardíaca aguda (embolização coronária, infarto miocárdico), os inibidores da ACE reduziram a elevada resistência periférica, diminuiram a pressão arterial e melhoraram o desequilíbrio na demanda/suprimento de oxigênio mediante o aumento do fluxo sangüíneo regional miocárdico. Em modelos *in vivo* de oclusão/reperfusão coronária, a incidência de fibrilação ventricular durante a reperfusão foi reduzida com alguns inibidores da ACE. Em modelos de insuficiência por baixo gasto cardíaco (rápido ritmo ventricular, constrição da veia cava inferior) e insuficiência por elevado gasto cardíaco (fistula aórtica-cava), tem-se observado que vários inibidores da ACE reduzem a pressão arterial, melhoram o equilíbrio de sódio e atenuam a esperada elevação na pressão da arteria pulmonar e a resistência periférica total. Nos ratos curados de infarto miocárdico e insuficiência cardíaca, o tratamento crônico com inibidores da ACE resulta numa melhor capacidade do coração para bombear sangue, menor aumento ventricular, dilatação preferencial miocárdica e renal, e melhor super-vivência a largo prazo. Os mecanismos precisos responsáveis em última análise pelo estado hemodinâmico melhorado dos animais tratados com inibidores da ACE são desconhecidos. Contudo, na base das respostas *in vivo* aos inibidores da ACE de vários modelos experimentais de insufiência cardíaca, agora é possível concluir-se que o sistema renina-angiotensina joga um papel cada vez mais dominante à medida que progressa o estado da insuficiência cardíaca.

RESUMEN

La formación de la angiotensina II (ANG II) constituye un importante ajuste compensatorio fisiológico en respuesta a la hipotensión que acompaña a algunos modelos experimentales de insuficiencia cardíaca e isquemia miocárdica. A medida que las enfermedades progresan, este importante mecanismo vasoconstrictor y de retención de sodio, en conjunción con otros mecanismos vasoconstrictores (por ejemplo, catecolaminas y vasopresina), aparentemente ayudan a la hemostasis cardiovascular a través de una compleja serie de interacciones. Sin embargo, en algún momento estos mecanismos vasoconstrictores juegan un papel cada vez más dominante y potencialmente nocivo. Se han empleado varios modelos animales *in vitro* e *in vivo* de isquemia miocárdica e insuficiencia cardíaca para descubrir el papel de la ANG II. Corazones isquémicos de rata aislados y tratados *in vitro* o *ex vivo* con dosis elevadas de inhibidores de la enzima convertidora de la angiotensina (ACE) presentan mejores propiedades mecánicas y de flujo coronario, y producen menos arritmias. En modelos de insuficiencia cardíaca aguda (embolización coronaria, infarto del miocardio), los inhibidores de la ACE redujeron la elevada resistencia periférica, disminuyeron la presión arterial y mejoraron el desequilibrio en la demanda/suministro de oxígeno mediante el incremento del flujo sanguíneo regional del miocardio. En modelos *in vivo* de oclusión/reperfusión coronaria, la incidencia de fibrilación ventricular durante la reperfusión fue reducida con algunos inhibidores de la ACE. En modelos de insuficiencia por bajo gasto cardíaco (rápido ritmo ventricular, constricción de la vena cava inferior) e insuficiencia por elevado gasto cardíaco (fistula aórtica-cava), se ha observado que varios inhibidores de la ACE reducen la presión arterial, mejoran el equilibrio de sodio y antenúan la esperada elevación en la presión de la arteria pulmonar y la resistencia periférica total. En las ratas curadas de infarto del miocardio e insuficiencia cardíaca, el tratamiento crónico con inhibidores de la ACE resulta en una mejor habilidad del corazón para bombear sangre, menor hipertrofia ventricular, dilatación preferencial miocárdica y renal, y mejor supervivencia a largo plazo. No se conocen todavía los mecanismos precisos que son responsables de la mejoría en el estado hemodinámico de los animales tratados con inhibidores de la ACE. Sin embargo, en base a las respuetas *in vivo* a los inhibidores de la ACE de varios modelos experimentales de insuficiencia cardíaca, se puede concluir que el sistema renina-angiotensina juega un papel cada vez más dominante a medida que progresa la insuficiencia cardíaca.

要約

アンジオテンシン II の生成は，低血圧に対する生理学的に重要な代償性適応現象の 1 つであり，このことはいくつかの心不全および心筋虚血の実験モデルで認められている。これらの疾患の進展に伴って，この重要な血管収縮および Na 保持機構が，他の血管収縮機構（たとえばカテコールアミンやバソプレシン）と共同し，複雑な相互作用を介して心血管系の恒常性維持に関与していると考えられる。しかし，ある点に達すると，これらの血管収縮機構はしだいに有害な作用が優位となってくる。アンジオテンシン II の役割を解明するために，in vitro および in vivo での心筋虚血や心不全の各種の動物モデルが用いられてきた。

心筋虚血ラットの単離心臓を用いて in vitro および ex vivo でアンジオテンシン変換酵素（ACE）阻害薬の高用量を作用させると，良好な機能と冠血流状態が保たれ，不整脈をほとんど誘発しない。急性心不全（冠動脈血栓，心筋梗塞）モデルでは，ACE 阻害薬が上昇していた末梢血管抵抗を低下させ，血圧を下げ，局所の心筋血流量を増加させて酸素需給のアンバランスを改善する。In vivo での冠動脈閉鎖/再灌流モデルでは，再灌流時の心室細動の頻度がいくつかの ACE 阻害薬により減少した。低心拍出量性心不全（速い心室ペーシング，下大静脈の結紮）モデルおよび高心拍出量性心不全（大動脈-大静脈瘻）モデルでは，種々の ACE 阻害薬が血圧を下げ，Na バランスを改善し，予想される肺動脈圧と総末梢血管抵抗の上昇を軽減すると報告されている。心筋梗塞治癒後で心不全のラットにおいては，ACE 阻害薬の長期投与により，良好なポンプ機能，心室肥大の抑制，好ましい腎の状態，心筋拡大，長期生存率の改善などがもたらされる。

ACE 阻害薬で治療した動物において，血行動態の改善を最終的にもたらした正確な機序については不明である。しかし，種々の実験的心不全モデルの in vivo での ACE 阻害薬への反応に基づいて考えると，心不全状態が進行するとレニン-アンジオテンシン系がしだいに優先的な役割を演じるようになると，現時点では結論できよう。

Cardiac and Renal Failure: An Expanding Role for ACE Inhibitors, edited by C. T. Dollery and L. M. Sherwood, Hanley & Belfus, Inc., Philadelphia.

DISCUSSION

PETERS: Have there been any attempts to develop immunological models of heart failure? They might provide the basis for a model of diffuse heart disease.

SWEET: There are laboratories working on immunologically-induced cardiomyopathy. In addition, there are also models in which diffuse disease has been produced by adriamycin. However, I have not had much experience with them.

MEZEY: Could these models be used in studies of sudden death? I am thinking particularly of the changes that might occur in sodium transport in the myocardium.

SWEET: Good animal models are needed to assess experimental compounds for their ability to protect against a sudden death. One canine model of sudden death has been used to demonstrate the efficacy of bretylium tosylate.

SONNENBLICK: In your work and that of Pfeffer, using animal models, we see that ventricular dilatation correlates with death. In Pfeffer's SAVE study in man, administration of an ACE inhibitor is started later after an infarction, but the mechanisms leading to hypertrophy and dilatation occur early.

SWEET: Studies of enalapril in man very early after myocardial infarction might be of considerable interest.

Cardiac and Renal Failure: An Expanding Role for ACE Inhibitors, edited by C. T. Dollery and L. M. Sherwood, Hanley & Belfus, Inc., Philadelphia.

Clinical Assessment of Chronic Heart Failure: Origin of Symptoms and Role of Exercise Testing

Philip A. Poole-Wilson

The term heart failure is used to describe many clinical entities that have in common a diminished ability of the heart to function as a pump. Numerous adjectives[1,2] are used in association with the words heart failure and are useful indicators to doctors of the expected pattern of symptoms, physical signs, and treatment. This medical notation does not always have a physiological or biochemical basis. In this article I shall discuss only chronic heart failure, by which I mean that the patient has left ventricular dysfunction, symptoms, and some evidence, past or present, of sodium and water overload.

CLINICAL ASSESSMENT

The history, symptoms, and physical signs of patients with chronic heart failure are well-described elsewhere. Necessary, even obligatory, investigations include full blood count, electrolytes and urea, chest x-ray and an electrocardiogram. In Britain more than 85% of patients in the community with heart failure undergo these investigations (unpublished data). Thyroid function may be measured in selected patients. Echocardiography should be performed in most patients with heart failure, since it greatly assists in establishing the etiology of heart failure, but in practice the procedure is undertaken in only 30% of patients.

Further investigations, such as the measurement of ejection fraction at rest or on exercise, exercise testing, and cardiac catheterization are only indicated in selected patients and do not yet (at least in Britain) form part of the essential investigations of the patient with heart failure either young or old.

The purpose of investigations is to establish the cause of heart failure so that it may be prevented or at least the progress of damage to the myocardium delayed, to establish the severity of heart failure, to assess the degree of sodium and water overload, because that will influence the nature of the initial therapy, to understand the nature of the functional abnormality of the heart, and to determine the likely prognosis.

EXTRACELLULAR AND CELLULAR HEART FAILURE

There are many causes of chronic heart failure. Conventionally, physicians have classified patients into those with one of the many manifestations of atheromatous coronary artery disease or into a group with the generic term cardiomyopathy. Cardiomyopathy is subclassified as hypertrophic, restrictive or dilated on the basis of clinical criteria. This classification has no particular merit or physiological basis. The word cardiomyopathy has often concealed ignorance of underlying etiology behind descriptive classification. An alternative classification is to consider heart failure as due to extracellular abnormalities of the heart (architecture, shape, size and fibrosis), incoordinate contractility, or cellular abnormalities. Cellular abnormalities can be either systolic or diastolic (Table I).

Results from several groups of investigators have indicated that, at least under resting conditions, the shortening of isolated myocardial cells or the tension generated by trabeculae or papillary muscles from man is normal.[3,4,5,6] A reduction in peak shortening or the peak rate of shortening or in the rate of decline of developed tension may be detected when the muscle is stressed either by an increase in stimulation rate or by an inotropic agent. Thus in many forms of heart failure the evidence for an abnormality of contraction of the myocardial tissue is poor. An alternative cause for malfunction of the heart as a pump may be alterations in the architecture of the heart[7] (Table I). These abnormalities include the shape of the ventricle (round rather than elliptical), the size of the ventricle, slippage of cells in relation to each other, and fibrosis and other alterations in the extracellular matrix

TABLE I. *Underlying causes of chronic heart failure*

1. Extracellular	Fibrosis and extracellular architecture
	Ventricular size — slippage of cells
	Ventricular shape — orientation of cells
2. Indoordinate contraction	
3. Cellular	Diastolic dysfunction
	Hypertrophy
	Ischemia
	Systolic dysfunction
	Down regulation of receptors
	Reduced c-AMP
	Abnormal sarcoplasmic reticulum
	Abnormal contractile proteins

linking cells. This may be the dominant pathology in many patients and it is not then logical to advocate the use of drugs designed to alter either the contraction or relaxation of the myocyte; an entirely novel approach is needed.

SYSTOLIC AND DIASTOLIC HEART FAILURE

Cellular abnormalities of the heart alter either systolic or diastolic function. Recently there has been a revival of interest in diastolic function of the heart.[8-12] In part this may be because some recent technologies, particularly radionuclide ventriculography[12] and Doppler echocardiography,[13] have allowed the simple measurement of the rapid rate of filling of the left ventricle and flow velocity through the mitral valve. Diastolic dysfunction is an old concept and has been known to be a key functional abnormality in patients with hypertrophy of any origin, hypertrophy associated with hypertension, cardiac function following aortic valve surgery for aortic stenosis, myocardial ischemia, and many other conditions. Most reports have made measurements of cardiac function in the resting state and emphasized the presence of a diastolic abnormality in the absence of a systolic abnormality. The presence of a defect at rest does not necessarily indicate the nature of the prime abnormality on exercise. Furthermore, the measure of diastolic cardiac function is commonly the rapid rate of left ventricular filling. Diastole is comprised of at least four components: (1) isovolumic relaxation, (2) rapid filling, (3) passive filling, and (4) atrial systole. It is by no means clear as to the relationship between rapid ventricular filling to the ventricular volume at end diastole and how these variables are altered on exercise and related to symptoms limiting exercise capacity.

Symptoms

In acute heart failure shortness of breath is related to the left atrial pressure. Reduction of the left atrial pressure leads to a rapid improvement in the symptoms. This has led to the widely held belief that the symptoms of fatigue and shortness of breath in patients with chronic heart failure are related to a reduced cardiac output and lower left atrial pressure, respectively. Recent work has shown this simple idea to be untrue. In patients with chronic heart failure treated with diuretics, peak oxygen consumption on exercise is not related to the left atrial pressure on exercise.[14] Different forms of exercise tests result in the tests being terminated by different symptoms, but the left atrial pressure remains the same.[15] Drugs can be used to lower the left atrial pressure but exercise capacity is not improved.[4]

The origin of symptoms on exercise in chronic heart failure is complex and almost certainly multifactorial (Table II). Abnormalities in the lung are con-

TABLE II. *Origin of symptoms on exercise in chronic heart failure*

1. Lung abnormalities	Increased stiffness due to raised venous pressure and lymphatic distension
	Increased left atrial pressure
	Increased physiological dead space
	Increased respiratory rate
2. Circulation	Reduced blood flow to skeletal muscle
	Increased production of metabolites
3. Skeletal muscle	Rest atrophy
	Ischemic atrophy
	Specific abnormality

tributory, and perhaps the major factor is the increased physiological dead space that is present.[16] Patients with heart failure have an increased ventilation in comparison to normal persons for a given workload or carbon dioxide production rate. The arterial blood gases are usually normal. This implies that there is considerable ventilation perfusion mismatch. The pathophysiological cause is not understood.

The exercise systolic blood pressure in patients with heart failure is not greatly reduced, but the femoral vein oxygen content is low.[17] This implies that most of the blood to the exercising legs is directed not to the skin but to the muscle and that the extraction of oxygen by skeletal muscle is almost maximal. The resistance in the vascular bed of exercising skeletal muscle is increased up to five-fold. The cause is not clear and is not related directly to activation of the neuroendocrine systems, since it is not greatly reduced by alpha blockers or inhibitors of renin angiotensin system. In addition several groups have identified abnormalities of skeletal muscle itself. Muscle mass is reduced and there is cell atrophy. Abnormalities of function,[18,19] histology,[19] and biochemistry[20] have been reported. The combination of a restricted blood flow to exercising muscle and abnormalities of the muscle itself may give rise to signals that are interpreted by the brain as shortness of breath or fatigue.

Treatment

Diuretics are the essential group of drugs used in the treatment of chronic heart failure. The benefit from thiazides was reported over 30 years ago.[21] Digoxin is appropriate in the presence of atrial fibrillation and is still used by some physicians in patients with sinus rhythm. Diuretics not only eliminate edema but prevent its recurrence. Careful clinical assessment allows the physician to select the dose of diuretic that normalizes the body fluid compartments.[22] Whether increase of the dose of diuretics until body fluid compartments are similar to those in normal persons results in the greatest improvement of symptoms is not known; there is a danger of over-diuresis and some expansion of the extracellular volume could be advantageous to patients. Furthermore, stimulation of the renin-angiotensin system in mild heart failure is largely a consequence of diuretic therapy and not a feature of heart failure per se.[23] An elevated renin can be regarded as a side effect of diuretic therapy. An argument exists that angiotensin-converting enzyme inhibitors should be used earlier in the treatment of heart failure to prevent activation of the renin-angiotensin system. In severe heart failure the renin-angiotensin system is stimulated even in untreated patients (unpublished data).

Many patients continue to have unacceptable symptoms despite treatment and the key question arises as to what further treatment they should receive or whether further treatment should be initiated at the time that diuretic therapy is begun. The answer rests on an understanding of the cause of symptoms in chronic heart failure.[14,24,25]

Exercise Testing

One major objective in assessing patients with heart failure is the determination of the prognosis. Almost all clinical variables that are indicative of heart failure have some predictive power. Several recent studies have sought to determine which of these variables are the most powerful predictors and have independent predictive value.[26-31] Physicians are familiar with patients who have enlarged hearts, possibly the consequence of damage earlier in life, and who seem to lead an almost normal life. But cardiac size has been shown to be a predictor of prognosis.[32] In our experience, and in that of others, the combination of peak oxygen consumption, ejection fraction at rest (a measure of left ventricular end diastolic size), and plasma sodium are the three best predictors of prognosis in patients who already have severe heart failure.

The purpose of exercise testing in chronic heart failure is to confirm the severity of the disability, to categorize the severity of heart failure, to predict prognosis, and to assess the efficacy of treatment. It is this latter indication that has received the most attention because of the desire of the pharmaceutical industry for a practical means of assessing new drug therapies.

The difficulties of exercise testing are well known and indicated in Table III. Much has been made of the so-called placebo effect. It is my opinion that the placebo effect would be more accurately described as a consequence of the training of doctors in performing exercise tests in patients with heart failure. In general cardiologists have been instructed in the use of exercise testing in the context of angina. Exercise tests are stopped when the patient becomes uncomfortable. If this approach is applied to the measurement of maximal exercise capacity in heart failure, exercise duration will increase as the confidence of the patient and experience of the doctor increases. A further consideration is the duration of the exercise test. Once exercise tests extend beyond

TABLE III. *Difficulties encountered in exercise testing in heart failure*

1. Type of exercise (bicycle or treadmill)
2. Boredom during protracted exercise tests
3. Design of exercise protocol
4. Reproducibility
5. Sensitivity
6. Subjective or objective endpoint
7. Placebo effect
8. Fitness effect
9. Training of doctors
10. Varying symptoms terminating exercise test

15 minutes, boredom becomes an important determinant of the exercise performance. The two major requirements for an effective exercise test are reproducibility and sensitivity. This latter requirement is not always fulfilled, particularly when the exercise test is based on some of the common protocols such as the Bruce protocol.

Most exercise tests have been adapted from those used for the investigation of patients with coronary artery disease. Measurements have been made at peak exercise. The moment of peak exercise is not an objective measurement but depends on the interaction between the patient and the doctor. Oxygen consumption at peak exercise has been widely used to assess function.[33,34] This is determined not only by the amount of exercise that the patient can perform and cardiovascular fitness, but also by muscle mass. In order to avoid some of these difficulties, some authors have attempted to measure what has been called the anaerobic threshold. Usually the relationship between oxygen consumption and CO_2 production is curvilinear; the data do not fit two straight lines. The anaerobic threshold is difficult to measure and may well be an erroneous concept, since increasing exercise is associated with recruitment of further muscle fibers, and the leg muscles contain both type I and type II fibers. We have used a different approach to this problem and have analyzed the relationship between oxygen consumption and CO_2 production as a curvilinear relationship.[35] It is then possible to predict the shape of the curve, provided the patient has reached the stage of the exercise where the respiratory quotient is greater than one and the duration of the test is approximately 70% of that which could be achieved maximally. With this approach a maximal test is not necessary, the test is truly objective, and weight is given to all the data not just that obtained in the last moments of the exercise test.

Exercise tests have traditionally used a protocol whereby the severity of exercise is increased during the test. That may be a poor measure of patients' activities and certainly a poor measure of the usual functions of the patients such as walking to the shops or undertaking household tasks. The 6-minute walking test was originally introduced to assess patients with lung disease but has now been applied to heart failure.[36,37] In this test the distance walked in a given period of time is measured rather than the maximum achievable level of exercise. We have recently adapted this test using a self-powered treadmill and shown that the distance walked on this apparatus correlates closely with the peak oxygen consumption but is a more sensitive test. Patients exercise at approximately 80% of their maximal oxygen consumption. An alternative way of undertaking this test would be to measure the distance walked when a treadmill is set to conditions where patients reach 80% of their maximal oxygen consumption.

The measurement of exercise capacity in one form or another remains the best means of assessing patients with heart failure. Further research is needed to establish the most sensitive and reproducible protocol. This will then provide an objective means of assessing patients so that the efficacy of new therapies can be properly assessed.

REFERENCES

1. Poole-Wilson PA. The management and treatment of chronic heart failure. *Recent Advances in Medicine.* 1987; **20**:161–175.
2. Poole-Wilson PA. Treatment of intractable heart failure. In Sheppard MC, ed. *Advanced Medicine.* London, Bailliere-Tindall, 1988, pp 321–332.
3. Ginsburg R, Bristow MR, Billingham ME, Stinson EB, Schroeder JS, Harrison DC. Study of the normal and failing isolated human heart: decreased response of failing heart to isoproterenol. *Am Heart J* 1983; **106**:535–540.
4. Harding SE, Jones SM, O'Gara P, Poole-Wilson PA. Human and rabbit ventricular cells—comparison of inotropic responses to calcium and isoprenaline. *J Mol Cell Cardiol* 1988; **20 (suppl 5)**:162.
5. Brown L, Lorenz B, Erdmann E. Reduced positive inotropic effects in diseased human ventricular myocardium. *Cardiov Res* 1986; **20**:516–520.
6. Feldman MD, Copelas L, Gwathmey JK, Phillips P, Warren SE, Schoen FJ, Grossman W, Morgan JP. Deficient production of cyclic AMP: pharmacologic evidence of an important cause of contractile dysfunction in patients with end-stage heart failure. *Circulation* 1987; **75**:331–339.
7. Linzbach AJ. Heart failure from the point of view of quantitative anatomy. *Am J Cardiol* 1960; **5**:370–380.
8. Katz AM. Role of the basic sciences in the practice of cardiology. *J Mol Cell Cardiol* 1987; **19**:3–17.
9. Soufer R, Wohlgelernter D, Vita NA, Amuchestegui M, Sostman D, Berger HJ, Zaret BL. Intact systolic left ventricular function in clinical congestive heart failure. *Am J Cardiol* 1985; **55**:1032–1036.
10. Gaasch WH. Diastolic mechanisms in heart failure. *Heart Failure* 1985; **1**:195–202.
11. Dougherty AH, Naccarelli GV, Gray EL, Hicks CH, Goldstein RA. Congestive heart failure with normal systolic function. *Am J Cardiol* 1984; **54**:778–782.
12. Lavine SJ, Krishnaswami V, Shreiner DP, Amidi M. Left ventricular diastolic filling in patients with left ventricular dysfunction. *Int J Cardiol* 1985; **8**:423–436.
13. Labowitz AJ, Pearson AC. Evaluation of left ventricular diastolic function: clinical relevance and recent Doppler echocardiographic insights. *Am Heart J* 1987; **114**:836–851.
14. Lipkin DP, Poole-Wilson PA. Symptoms limiting exercise in chronic heart failure. *Br Med J* 1986; **292**:1030–1031.
15. Lipkin DP, Canepa-Anson R, Stephens MR, Poole-Wilson PA. Factors determining symp-

toms in heart failure: comparison of fast and slow exercise tests. *Br Heart J* 1986; **55**:439–445.

16. Sullivan MJ, Higginbotham MB, Cobb FR. Increased exercise ventilation in patients with chronic heart failure: intact ventilatory control despite hemodynamic and pulmonary abnormalities. *Circulation* 1988; **77**:552–559.

17. LeJemtel TH, Maskin CS, Lucido D, Chadwick BJ. Failure to augment limb blood flow in response to one-leg versus two-leg exercise in patients with severe heart failure. *Circulation* 1986; **74**:245–251.

18. Buller NP, Jones D, Poole-Wilson PA. Evidence for an intrinsic defect of skeletal metabolism in patients with chronic heart failure. *Clin Sci* 1987; **72 (suppl 16)**:60P.

19. Lipkin DP, Jones DA, Round JM, Poole-Wilson PA. Abnormalities of skeletal muscle in patients with chronic heart failure. *Int J Cardiol* 1988; **18**:187–195.

20. Massie BM, Conway M, Rajagopalan B, Yonge R, Frostick S, Ledingham J, Sleight P, Radda G. Skeletal muscle metabolism during exercise under ischaemic conditions in congestive heart failure. Evidence for abnormalities unrelated to blood flow. *Circulation* 1988; **78**:320–326.

21. Slater JDH, Nabarro JDN. Clinical experience with chlorothiazide. *Lancet* 1958; **1**:124–126.

22. Anand IS, Veall N, Kalra GS, Ferrari R, Sutton G, Harris P, Poole-Wilson PA. Treatment of heart failure with diuretics: body compartments, renal function and plasma hormones. *Eur Heart J* (in press).

23. Bayliss J, Norell M, Canepa-Anson R, Sutton G, Poole-Wilson P. Untreated heart failure: clinical and neuroendocrine effects of introducing diuretics. *Br Heart J* 1987; **57**:17–22.

24. Poole-Wilson PA, Buller NP, Lipkin DP. Regional blood flow, muscle strength and skeletal muscle histology in severe congestive heart failure. *Am J Cardiol* 1988; **62**:49E–52E.

25. Poole-Wilson PA. The origin of symptoms in patients with chronic heart failure. *Eur Heart J* 1988; **9 (suppl H)**:49–53.

26. Cohn JN, Archibald DG, Francis GS, Ziesche S, Franciosa JA, Harston WE, Tristani FE, Dunkman WB, Jacobs W, Flohr FH, Goldman S, Cobb FR, Shah PM, Saunders R, Fletcher RD, Loeb HS, Hughes VC, Baker B. Veterans Administration Cooperative study on vasodilator therapy of heart failure: influence of prerandomisation variables on the reduction of mortality by treatment with hydralazine and isosorbide dinitrate. *Circulation* 1987; **75 (suppl 4)**:49–54.

27. Szlachic J, Massie BM, Kramer BL, Topic N, Tubau J. Correlates and prognostic implication of exercise capacity in chronic congestive heart failure. *Am J Cardiol* 1985; **55**:1037–1042.

28. Likoff MJ, Chandler SL, Kay HR. Clinical determinants of mortality in chronic congestive heart failure secondary to idiopathic dilated or to ischaemic cardiomyopathy. *Am J Cardiol* 1987; **59**:634–638.

29. Cleland JGF, Dargie HJ, Ford I. Mortality in heart failure: clinical variables of prognostic value. *Br Heart J* 1987; **58**:572–582.

30. Diaz RA, Obasohan A, Oakley CM. Prediction of outcome in dilated cardiomyopathy. *Br Heart J* 1987; **58**:393–399.

31. Glover D, Littler WA. Factors influencing survival and mode of death in severe chronic ischaemia cardiac failure. *Br Heart J* 1987; **57**:125–132.

32. Packer M, Meller J, Medina N, Gorlin R, Herman MV. Importance of left ventricular size in determining the response to hydralazine in severe chronic heart failure. *N Engl J Med* 1980; **303**:250–255.

33. Lipkin D. The role of exercise testing in chronic heart failure. *Br Heart J* 1987; **58**:559–566.

34. Lipkin DP, Perrins J, Poole-Wilson PA. Respiratory gas exchange in the assessment of patients with impaired ventricular function. *Br Heart J* 1985; **54**:321–328.

35. Buller NB, Poole-Wilson PA. "Extrapolated maximum oxygen consumption"; A new method for the objective analysis of respiratory gas exchange during exercise. *Br Heart J* 1988; **59**:212–217.

36. Lipkin DP, Scriven AJ, Crake T, Poole-Wilson PA. Six minute walking test for assessing exercise capacity in chronic heart failure. *Br Med J* 1986; **292**:653–655.

37. Guyatt GH, Sullivan MJ, Thompson PJ, Fallen EL, Pugsley SO, Taylor BW, Berman LB. The 6-minute walk: a new measure of exercise capacity in patients with chronic heart failure. *Can Med Assoc J* 1985; **132**:919–923.

SUMMARY

Chronic heart failure is defined as the presence of left ventricular dysfunction, symptoms, and evidence, past or present, of sodium and water retention. Clinical assessment and investigations are undertaken to establish the cause of heart failure (in order that the progress of damage to the myocardium can be delayed), to establish the severity of heart failure, to assess the degree of sodium and water overload (because this will determine the initial choice of therapy), and to determine the probable prognosis. There are many causes of heart failure and some of the different manifestations of heart failure (extracellular and cellular heart failure, and systolic and diastolic heart failure) require specific treatment. Determination of prognosis is a major objective when assessing patients with heart failure. Exercise testing is used to determine the severity of heart failure, to predict prognosis, and to assess the efficacy of treatment. Traditional exercise tests have numerous limitations and newer tests, such as the 6-minute walking test, have important advantages. More research is needed to establish the most sensitive and reproducible method of exercise testing. This should provide a test which gives an objective means of assessing patients so that the efficacy of new therapies can be properly measured.

RÉSUMÉ

La présence d'une insuffisance ventriculaire gauche, les symptômes et l'évidence, passée ou actuelle, d'une rétention hydrosaline sont les caractéristiques d'une insuffisance cardiaque chronique. On procède à une évaluation et à des investigations cliniques pour déterminer la cause de l'insuffisance cardiaque (afin de retarder la progression de la détérioration du myocarde), pour déterminer la séverité de l'insuffisance cardiaque, pour évaluer le degré d'excès de sodium et d'eau (parce que cela déterminera la stratégie thérapeutique à envisager intitialement), et pour déterminer le pronostic probable. Beaucoup de causes sont à l'origine des insuffisances cardiaques et certaines des différentes manifestations d'insuffisance cardiaque (insuffisance cardiaque extracellulaire et cellulaire, insuffisance cardiaque systolique et diastolique) exigent un traitement particulier. La détermination du pronostic est un objectif majeur lorqu'on évalue les patients atteints d'insuffisance cardiaque. On utilise des tests de performance physique pour déterminer la séverité de l'insuffisance cardiaque, pour pronostiquer et pour évaluer l'efficacité du traitement. Les épreuves traditionnelles de performance physique sont tres limitées et de nouveaux tests, tel l'epreuve de marche de 6 minutes, présentent de gros avantages. D'autres travaux de recherche doivent être menés afin d'établir la méthode de performances physiques la plus sensible et la plus reproductible. Ceci devrait donner une épreuve qui permette une evaluation objective des patients de façon à pouvoir mesurer l'efficacité de nouvelles stratégies thérapeutiques.

ZUSAMMENFASSUNG

Chronische Herzinsuffizienz ist definiert als Vorliegen einer Dysfunktion der linken Herzkammer und der Symptome und Anzeichen von Natrium- und Wasserretention in der Vergangenheit oder Gegenwart. Klinische Beobachtungen und Untersuchungen beschäftigen sich mit den Gründen für Herzinsuffizienz (mit dem Ziel, den Fortschritt des Schadens am Herzmuskel zu verzögern), mit dem Ausmass an Herzversagen, mit Messungen der Natrium- und Wasserüberbelastung (denn dies wird die Wahl der Anfangstherapie beeinflussen), und mit der Bestimmung der wahrscheinlichen Prognose. Herzinsuffizienz hat viele Gründe, und einige der veschiedenen Auswirkungen von Herzinsuffizienz verlangen eine spezifische Behandlung (extrazelluläres und zellulares Herzversagen und systolische und diastolische Herzinsuffizienz). Die Bestimmung der Prognose ist ein sehr wichtiges Ziel der Beurteilung von Patienten mit Herzinsuffizienz. Bewegunstests werden verwendet zur Bestimmung der Schwere des Herzversagens, zur Vorausbestimmung der Prognose und zur Feststellung der Wirksamkeit der Behandlung. Traditionelle Bewegungstests unterliegen zahllosen Grenzen, und neuere Tests, wie der 6-Minuten-Wandertest, haben wichtige Vorteile. Weitergehende Forschung ist notwendig, um die empfindlichste und reproduzierbarste Methode für Bewegungstests festzustellen. Man hofft auf die Entwicklung eines Tests als objektives Messinstrument für Patienten, so dass die Wirksamkeit neuer Therapien angemessen festgestellt werden kann.

RIASSUNTO

L'insufficienza cardiaca cronica viene definita come la presenza di disfunzione ventricolare sinistra, sintomi e segni, passati o presenti, di ritenzione di sodio e d'acqua. Valutazione ed investigazioni cliniche vengono intraprese per stabilire la causa dell'insufficienza cardiaca (al fine di poter ritardare il progresso dei danni al miocardio), per stabilire la gravita dell'insufficienza cardiaca, per valutare il livello di sovraccarico di sodio e d'acqua (perché ciò determinerà la scelta iniziale della terapia) e per determinare la prognosi probabile. Esistono molte cause d'insufficienza cardiaca ed alcune delle sue diverse manifestazioni (insufficienza extracellulare e cellulare, insufficienza sistolica e diastolica) richiedono cure specifiche. La determinazione della prognosi è l'obiettivo principale nella valutazione di pazienti con insufficienza cardiaca. I test d'esercizio fisico vengono usati per determinare la severità dell'insufficienza, elaborare la prognosi e valutare l'efficacia della cura. I test d'esercizio fisico tradizionali avevano molte limitazioni e quelli più nuovi, quali il test di marcia di 6 minuti, presentano vantaggi considerevoli. Sono necessarie maggiori ricerche per stabilire il metodo di test d'esercizio fisico più sensibile e riproducibile. Ciò dovrebbe portare ad un test che dia dei mezzi obiettivi per valutare i pazienti in modo da poter misurare correttamente l'efficacia delle terapie.

SUMÁRIO

A insuficiência cardíaca crónica define-se como a presença de disfunção do ventrículo esquerdo, sintomas e evidências, passadas ou presentes, de retenção de água e sódio. Efetuam-se a avaliação e investigações clínicas para estabelecer a causa de insuficiência cardíaca (com o fim de atrasar o progresso da lesão ao miocárdio), para estabelecer a severidade da insuficiência cardíaca, para avaliar o grau de sobrecarga de sódio e água (porque isto determina a escolha inicial de terapia), e para determinar o prognóstico provável. Existem várias causas para a insuficiência cardíaca e algumas das diferentes manifestações da mesma (insuficiência cardíaca extracelular e celular, e insuficiência cardíaca sistólica e diastólica) requerem um tratamento específico. A determinação do prognóstico é um dos objetivos principais na avaliação de pacientes com insuficiência cardíaca. Utilizam-se testes de exercício para determinar a severidade da insuficiência cardíaca, para estabelecer o prognóstico e para avaliar a eficácia do tratamento. Os testes de exercício tradicionais têm muitas limitações e os testes mais modernos, tais como o teste de caminhar 6 minutos, têm importantes vantagens. Precisa-se mais pesquisa para estabelecer o método de testes de exercício que é o mais sensível e reproduzível. Com isto, obterá-se uma prova que proporcione um meio objetivo de avaliar os pacientes, de maneira que a eficácia de novas terapias pode estabelecer-se apropriadamente.

RESUMEN

La insuficiencia cardíca crónica se define como la presencia de disfunción del ventículo izquierdo, síntomas y evidencias, pasadas o presentes, de retención de agua y sodio. Se efectúan investigaciones y reevaluación clínica para establecer la causa de insuficiencia cardíaca (con el fin de demorar el progreso de la lesión al miocardio), para establecer la gravedad de la insuficiencia cardíaca, para determinar el grado de sobrecarga de sodio y agua (porque esto determinará la elección inicial de la terapia), y para determinar la prognosis probable. Existen varias causas para la insuficiencia cardíaca y algunas de las diferentes manifestaciones de la misma (insuficiencia cardíaca extracelular y celular, e insuficiencia cardíaca sistólica y diastólica) requieren un tratamiento específico. La determinación de la prognosis es uno de los objetivos principales al evaluar a pacientes con insuficiencia cardíaca. Se emplean ejercicios para determinar la gravedad de la insuficiencia cardíaca, para establecer la prognosis y evaluar la eficacia del tratamiento. Las pruebas de ejercicios tradicionales tienen numerosas limitaciones y los ejercicios más modernos, tales como la prueba de caminar 6 minutos, tienen importantes ventajas. Se necesitan más investigaciones para establecer los tipos de ejercicios que son más sensibles y capaces de reproducirse. Con esto se obtendrá una prueba que brinde un medio objetivo de evaluar a los pacientes, de modo que la eficacia de nuevos tratamientos pueda establecerse apropiadamente.

要約

　慢性心不全は，左室機能障害，症状，過去あるいは現在の Na および水分貯留の所見の存在によって定義づけられる。心不全の原因の究明（これにより障害が心筋に進展するのを遅らせることができる），心不全の重症度の判定基準の確立，Na および水分の過剰の程度の評価（これにより治療法の第一選択が決定できよう），さらにきたるべき予後の判定などのために，臨床的な評価や検査が行われる。

　心不全には多くの原因があり，いくつかの異なる病型（細胞外および細胞性心不全，あるいは収縮性および拡張性心不全）ごとに特異的な治療法が要求される。予後の判定は心不全患者を評価するうえで主要な課題である。運動負荷試験は，心不全の重症度，予後の予測，治療効果の評価などのために行われる。従来の運動負荷試験には多くの制約があったが，6分間歩行試験のような新しい試験法には大きな利点がある。感度と再現性の最も高い運動負荷試験法を確立するには，さらに研究が必要である。もしそれが確立されれば，患者評価の客観的な手段・指標となり，新しい治療法の効果が的確に測定できるようになろう。

Cardiac and Renal Failure: An Expanding Role for ACE Inhibitors, edited by C. T. Dollery and L. M. Sherwood, Hanley & Belfus, Inc., Philadelphia.

DISCUSSION

JOHNSTON: What prevents the people in your trial from walking if they are only going at 80% capacity?

POOLE-WILSON: Volunteers and patients undertook a trial test. They attempted to pace themselves so as to last the 12 minutes. They could stop, rest and start again, although they tended not to do that. In the last few moments, as they can see the clock, there is a temptation to try to go further. For me the limiting factor was exhaustion.

DOLLERY: Are you saying that your definition of heart failure is somebody who can only walk 600 m on your treadmill with a respiratory quotient [RQ] of > 1 when they stop?

POOLE-WILSON: The last point is very important. If a person is limited on exercise without an $RQ > 1$, the diagnosis of heart failure as the limiting factor on exercise should be reconsidered. The question of how far they walk is irrelevant and has no absolute significance. It is merely a technique that can be applied to clinical trials.

SMITH: Some studies suggest that a submaximal exercise test is more sensitive than a maximal exercise test in response to specific therapy for heart failure. Is that your experience?

POOLE-WILSON: Yes. One does have to be careful to identify the type of test. We are measuring the distance walked in a given time. Others are measuring the time you can walk at approximately 80% of your measured maximum. Those are different. I am not sure if the differences are important. They may be.

COHN: Our experience with submaximal tests has not been good, because we do not have a good end point. It is not discriminatory in our hands.

POOLE-WILSON: That is why we went for this type of test.

SONNENBLICK: With my associate, Dr. Thierry Le Jemtel, we have been using an exercise level 80% of maximal while studying the lactate levels. If you can sustain 80% of maximum with a lower lactate level, it means you have a better working metabolism. With regard to fatigue, we have found respiratory muscle fatigue to be important and correlates with a rising lactate.

You said that your patients all had an ejection fraction of 17%. Did they not also have heart failure? Would it be advisable to distinguish between heart failure and congestive failure? Otherwise you could argue that a man with no heart has no heart failure as long as he can exercise. Since there is no correlation between exercise and ejection fraction you could have no heart and good exercise performance and vice versa. It is dangerous to define heart failure as an exercise test.

POOLE-WILSON: I no longer refer to "adjectival" heart failure, because usually we don't know what the adjective means. Heart failure, to me, is left ventricular dysfunction, symptoms, and treatment with diuretics. Otherwise I call it left ventricular dysfunction.

SONNENBLICK: If the patient has no symptoms, an ejection fraction of 20%, no edema, no limitation, and normal exercise performance, he will still be dead within 2 years. And yet, he may need no therapy that will be useful. Diuretics might even kill him. He has *heart failure* but not *congestive failure.*

POOLE-WILSON: A good example of left ventricular dysfunction!

Cardiac and Renal Failure: An Expanding Role for ACE Inhibitors, edited by C. T. Dollery and L. M. Sherwood, Hanley & Belfus, Inc., Philadelphia.

Therapy of Heart Failure: Two Centuries of Progress

Thomas W. Smith

Despite major advances in many areas of cardiovascular therapeutics in the past few decades, any discussion of the treatment of congestive heart failure (CHF) must begin with the admission that the prognosis of patients with overt congestive heart failure remains guarded. The 50% mortality level is reached within about 5 years for groups of patients with relatively mild failure[1] and within only 6 months or less in groups with severe and relatively refractory CHF.[2] Thus, a compelling case exists for appropriate emphasis to be placed upon *prevention* of end-stage heart disease with CHF. The more restricted aim of this discussion is to consider the current status of the use of digitalis and diuretics in the management of CHF. The use of vasodilators is considered in some detail elsewhere in this volume.

Three general types of approaches are used in the contemporary management of CHF. The first priority is removal of underlying causes of heart failure, including surgical correction of valvular lesions or congenital malformations. Effective medical treatment of hypertension or infective endocarditis would also potentially fit in this category.

Second, the removal of precipitating causes is of major importance, since the initial development or exacerbation of heart failure is frequently related to a superimposed stress, rather than worsening of the underlying cardiac condition. Thus, causes of increased demand for cardiac work such as anemia, fever, infection, fluid overload, thyrotoxicosis, and many other intercurrent problems require immediate attention. Cardiac rhythm disturbances, pulmonary embolism, poor compliance with the therapeutic regimen, and certain drugs are additional well-known precipitating causes of heart failure.

Finally, treatment of the clinical manifestations of heart failure comprises the third category. This may, in turn, be divided into the following measures:

1. Interventions to enhance the pump performance of the failing ventricle (e.g., digitalis glycosides; sympathomimetic drugs; other positive inotropic drugs; pacemakers).

2. Reduction of cardiac workload (e.g., physical and emotional rest; correction of obesity; vasodilator drugs; assisted circulation, such as with intra-aortic balloon counterpulsation).

3. Control of salt and water retention (e.g., restriction of salt intake; diuretics; mechanical removal of fluid).

In considering the general strategy of heart failure management, it is frequently and appropriately stated that the diverse etiologies and degrees of severity of CHF require an individualized approach in each case. A scheme showing the typical sequence of measures employed is shown in Table I.

TABLE I. *Steps in the management of chronic congestive heart failure*

	Functional Class		
Steps	*II*	*III*	*IV*
A	Restrict physical activity: limit competitive sports and heavy labor	Reduce work schedule; rest periods during day	Limit to house and finally to bed and chair
B	Dietary sodium restriction: eliminate salt shaker and heavily salted foods	Eliminate salt in cooking and at table (Na intake 1.2–1.8 g or 50–80 mmol/day)	As in III, plus low-sodium foods (Na intake <1 g or 40 mmol/day)
C	Diuretics: thiazide or low-dose loop diuretic	Loop diuretic (progressive doses); consider adding distally acting (K$^+$-sparing) diuretic	Loop diuretic with distally acting (K$^+$-sparing) and/or thiazide diuretic
D	Digitalis glycosides: conventional maintenance doses	──────────────────→	Dose to maintain serum digoxin level in 1.5 ng/ml range
E	Vasodilators: hydralazine and isosorbide dinitrate or angiotensin-converting enzyme inhibitor	──────────────────→	Intravenous nitroprusside
F			Other inotropic drugs (intravenous): dopamine, dobutamine, amrinone
G			Consider cardiac transplantation; thoracentesis, paracentesis; dialysis, assisted circulation (e.g., intra-aortic balloon pump)

Modified from Smith TW,[3] with permission from the publisher.

CARDIAC GLYCOSIDES

Digitalis has been employed in the treatment of heart failure for more than 200 years. It remains the only class of drugs with a positive inotropic effect currently available for chronic ambulatory use. Following several decades of active controversy, the fundamental cellular mechanism by which the cardiac glycosides exert their positive inotropic effect is now generally agreed to be the following sequence:

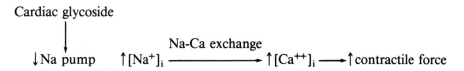

Cardiac glycoside

$\downarrow$ Na pump $\uparrow [Na^+]_i$ ——Na-Ca exchange——→ $\uparrow [Ca^{++}]_i$ ——→$\uparrow$ contractile force

This is summarized, together with some additional features of the cellular mechanism, in Figure 1. Cardiac glycosides bind to the domain of NaK-ATPase that faces the external cell surface, completely inhibiting each "sodium pump" site so occupied. When a fraction of sodium pump sites on a cardiac myocyte are inhibited, the intracellular sodium concentration rises, leading to augmentation of intracellular calcium content through the mechanism of Na^+-Ca^{++} exchange. The enhanced intracellular Ca^{++} store produces an increased contractile state in both normal and failing myocardium. Car-

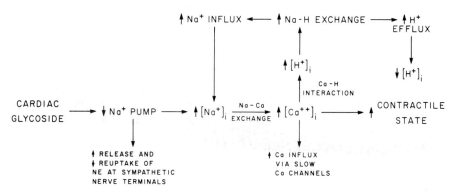

FIG. 1. Mechanisms of modulation of myocardial function by cardiac glycosides. In addition to the horizontal sequence leading from cardiac glycoside-induced inhibition of the sodium-ion pump to enhanced myocardial contractile state, three ancillary processes are shown: enhanced norepinephrine (NE) release and reduced reuptake at cardiac sympathetic-nerve terminals, which may occur in experimental circumstances but has doubtful clinical relevance; an enhanced slow inward calcium current with increased calcium influx through slow calcium channels in response to an increased concentration of intracellular calcium ions over a limited range of values for these ions[4]; and decreased intracellular pH (increased [H^+]) in response to increased intracellular calcium, leading to enhanced sodium-hydrogen exchange and hence augmentation of the rise in intracellular sodium ([Na^+]) caused by sodium-pump inhibition.[5] Reproduced, with permission, from Smith TW. *N Engl J Med* 1988; **318**:358–365.[6]

diac rhythm disturbances frequently encountered in patients who have received excessive digitalis doses appear to result from a further extension of the same basic mechanism of NaK-ATPase inhibition. Thus, intracellular Ca^{++} overload has been implicated as a major contributing factor in causing the cardiac manifestations of digitalis toxicity. The favorable electrophysiologic effects of digitalis in supraventricular tachyarrhythmias are exerted in large part through enhancement of vagal tone. These electrophysiologic effects of digitalis will not be further discussed here.

The positive inotropic effects that underlie the favorable hemodynamic changes in patients with heart failure can be observed in isolated cardiac muscle or in single cardiac muscle cells, as well as in the intact heart. It is useful to examine the effect of cardiac glycosides on the intact circulation in terms of the ventricular function curves illustrated in Figure 2. In contrast to diuretics, which shift ventricular function to the left along a given ventricular function curve, as shown in Figure 2, cardiac glycosides tend to shift cardiac function upward and to the left, resulting in improved cardiac output at any given ventricular filling pressure or volume.

Details of pharmacokinetics, bioavailability, and dosage considerations of cardiac glycosides are discussed in detail elsewhere.[7] Other general aspects of the pharmacological management of heart failure are also considered in detail in standard texts.[8] This presentation concentrates on recent data bearing on the efficacy of digitalis glycosides in patients with congestive heart failure.

During the decade beginning in the late 1960s, a number of authors reported clinical observations that cast doubt on the clinical efficacy of cardiac glycosides in the treatment of congestive heart failure.[9] Most of these studies were uncontrolled but did serve to demonstrate convincingly that substantial numbers of patients were being treated with digitalis who appeared to be receiving little demonstrable benefit despite the appreciable risk of toxicity accompanying the use of these drugs. More recent studies have, however, provided valuable data supporting the efficacy of digitalis in patients with dilated ventricles and systolic ventricular dysfunction. This group of patients is to be carefully distinguished from the subset of patients with preserved systolic function, but with signs and symptoms of heart failure due to "diastolic dysfunction," with reduced left ventricular compliance resulting in elevated left ventricular filling pressures and pulmonary vascular congestion. Thus, Lee *et al.* found that the hallmark of a dilated, poorly contracting ventricle, an S_3 gallop, was a good predictor of a favorable therapeutic response to digoxin.[10]

It is important to emphasize that favorable hemodynamic effects of digoxin are additive to those of vasodilators such as captopril, as shown in Figure 3.[11] Gheorghiade and colleagues[12] found that patients with severe heart failure and sinus rhythm given optimal doses of diuretics and vasodilators responded to the addition of digoxin to the regimen with a further mean increase of 27% in cardiac output, an increase of 59% in left ventricular stroke work index,

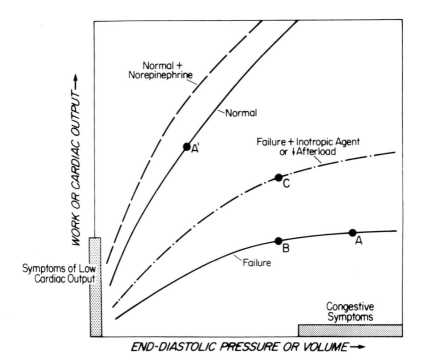

FIG. 2. Schematic diagram demonstrating the relationship between ventricular end-diastolic pressure or volume and cardiac index in a normal and a failing heart. The normal left ventricle increases its stroke output as preload (often measured clinically as pulmonary capillary wedge pressure) increases, moving up the ascending limb of the curve until reserve is exhausted. In heart failure, the ventricular function curve is displaced downward and to the right. An increase in contractility, as after administration of norepinephrine or digitalis, displaces the curve to the left; i.e., a larger stroke output is accomplished at any given filling pressure. A and A' represent the operating points at rest of a hypothetical patient with heart failure and of a normal person, respectively. Reduction of physical activity allows the failing heart to meet the demands of the metabolizing tissues. Treatment of heart failure by a reduction in preload (e.g., with a diuretic or a vasodilator acting predominantly on the venous bed) causes a shift from point A to B on the same ventricular function curve. Administration of a positive inotropic agent or a vasodilator producing afterload reduction will shift the curve as shown, resulting in improvement of the circulatory state in the direction shown by a shift from point A to C. Reproduced with permission, from Smith TW. In *Cecil Textbook of Medicine*, 1987.[3]

and a 29% decrease in pulmonary capillary wedge pressure. The left ventricular ejection fraction increased from an average of 21% to 29% in response to digoxin administration. Of particular interest was the observation, summarized in Figure 4, that patients with residual abnormalities of left ventricular function after optimal doses of diuretics and vasodilators had been given responded with substantially greater hemodynamic improvement in response to digoxin than those patients who had already achieved relatively normal filling pressures and cardiac index values on diuretics and vasodilators alone.

The recent study of Guyatt *et al.*[13] compared digoxin with placebo in 20

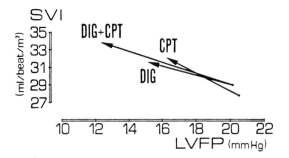

FIG. 3. Combined hemodynamic effects of digoxin (DIG) and captopril (CPT) in patients with left ventricular failure. SVI = stroke volume index; LVFP = left ventricular filling pressure. Reproduced, with permission, from Cantelli I, et al. *Curr Ther Res* 1984; **36**:323–331.[11]

patients with chronic congestive heart failure. In this double-blind crossover trial, seven instances of worsening heart failure occurred when digoxin was switched to placebo compared to no instances of worsening when placebo was switched to digoxin (p < 0.05). In addition, improvement in dyspnea, walking test score, clinical assessment of CHF, and left ventricular ejection fraction were documented during the digoxin phase of the study compared to placebo.

Noteworthy advances in diuretic and vasodilator therapy have obviated the need to use the maximum dose of digitalis that can be tolerated without the emergence of signs or symptoms of digitalis intoxication. It is likely that little, if any, incremental benefit can be expected in patients with normal sinus rhythm from increasing the digoxin dose to levels that produce serum concentrations above the 1.5–2.0 ng/ml range.

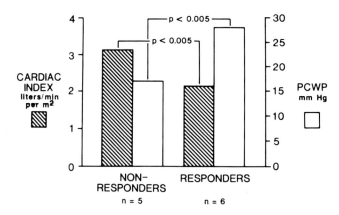

FIG. 4. Baseline differences in cardiac index and pulmonary capillary wedge pressure (PCWP) between five nonresponders and six responders, immediately before the administration of digoxin. Reproduced, with permission, from Gheorghiade M, *et al. J Am Coll Cardiol* 1987; **9**:849–857.[12]

DIURETICS

The retention of salt and water leading to increased intravascular and interstitial fluid is a characteristic abnormality in chronic congestive heart failure. Elimination of such excessive salt and water retention is a principal goal in the treatment of heart failure, and will ameliorate many of the common signs and symptoms.

Diuretic use involves first the elimination of accumulated excess salt and water, followed by maintenance of optimal fluid balance. In general, the mildest diuretic program that achieves and maintains appropriate fluid balance is desirable. Severe salt restriction is not usually necessary and may lead to impaired nutritional status or to hypovolemia with impaired renal function, oliguria, and prerenal azotemia in patients with relatively severe heart failure.

Diuretics ameliorate the abnormalities of heart failure by decreasing the reabsorption of Na^+ and water by the renal tubule. Thiazide diuretics are widely used because of their ease of oral administration, predictable effects, and relative freedom from toxicity. All agents in this class inhibit NaCl reabsorption in the distal tubule. Thus, dilution of tubular fluid is preserved and there is enhanced delivery of solute and water to the H^+- and K^+-secreting sites in the collecting duct. The efficacy of the thiazides is limited by avid solute reabsorption in the proximal nephron in patients with glomerular filtration rates (GFRs) less than about 30 ml/min. A number of potentially troublesome metabolic side effects deserve mention, including K^+ depletion, hyperuricemia, glucose intolerance, and plasma lipid elevations.

Loop diuretics are the most potent diuretics in routine clinical use and can induce a natriuresis (at least transiently) of as much as 20% of the filtered load of sodium ions. They are frequently used intravenously in acute pulmonary edema, and are also of value in severe or refractory heart failure or when renal functional impairment is present. The agents in this class (furosemide, ethacrynic acid, bumetanide, and piretanide) act to inhibit the Na/K/Cl cotransport system in the thick ascending limb of the loop of Henle. The absorption of furosemide from the gastrointestinal tract is variable, averaging about 60%. This tends to decrease when the drug is given with meals and may also be reduced in the presence of congestive heart failure. Nonsteroidal anti-inflammatory drugs, including aspirin, tend to blunt the usual response to loop diuretics and may account for worsening heart failure.

Potassium-sparing diuretics include the aldosterone antagonist, spironolactone, and those drugs that directly inhibit Na^+ permeability in the collecting duct (amiloride and triamtrene). All of these drugs reduce renal K^+ secretion, and are of use in combination with thiazides or loop diuretics that tend to increase K^+ excretion. They are all capable of producing clinically significant hyperkalemia, particularly in patients with renal insufficiency.

In patients with advanced and refractory heart failure, combined use of diuretics is frequently helpful. Appropriate combinations will tend to avoid electrolyte disturbance that may occur with the use of a powerful loop diuretic alone, and appropriately chosen combinations will tend to augment salt and water excretion in patients with refractory edema. Thus, combined use of K^+-sparing diuretics with more proximally-acting agents such as thiazides or loop diuretics limits K^+ and H^+ loss. Combined use of loop diuretics with a thiazide or metolazone often results in a synergistic enhancement of Na^+ and water excretion, but must be used with great care because of the propensity of this combination to produce marked intravascular volume depletion and K^+ loss.

A useful rule of thumb is to avoid sudden volume shifts or intravascular volume depletion by aiming at no more than about 1 kg of fluid loss per day. Further details of diuretic use in congestive heart failure may be found in the discussion of Smith *et al.*[8]

CONCLUSIONS

The therapeutic choices in the treatment of CHF have become broader and more effective in recent years. The recognition of an important subset of patients with diastolic rather than systolic dysfunction demands that appropriate attention be paid to the underlying pathophysiology producing the signs and symptoms of CHF. When impaired diastolic function due to left ventricular hypertrophy or ischemia produces markedly elevated filling pressures despite reasonably well-preserved systolic function, emphasis should be placed on treating the underlying causes of reduced ventricular compliance rather than on inotropic support with digitalis glycosides. The treatment of patients with dilated ventricles and impaired systolic contractile function should seek to correct abnormalities of preload and afterload by means of diuretics and vasodilators. The angiotensin-converting enzyme inhibitors are particularly valuable in producing a balanced vasodilator response. As noted earlier, the combined effect of digoxin and angiotensin-converting enzyme inhibitors has been particularly impressive when compared with either agent alone.[11,12]

Finally, although this discussion has considered approaches to the symptom complex resulting from elevated ventricular filling pressures and reduced cardiac output, two additional major problems are frequently encountered in patients with overt heart failure: high-grade ventricular arrhythmias are commonly encountered, and deserve attention even though the efficacy of anti-arrhythmic drug therapy in this setting remains to be proven;[14] and pulmonary and systemic thromboemboli also produce substantial morbidity and mortality, and anticoagulation deserves consideration in patients with severely reduced left ventricular ejection fractions.

REFERENCES

1. McKee PA, Castelli WP, McNamara PM, Kannel WB. The natural history of congestive heart failure: the Framingham study. *N Engl J Med* 1971; **285**:1441–1446.

2. Massie BM, Conway M. Survival of patients with congestive heart failure: past, present and future prospects. *Circulation* 1987; **75 (suppl IV)**:Iv-11-IV-19.
3. Smith, TW. Heart failure. In Wyngaarden J, Smith LH Jr, eds. *Cecil Textbook of Medicine*, 18th edition. Philadelphia, WB Saunders Co, 1987.
4. Eisner DA, Lederer WJ, Vaughan-Jones RD. The quantitative relationship between twitch tension and intracellular sodium activity in sheep cardiac Purkinje fibers. *J Physiol (Lond)* 1984; **355**:251-266.
5. Kim D, Cragoe EJ Jr, Smith TW. Relations among sodium pump inhibition, Na-Ca and Na-H exchange activities, and Ca-H interaction in cultured chick heart cells. *Circ Res* 1987; **60**:185-193.
6. Smith TW. Digitalis. mechanisms of action and clinical use. *N Engl J Med* 1988; **318**:358-365.
7. Smith TW, ed. *Digitalis Glycosides*. Orlando, Grune & Stratton, 1986.
8. Smith TW, Kelly RA, Braunwald E. The management of heart failure. In Braunwald E, ed. *Heart Disease*, 3rd edition. Philadelphia, WB Saunders Co, 1988, 485-543.
9. Smith TW. Medical treatment of advanced congestive heart failure: Digitalis and diuretics. In Braunwald E, Mock MB, Watson JR, eds. *Congestive Heart Failure*. New York, Grune & Stratton, 1982, 261-278.
10. Lee DC-S, Johnson RA, Bingham JB, et al. Heart failure in outpatients: a randomized trial of digoxin versus placebo. *N Engl J Med* 1982; **306**:699-705.
11. Cantelli I, Vitolo A, Lombardi G, Bomba E, Bracchetti D. Combined hemodynamic effects of digoxin and captopril in patients with congestive heart failure. *Curr Ther Res* 1984; **36**:323-331.
12. Gheorghiade M, St. Clair J, St. Clair C, Beller GA. Hemodynamic effects of intravenous digoxin in patients with severe heart failure initially treated with diuretics and vasodilators. *J Am Coll Cardiol* 1987; **9**:849-857.
13. Guyatt GH, Sullivan MJJ, Fallen EL, et al. A controlled trial of digoxin in congestive heart failure. *Am J Cardiol* 1988; **61**:371-375.
14. Bigger JT Jr. Why patients with congestive heart failure die: arrhythmias and sudden cardiac death. *Circulation* 1987; **75 (suppl IV)**:IV-28-IV-35.

SUMMARY

Despite major advances in many areas of cardiovascular therapeutics in the past few decades, the prognosis for patients with overt congestive heart failure (CHF) remains quite poor. There is, therefore, a compelling case for prevention of end-stage heart failure with CHF. The three types of approaches used in the contemporary management of CHF are (1) the removal of the underlying causes of heart failure, (2) the removal of the precipitating causes, and (3) treatment of the clinical manifestations of heart failure. This third category includes interventions to enhance pump performance (e.g., the use of digitalis glycosides and sympathomimetic drugs), the reduction of work load, and the control of salt and water retention (e.g., restriction of salt intake, use of diuretics). The history of the use of cardiac glycosides and diuretics in heart failure is traced, and some recent studies are reviewed. It is emphasized that the diverse etiologies and degrees of severity of heart failure require an individualized approach in each case. The therapeutic choices in the treatment of CHF have become wider in recent years, and the recognition of different subsets of patients with CHF is enabling more appropriate selection of treatment to be made.

RÉSUMÉ

Le traitement médical des insuffisances cardiaques a beaucoup évolué au cours de ces vingt dernières années, cependant le pronostic pour les patients atteints d'insufissance cardiaque congestive demeure assez mauvais. Il est donc impératif de prendre des mesures préventives contre la phase finale de l'insuffisance cardiaque dans le cas d'insuffisance cardiaque congestive. On discute ici des trois schémas thérapeutiques utilisés actuellement dans le traitement des insuffisances cardiaques. Ce sont:
1. la suppression des causes fondamentales d'insuffisance cardiaque
2. la suppression des causes précipitantes
3. le traitement des manifestations cliniques d'insuffisance cardiaque.
Cette troisième catégorie comprend les traitements qui ont pour objectif d'accroître la performance cardiaque (d'où l'utilisation de glucosides digitaliques et la prescription de médicaments sympathomimétiques), la réduction des heures de travail et le contrôle de la rétention hydrosodée (d'où restriction de sel dans le régime alimentaire et utilisation de diurétiques). On retrace l'histoire de l'utilisation des glucosides cardiaques et des diurétiques dans les cas d'insuffisance cardiaque et on fait le point sur les études les plus récentes. On insiste sur le fait que l'on doit tenir compte de la diversité des étiologies et du degré de sévérité des insuffisances cardiaques et envisager des traitments thérapeutiques individualisés dans chaque cas. Ces dernières années on a disposé d'un choix beaucoup plus grand de traitements médicaux et le fait d'avoir établi différents sous-groupes de patients atteints d'insuffisance cardiaque congestive permet un choix plus approprié des traitements.

ZUSAMMENFASSUNG

Trotz grosser Fortschritte auf vielen Gebieten der Herzgefässtherapie in den letzten paar Jahrzehnten bleibt die Prognose für Patienten mit offenbarer hyperhämischer Herzinsuffizienz (CHF) relativ schlecht. Die Verhütung des Endstadiums der Herzinsuffizienz CHF ist daher zwingend. Diese Veröffentlichung diskutiert die drei Methoden, die gegenwärtig in der Behandlung des CHF angewendet werden. Diese sind folgende: 1. Entfernung der Gründe für die Herzinsuffizienz, 2. Entfernung der auslösenden Faktoren, und 3. Behandlung der klinischen Auswirkungen der Herzinsuffizienz. Diese dritte Kategorie schliesst Bemühungen ein, die Pumpenleistung zu verbessern (zum Beispiel die Verwendung von Digitalis-Glykosiden und sympathikomimetischen Drogen), die Reduktion der Arbeitsbelastung und die Kontrolle der Salz- und Wasserretention (zum Beispiel Beschränkung der Salzaufnahme, Anwendung von Diuretika). Es folgt die Entwicklungsgeschichte der Verwendung von Herzgefäss-Glykosiden und Diuretika und eine Besprechung einiger neuerer Veröffentlichungen. Der Autor betont, dass die diversen Äthiologien und die Schwere der Herzinsuffizienz eine individuelle Behandlung jedes Falls fordern. In den letzten Jahren sind die therapeutischen Möglichkeiten der Behandlung von CHF ausgeweitet worden, und das Erkennen von diversen Untergruppen von Patienten mit CHF macht eine angemessenere Auswahl der Behandlungsmethode möglich.

RIASSUNTO

Malgrado importanti passi avanti in molti campi della terapeutica cardiovascolare negli ultimi decenni, la prognosi per pazienti con manifesta insufficienza cardiaca congestizia rimane scadente. E'quindi estremamente importante prevenire il manifestarsi dello stadio finale dell'insufficienza cardiaca congestizia. Vengono discussi i tre tipi di metodi usati attualmente per gestire l'insufficienza cardiaca congestizia. Essi sono: 1) la rimozione delle cause soggiacenti dell'insufficienza cardiaca; 2) la rimozione delle cause che la fanno precipitare; e 3) cura delle manifestazioni cliniche dell'insufficienza cardiaca. La terza categoria comprende gli interventi per migliorare le prestazioni di pompaggio (p. es.: l'uso di digitalis glucosides e di farmaci simpatomimetici), la riduzione del carico di lavoro ed il controllo della ritenzione di sale e d'acqua (per es.: limitazione del consumo di sale, uso di diuretici). Viene ripercorsa la storia dell'uso di glicosidi cardiaci e di diuretici per l'insufficienza cardiaca e vengono passati in rassegna alcuni studi recenti. Viene sottolineato che le diverse eziologie ed il diverso grado di gravità dell'insufficienza cardiaca richiedono un approccio individualizzato per ogni caso. Le scelte terapeutiche nella cura dell'insufficienza cardiaca congestizia si sono allargate negli ultimi anni e il riconoscimento di diversi sottogruppi di pazienti affetti da insufficienza cardiaca congestizia permette di fare una scelta più appropriata della cura.

SUMÁRIO

Apesar de importantes avanços em muitas áreas da terapia cardiovascular nas últimas décadas, o prognóstico para pacientes com insuficiência cardíaca congestiva (CHF) manifesta fica bastante má. Portanto, há um caso convincente para a prevenção das últimas etapas da insuficiência cardíaca congestiva. Discutem-se três tipos de enfoque utilizados no manejo contemporâneo da CHF. Estos são: 1) a remoção das causas básicas da insuficiência cardíaca, 2) a remoção das causas precipitantes, 3) o tratamento das manifestações clínicas da insuficiência cardíaca. Esta terceira categoria inclui as intervenções para aumentar o bombeamento de sangue (por exemplo, o uso de glicósidos digitálicos e drogas simpatomiméticas), a redução da carga cardíaca e o controle da retenção de água e sal (por exemplo, restrição de ingestão de sal, uso de diuréticos). Esboça-se a história do uso de glicósidos cardíacos e diuréticos na insuficiência cardíaca, e revisam-se alguns estudos recentes. Enfatiza-se que as diversas etiologias e grau de severidade da insuficiência cardíaca requerem um enfoque individualizado em cada caso. Nos últimos anos, tem sido um aumento no número de possíveis tratamentos da CHF, e o reconhecimento dos diferentes subconjuntos de pacientes com CHF permite uma seleção mais apropriada do tratamento.

RESUMEN

A pesar de importantes avances en muchas áreas de la terapia cardiovascular en las últimas décadas, la prognosis para pacientes con insuficiencia cardíaca congestiva manifiesta (CHF) es bastante mala. Por lo tanto, esto representa un claro caso para la prevención de las últimas etapas de la insuficiencia cardíaca congestiva. Se discuten tres de enfoque empleados en el manejo contemporáneo de la CHF. Estos son: 1) la remoción de las causas básicas de la insuficiencia cardíaca, 2) la remoción de las causas precipitantes, y 3) el tratamiento de las manifestaciones clínicas de la insuficiencia cardíaca. Esta tercera categoría incluye las intervenciones para mejorar el bombeo de sangre (por ejemplo, el empleo de glucósidos digitálicos y fármacos simpatomiméticos), la reducción de la carga cardíaca y el control de la retención de agua y sal (por ejemplo, restricción de ingestión de sal, empleo de diuréticos). Se bosqueja la historia del empleo de glucósidos cardíacos y diuréticos en la insuficiencia cardíaca, y se repasan algunos estudios recientes. Se enfatiza que las diversas etiologías y grado de severidad de la insuficiencia cardíaca requieren un enfoque individualizado en cada caso. En los últimos años ha habido un incremento en el número de posibles tratamientos de la CHF, y el reconocimiento de los diferentes tipos de pacientes con CHF permite una selección más apropiada del tratamiento.

要約

過去数十年間に，心血管治療法の多くの分野での大きな進歩にもかかわらず，明白なうっ血性心不全（CHF）患者の予後はきわめて不良のままである。そこで，CHF の最終段階に至るのを予防せざるをえない場合が生じてくる。

ここでは，CHF 治療に現在用いられている 3 タイプの方法について考察する。すなわち，心不全の根本原因の除去，促進要因の除去，および臨床症状に対する治療の 3 つである。第 3 の範疇には，ポンプ機能亢進のための治療（たとえばジギタリス，交感神経刺激薬），仕事負荷の軽減，および食塩・水分貯留のコントロール（たとえば食塩摂取の制限，利尿薬の使用）などが含まれる。

心不全における強心配糖体および利尿薬の使用の歴史をふりかえり，いくつかの最近の研究についても概説する。とくに，各症例ごとに個別的なアプローチを行うためには，種々の病因学的検討と心不全の重症度判定が必要であるという点を強調したい。CHF 治療法の選択の幅は近年広がりつつあり，CHF 患者の異なる亜群をみきわめることによって，より適切な治療法の選択が可能になりつつある。

Cardiac and Renal Failure: An Expanding Role for ACE Inhibitors, edited by C. T. Dollery and L. M. Sherwood, Hanley & Belfus, Inc., Philadelphia.

Vasodilator Therapy of Heart Failure

Jay N. Cohn

Vasodilator drugs have achieved acceptance in the management of heart failure based on physiologic considerations buttressed by a wide array of clinical studies carried out over the past 15 years. We shall briefly review these data and consider future directions for research into clinical applications of this approach to the management of left ventricular dysfunction.

AORTIC IMPEDANCE AND LEFT VENTRICULAR FUNCTION

The role of aortic impedance in the control of left ventricular dysfunction was neglected in early studies that defined ventricular function as dependent on filling pressure and contractility.[1] Since the normal ventricle appeared capable of adjusting its performance to match imposed changes in outflow resistance,[2] it was assumed that resistance to ejection was not a dominant factor in the impaired ventricular performance of heart failure. However, when studies were performed in animal models of myocardial failure or in patients with clinical heart failure, the important influence of impedance on left ventricular performance became apparent.[3,4]

Early clinical studies demonstrated a dramatic, favorable hemodynamic response to intravenous infusions of sodium nitroprusside or phentolamine in patients with severe left ventricular failure.[5,6] The favorable effect of nitroprusside on stroke volume and cardiac output could be attributed largely to the arterial dilating action of the drug. The accompanying reduction in left ventricular filling pressure implied, in addition, an acute redistribution of vascular volume out of the heart and lungs and into the peripheral vascular reservoir. This volume redistribution is dependent largely on relaxation of venous capacitance vessels.[7]

The arterial effects of many vasodilators, including nitroprusside, involve an action on arterial compliance as well as arteriolar resistance. In recent studies we have utilized a diastolic pulse wave analysis technique to quantitate proximal and distal arterial compliance on the basis of a modified

185

windkessel model of the circulation.[8] Distal compliance is strikingly reduced in heart failure, and nitroprusside infusion results in a prominent rise in both proximal and distal compliance, as well as a fall in arteriolar resistance.[9] Thus, the vascular contribution to pulsatile flow phenomena may play a critical role in the hemodynamic response to drugs in patients with heart failure.

MECHANISM OF VASOCONSTRICTION

The favorable hemodynamic response to vasodilator drugs in heart failure implies that the vasculature is inappropriately vasoconstricted in this syndrome. We have sought to define the mechanism of this vasoconstriction by assessing the neurohormonal response to heart failure. Plasma concentration of norepinephrine, an index of sympathetic nervous system activation, is almost always increased in heart failure.[10] Plasma renin activity, an index of activity of the renin-angiotensin-aldosterone system, is frequently elevated, sometimes to exceedingly high levels.[10] Plasma arginine-vasopressin also is frequently elevated.[11] These three endogenous vasoconstrictor systems, therefore, appear to be activated adequately to account for intense vasoconstriction in the syndrome.

Despite the evidence for neurohormonal activation, however, the degree of vasoconstrictor hormone release does not appear to correlate well with the severity of systemic vasoconstriction assessed by hemodynamic measurements.[10] Furthermore, levels of atrial natriuretic peptide, which may function as a vasodilator, also are increased in heart failure.[12] This hormone may, therefore, tend to counteract some of the vasoconstrictor effect of the other systems. Indeed, it is likely that a variety of other local or circulating hormonal systems may be activated in heart failure and contribute to the net vascular tone. Alterations in endothelial relaxing and constricting factors could also influence local vascular tone.

Although the correlation between neurohormonal stimulation and hemodynamic derangement is poor, the degree of sympathetic activation appears to be a useful guide to prognosis in heart failure. Plasma norepinephrine serves as a sensitive predictor of long-term mortality in the syndome.[13] It is unknown whether this relationship between sympathetic activation and mortality is indicative of a direct deleterious effect of sympathetic stimulation or merely suggests that the sympathetic activation is a marker for the severity of the disease.

CLINICAL RESPONSE TO VASODILATOR THERAPY

The physiological rationale and hemodynamic response to vasodilator drugs in heart failure do not necessarily mean that the drugs will have a long-term beneficial effect in the syndrome. Over the past 10 years a large number of clinical trials have been carried out to address the question of clinical efficacy. These studies have been hindered by the absence of a clear-cut end-point that can be used as an index of clinical response. In most studies, exercise tolerance has served as the primary end-point because exercise intolerance is a primary symptom in most patients with congestive heart failure. However, selection of an appropriate exercise test protocol that is reproducible and sensitive to therapeutic intervention has been a formidable problem. Most studies have utilized a gradually progressive exercise test that is terminated by dyspnea, fatigue, or a metabolic index of anaerobiosis, usually a rise in the respiratory exchange ratio of CO_2 and O_2. The end-point of such tests has been either duration of exercise or the peak oxygen consumption (VO_2) achieved.

Results of controlled studies utilizing exercise tolerance to assess this chronic response to vasodilator drugs have been quite variable. In some studies the drugs have been reported to significantly improve exercise tolerance;[14,15] in others there has been no apparent efficacy;[16] and in still others the results have been equivocal.[17] Among the problems in these studies is the fact that the duration of the exercise test may be determined subjectively by both the patient and the physician, and that a large placebo effect is often apparent. It is clear that there is need for the development of a more objective and discriminating test of exercise performance in patients with heart failure.

Other clinical end-points for efficacy of vasodilator therapy have not been well-standardized or well-accepted. Perhaps the most attractive is the attempt to assess quality of life.[18] Since the only goals of therapy are to increase the quality of life or the duration of life, exercise tolerance can at best serve as a surrogate for quality of life. The reason for choosing this surrogate is that quality of life assessments are generally viewed as too subjective and too qualitative to serve as a useful primary therapeutic end-point. However, the problems encountered with quantitative exercise testing, and the development of validated and sensitive questionnaires to assess disease-specific effects on life quality may lead to a reassessment of this view.

We have developed a "Living With Heart Failure" questionnaire that has been assessed in a growing number of patients with left ventricular dysfunction and heart failure.[19] Our preliminary data suggest that the scores on this questionnaire provide a reproducible guide to the severity of heart failure and that the scores may provide a sensitive index of therapeutic efficacy.

EFFECT OF VASODILATORS ON MORTALITY

The improvement in left ventricular function accompanying vasodilator therapy of heart failure was, until recently, viewed by most as a "cosmetic" response that would not alter the natural history of the disease. That concept has now undergone revision as a result of two recent clinical trials demonstrating that chronic administration of vasodilator drugs to patients already treated with digitalis and diuretics can significantly prolong life. The first of these trials, the Veterans Administration Vasodilator-Heart Failure Trial (V-HeFT), studied the effect of hydralazine and isosorbide dinitrate vs. prazosin and vs. placebo in a three-armed study in patients with mild-to-moderate (Class II–III) heart failure.[20] The other trial from Northern Scandinavia (CONSENSUS) studied the effect of enalapril in severe (Class IV) heart failure.[21] The V-HeFT was carried out over more than 5 years, whereas the CONSENSUS study was terminated after 1 year because of the high event rate in the severely ill group of patients. A similar reduction in mortality was observed at the 1-year time point common to the two studies. In the V-HeFT, the 1-year mortality was reduced by 38% and in CONSENSUS by 31%. Interestingly, the other vasodilator in the V-HeFT, prazosin, exerted no favorable effect on survival. Thus, all vasodilators may not be equally effective in altering the natural history of heart failure.

The favorable effects of the nonspecific vasodilators, hydralazine and isosorbide dinitrate, and of the converting-enzyme inhibitor enalapril, now raise the issue as to whether neurohormonal inhibition or direct vasodilation is the preferable approach to therapy. Indeed, perhaps a nonspecific vasodilator regimen plus an ACE inhibitor would be an even more effective therapy. V-HeFT II is now comparing enalapril and hydralazine-nitrate in the same patient population. Study of combined therapy must await subsequent trials.

PREVENTION OF HEART FAILURE

The beneficial effects of vasodilators in symptomatic heart failure have now raised the possibility that interference with the vicious cycle of vasoconstriction could have a favorable effect on the natural history of left ventricular dysfunction when therapy is introduced in the asymptomatic or presymptomatic phase of the disease. The overriding concept behind this approach is that prevention of heart failure is infinitely more desirable than treating it.

Two current studies are exploring the use of ACE inhibitors in patients with left ventricular dysfunction who are not necessarily symptomatic. One study sponsored by the National Heart Lung and Blood Institute (known as SOLVD) is utilizing enalapril vs. placebo in the therapeutic regimens. The other trial sponsored by industry is utilizing captopril vs. placebo. An answer to this important question will likely not become available from these studies before 1991.

Thus, the concept of vasodilator therapy for the failing heart has moved rather quickly from the laboratory to the clinic and to large-scale trials. These drugs now appear to form a cornerstone of therapy for heart failure. But further and more detailed proof of efficacy, and the need for better drugs and drug combinations should keep clinical investigators busy for the next decade.

REFERENCES

1. Sarnoff SJ, Berglund E. Ventricular function. I. Starling's law of the heart studies by means of simultaneous right and left ventricular function curves in the dog. *Circulation* 1954; 9:706.
2. Sarnoff SJ, Mitchell JH, Gilmore JP, Remensnyder JP. Homeometric autoregulation of the heart. *Circ Res* 1960; 8:1077.
3. Cohn JH. Vasodilator therapy for heart failure: The influence of impedance on left ventricular performance. *Circulation* 1973; 48:5-8.
4. Cohn JH, Mashiro I, Levine TB, Mehta J. Role of vasoconstrictor mechanisms in the control of left ventricular performance of the normal and damaged heart. *Am J Cardiol* 1979; 44:1019-1022.
5. Majid PA, Sharma B, Taylor SH. Phentolamine for vasodilator treatment of severe heart failure. *Lancet* 1971; 2:720.
6. Franciosa JA, Giuha NH, Limas CJ, Rodriguera E, Cohn JN. Improved left ventricular function during nitroprusside infusion in acute myocardial infarction. *Lancet* 1972; 1:650-654.
7. Franciosa JA, Pierpont G, Cohn JN. Hemodynamic improvement after oral hydralazine in left ventricular failure: A comparison with nitroprusside infusion in 16 patients. *Ann Intern Med* 1977; 86:388-393.
8. Watt B, Burrus C. Arterial pressure contour analysis for estimating human vascular properties. *J Appl Physiol* 1976; 40:171-176.
9. Finkelstein SM, Cohn JN, Collins RV, Carlyle PF, Shelley W. Vascular hemodynamic impedance in congestive heart failure. *Am J Cardiol* 1985; 55:423-427.
10. Levine TB, Francis GS, Goldsmith SR, Simon A, Cohn JN. Activity of the sympathetic nervous system and renin-angiotensin system assessed by plasma hormone levels and their relationship to hemodynamic abnormalities in congestive heart failure. *Am J Cardiol* 1982; 49:1659-1666.
11. Goldsmith SR, Francis GS, Cowley AW, Levine TB, Cohn JN. Increased plasma arginine vasopressin in patients with congestive heart failure. *J Am Coll Cardiol* 1983; 1:1385-1390.
12. Raine AEG, Erne P, Burgisser E, Müller FB, Bolli P, Burkart F, Bühler FB. Atrial natriuretic peptide and atrial pressure in patients with congestive heart failure. *N Engl J Med* 1986; 315:533-537.
13. Cohn JN, Levine TB, Olivari MT, Garberg V, Lura D, Francis GS, Simon A. Plasma norepinephrine as a guide to prognosis in patients with chronic congestive heart failure. *N Engl J Med* 1984; 311:819-823.
14. Captopril Multicenter Research Group. A placebo-controlled trial of captopril in refractory chronic congestive heart failure. *J Am Coll Cardiol* 1983; 2:755-763.
15. Franciosa JA, Goldsmith SR, Cohn JN. Contrasting immediate and long-term effects of isosorbide dinitrate on exercise capacity in congestive heart failure. *Am J Med* 1980; 69:559-566.
16. Franciosa JA, Jordan RA, Wilen MM, Reddy CL. Minoxidil in patients with chronic left heart failure: Contrasting hemodynamic and clinical effects in a controlled trial. *Circulation* 1984; 70:63.
17. Franciosa JA, Weber KT, Levin TB, Kinasewitz GT, Janicki JS, West J, Henis M, Cohn JN. Hydralazine in the long-term treatment of chronic heart failure: Lack of differences from placebo. *Am Heart J* 1982; 104:587-594.
18. Rector TS, Cohn JN. Quality of life and congestive heart failure: Implications for clinical care. *Quality of Life and Cardiovascular Care* 1986; 1:262-266.
19. Rector TS, Kubo SK, Cohn JN. Patient's self-assessment of their congestive heart failure. Part 2. Content, reliability and validity of a new measure, The Minnesota Living with Heart Failure Questionnaire. *Heart Failure* 1987; 3:198-209.
20. Cohn JN, Archibald DG, Ziesche S, Franciosa JA, Harston WE, Tristani FE, Dunkman WB, Jacobs W, Francis GS, Flohr KH, Goldman S, Cobb FR, Shah PM, Saunders R, Fletcher RD, Loeb HS, Hughes VC, Baker B. Effect of vasodilator therapy on mortality in chronic congestive heart failure. Results of a Veterans Administration Cooperative Study (V-HeFT). *N Engl J Med* 1986; 314:1547-1552.
21. The CONSENSUS Trial Study Group. Effects of enalapril on mortality in severe congestive heart failure. *N Engl J Med* 1987; 316:1429.

SUMMARY

Over the past 15 years, vasodilator drugs have been shown to produce a significant improvement in cardiac performance and have thus achieved wide acceptance in the management of heart failure. The efficacy of vasodilator therapy has been more difficult to establish. Recent attempts have been made to assess efficacy of vasodilator therapy through a measurement of quality of life, since improvement of quality of life is one of the main goals of treatment. Exercise tests have traditionally been used as a surrogate, but the results have been variable and more objective and discriminating tests for exercise performance are needed. A questionnaire entitled "Living with Heart Failure" has been developed to assess patients with left ventricular dysfunction and heart failure. Preliminary results suggest that it provides a reproducible guide to the severity of heart failure and a sensitive index of therapeutic efficacy. The effects of vasodilators on mortality have been examined in the Veterans Administration Vasodilator-Heart Failure Trial (V-HeFT) and the Northern Scandinavia (CONSENSUS) trial. The results indicate that vasodilator therapy can prolong life, but that not all vasodilators are equally effective in altering the natural history of heart failure. An unresolved question is whether inhibition of neurohormonal vasoconstriction or direct vasodilation is the better approach to therapy. The outcome of further trials is awaited. The possible advantages of using vasodilators in the prevention of heart failure, by early treatment of asymptomatic left ventricular dysfunction, is also under active study.

RÉSUMÉ

Au cours de ces quinze dernières années, l'utilisation des vasodilatateurs a montré une nette amélioration de la performance cardiaque. Ils sont donc maintenant bien acceptés dans le traitement des insuffisances cardiaques. Il a été plus difficile d'établir l'efficacité des agents vasodilatateurs. On a récemment essayé d'évaluer l'efficacité des vasodilatateurs en mesurant le confort de vie, étant donné que l'amélioration du confort de vie demeure l'un des principaux objectifs du traitement. On a traditionnellement utilisé des tests d'exercices physiques comme substituts mais on a obtenu des résultats variables. Il s'avère donc nécessaire de découvrir des tests plus objectifs et plus précis. On a rédigé un questionnaire intitulé: "Vivre avec une insuffisance cardiaque". L'objectif de ce questionnaire était d'évaluer les patients atteints d'une hypertrophie ventriculaire gauche et d'insuffisance cardiaque. Les premiers résultats font apparaître un guide reproductible du degré de sévérité des insuffisances cardiaques et un répertoire sensible de l'efficacité thérapeutique. L'étude des Vétérans aux Etats-Unis (Veterans Administration Vasodilator-Heart Failure Trials — V-HeFT) et l'étude Consensus en Scandinavie du nord ont démontré que les agents vasodilatateurs peuvent prolonger la vie, cependant tous les vasodilatateurs n'ont pas la même efficacité sur l'atération de l'histoire naturelle de l'insuffisance cardiaque. On se demande toujours si l'inhibition de vasoconstriction neurohormonale ou de vasodilatation directe est une meilleure stratégie thérapeutique. On attend les résultats d'études en cours. Des études sur les effets bénéfiques des vasodilatateurs en terme de prévention des insuffisances cardiaques, utilisés à un stade précoce du traitement de l'insuffisance ventriculaire gauche asymptomatique, sont actuellement en cours.

ZUSAMMENFASSUNG

Die letzten 15 Jahre haben gezeigt, dass gefässerweiternde Drogen eine deutliche Verbesserung der Herzleistung bewirken, was zu ihrer weitreichenden Verwendung in der Behandlung von Herzinsuffizienz geführt hat. Weit schwieriger ist es, die Wirksamkeit vasodilatorischer Therapien festzustellen. Kürzliche Versuche haben die Wirksamkeit vasodilatorischer Therapien festzustellen. Kürzliche Versuche haben die Wirksamkeit gefässerweiternder Therapie mit Messungen der Lebensqualität korreliert, da die Verbesserung der Lebensqualität eins der Hauptziele der Behandlung darstellt. Traditionell wurden Bewegungstests ersatzweise benutzt; aber die Resultate variierten, und objektivere und besser diskriminierende Bewegungstests werden benötigt. Ein Fragebogen mit dem Titel "Leben mit Herzinsuffizienz" ist entwickelt worden, um Patienten mit Dysfunktion der linken Herzkammer und Herzinsuffizienz auszuwerten. Die vorläufigen Ergebnisse zeigen, dass dieser Auswertungsbogen einen reproduzierbaren Hinweis auf die Schwere der Herzinsuffizienz liefert und ausserdem sensible Richtlinien für die therapeutische Wirksamkeit zur Verfügung stellt. Zwei Studien haben die Effekte von Vasodilatoren auf die Mortalitätsrate untersucht: der Veterans Administration Vasodilatoren-Herzinsuffizienzversuch (V-HeFT) und der Nord-Skandinavien-Versuch (CONSENSUS). Die Ergebnisse zeigen, dass gefässerweiternde Therapie die Lebensspanne verlängern kann; aber auch, dass nicht alle Vasodilatoren die gleiche Wirksamkeit in der Änderung des natürlichen Verlaufs des Herzversagens aufweisen. Die Frage, ob Inhibition der neurohormonalen Gefässkontraktion oder direkte Gefässerweiterung bessere therapeutische Effekte zeigt, ist ungeklärt. Gegenwärtige Forschungsprojekte beschäftigen sich aktiv mit den möglichen Vorteilen der Verwendung von Vasodilatoren in der präventativen Behandlung von Herzinsuffizienz durch frühzeitige Behandlung der asymptomatischen Dysfunktion der linken Herzkammer.

RIASSUNTO

Nel corso degli ultimi 15 anni, è stato dimostrato che i farmaci vasodilatatori producono un significativo miglioramento delle prestazioni cardiache e questi sono quindi stati generalmente accettati per la gestione delle insufficienze cardiache. L'efficacia della terapia a base di vasodilatatori è stata più difficile da stabilire. Sono stati fatti recentemente dei tentativi di valutare l'efficacia della terapia a base di vasodilatatori mediante una misurazione della qualità della vita, dato che il miglioramento della qualità della vita è uno degli scopi principali della cura. Tradizionalmente sono stati usati test d'esercizio fisico come surrogato, ma i risultati sono stati variabili e c'è l'esigenza di test più obiettivi e discriminatori per le prestazioni nell'esercizio fisico. E' stato preparato un questionario intitolato "Come vivere con l'insufficienza cardiaca" al fine di valutare i pazienti con disfunzione ventricolare sinistra e insufficienza cardiaca. I risultati preliminari fanno pensare che si tratta di una guida riproducibile alla gravità dell'insufficienza cardiaca ed un indice sensibile dell'efficacia terapeutica. Gli effetti dei vasodilatatori sulla mortalità sono stati esaminati nell'esperimento Vasodilatatore-Insufficienza cardiaca della Veterans Administration (V-HeFT) e nell'esperimento della Scandinavia del Nord (CONSENSUS). I risultati indicano che la terapia a base di vasodilatatori può prolungare la vita ma che non tutti i vasodilatatori sono ugualmente efficaci nell'alterare il progresso naturale dell'insufficienza cardiaca. Una questione irrisolta è se il miglior approccio alla terapia sia l'inibizione della vasocostrizione neuroormonale o la vasodilatazione diretta. Si attende il risultato di altri esperimenti. I possibili vantaggi dell'uso di vasodilatatori nella prevenzione dell'insufficienza cardiaca, mediante cura della disfunzione ventricolare sinistra asintomatica, sono anch'essi attivamente sotto studio.

SUMÁRIO

Nos últimos 15 anos, tem-se demonstrado que as drogas vasodilatadoras produzem uma melhoria significativa na função cardíaca e portanto tem-se conseguido ampla aceptação no manejo da insuficiência cardíaca. Tem sido mais difícil estabelecer a eficácia da terapia vasodilatora. Últimamente, têm-se realizado vários intentos de avaliar a eficácia da terapia vasodilatora mediante a medição da "qualidade de vida", já que a melhoria da qualidade de vida é uma das metas principais do tratamento. Os testes de exercício têm sido utilizados tradicionalmente como um substituto, mas os resultados têm sido variáveis e precisam-se testes mais objectivos e discriminatórios para os exercícios. Tem-se desenvolvido um questionário titulado "Vivendo com a insuficiência cardíaca" para avaliar pacientes com disfunção do ventrículo esquerdo e insuficiência cardíaca. Os resultados preliminares sugerem que este questionário proporciona uma guia reproduzível da severidade da insuficiência cardíaca e um índice sensível da eficácia terapêutica. Os efeitos dos vasodilatadores na mortalidade têm sido examinados no "Vasodilator-Heart Failure Trial" (V-HFT) da Administração de Veteranos dos E.U.A. e no teste CONSENSUS do Norte de Escandinávia. Os resultados indicam que a terapia vasodilatadora pode prolongar a vida, mas não todos os vasodilatadores são igualmente eficazes na alteração da história natural da insuficiência cardíaca. Uma questão não resolvida é se a inibição da vasoconstrição neurohormonal constituir um melhor enfoque que a vasodilatação direta. Esperam-se os resultados de outros testes. Também estuda-se atualmente as possíveis vantagens do uso de vasodilatadores na prevenção da insuficiência cardíaca mediante o tratamento precoce da disfunção assintomática do ventrículo esquerdo.

RESUMEN

En los últimos 15 años se ha demostrado que los fármacos vasodilatadores producen una mejoría significativa en la función cardíaca y por tanto han logrado amplia aceptación en el manejo de la insuficiencia cardíaca. Ha sido más difícil establecer la eficacia de la terapia vasodilatante. Ultimamente se han realizado varios intentos de evaluar la eficacia de la terapia vasodilatante mediante la determinación de la "calidad de vida", ya que la mejoría de la calidad de vida es uno de los objetivos principales del tratamiento. Los ejercicios se han empleado tradicionalmente como un método, pero los resultados son variables y se necesitan pruebas más objetivas y discriminatorias para los ejercicios. Se ha desarrollado un cuestionario titulado "Viviendo con la insuficiencia cardíaca" para evaluar a pacientes con disfunción del ventrículo izquierdo e insuficiencia cardíaca. Los resultados preliminares sugieren que este cuestionario proporciona una guía reproducible de la gravedad de la insuficiencia cardíaca y un índice sensible de la eficacia terapéutica. Los efectos de los vasodilatadores en la mortalidad han sido examinados en el "Vasodilator-Heart Failure Trial" (V-HeFT) de la Administración de Veteranos de los E.U.A.y en la prueba (CONSENSUS) del Norte de Escandinavia. Los resultados indican que la terapia vasodilatadora peude prolongar la vida, pero no todos los vasodilatadores son igualmente eficaces en la alteración de la historia natural de la insuficiencia cardíaca. Una cuestión no resuelta todavía es si la inhibición de la vasoconstricción neurohormonal constituye un mejor enfoque que la vasodilatación directa. Se esperan los resultados de otros ensayos. También se está estudiando actualmente las posibles ventajas del empleo de vasodilatadores en la prevención de la insuficiencia cardíaca, mediante el tratamiento temprano de la disfunción asintomática del ventrículo izquierdo.

要約

過去15年あまりの間に，血管拡張薬は心機能の著明な改善をもたらすことが明らかにされ，心不全治療に広く用いられるようになった。ただ，血管拡張薬治療の有効性を明確にすることは，かなり困難なことである。

　最近では，quality of life の改善こそが治療の主要な最終目標の1つであること
から，この quality of life を測定することにより，血管拡張薬の有効性を評価する
という試みがなされている。従来から，運動負荷試験がその代用として使用され
てきたが，結果は一定せず，より客観的で判別可能な試験法が必要である。そこ
で，左室機能障害および心不全患者を評価するために，「心不全とともに生きる」
と題した質問票が開発された。予備研究の結果，これは再現性のある心不全重症
度の指標，および感度の高い治療効果の指数になりうることが示唆されている。

　血管拡張薬の死亡率に対する効果が，Veterans Administration 血管拡張薬-心不
全試験（V-HeFT）と北スカンジナビア（CONSENSUS）試験で検討された。そ
の結果は，血管拡張薬治療は延命をもたらすが，すべての血管拡張薬が等しく心
不全の自然歴を変えるわけではないことを示した。

　神経ホルモン性血管収縮の抑制あるいは直接的血管拡張のいずれが優れた治療
法であるのかは，未解決の問題である。今後の治験成績の発表が待たれるところ
である。無症候性の左室機能障害を早期に治療することによって，心不全の予防
に血管拡張薬が有用性を発揮する可能性についても，目下検討が進められている。

Cardiac and Renal Failure: An Expanding Role for ACE Inhibitors, edited by C. T. Dollery and L. M. Sherwood, Hanley & Belfus, Inc., Philadelphia.

ACE Inhibitors in Heart Failure: Evolving Clinical Role

J. E. Rush and J. D. Irvin

It can now be stated emphatically that angiotensin-converting enzyme (ACE) inhibitors as a class are remarkably efficacious agents in the treatment of patients with heart failure who remain symptomatic despite therapy with digoxin and diuretics.[1-4] Primarily via their effect on the renin angiotensin-aldosterone system, ACE inhibitors decrease systemic vascular resistance resulting in decreased cardiac afterload and increased cardiac output. They also act on the venous side of the circulation by producing venous dilatation and a reduction in aldosterone secretion leading to decreased sodium and water retention and decreased preload. The ACE inhibitors improve hemodynamic parameters, exercise duration, and the signs and symptoms of heart failure.[5-8] In severe heart failure, enalapril has been shown to improve survival; studies are underway to evaluate whether this effect is also true for patients with moderate heart failure.[4]

ACE INHIBITORS AS ADJUNCTIVE THERAPY TO DIGOXIN AND DIURETICS IN HEART FAILURE

The first studies in heart failure were performed in patients still symptomatic despite the tried and true therapeutic regimen for heart failure, digoxin plus diuretics.

ACE inhibitors probably act in a number of ways to improve the hemodynamic status of patients with heart failure. It is true that many patients with heart failure have evidence of activation of the renin-angiotensin system, although patients without this evidence may respond to ACE inhibitors as well.[9] By interfering with the production of angiotensin II (ANG II), ACE inhibitors reduce systemic vasoconstriction in patients with congestive heart failure, thereby reducing afterload and allowing better myocardial performance (Figure 1). Cardiac output and stroke volume thus increase. The reduc-

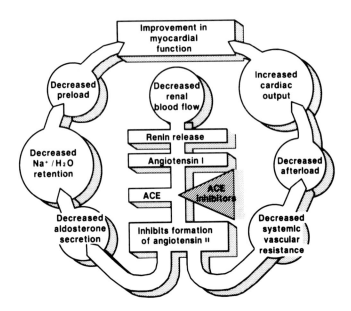

FIG. 1. Mechanism of action of ACE I in heart failure.

tion in preload noted after ACE inhibitor therapy is more difficult to explain because it is not clear that angiotensin acts as a vasoconstrictor in the venous circulation.[10] A number of mechanisms have been invoked in order to explain the observed preload reducing property. Some reduction in preload may be due to the reduction in afterload, with resultant improvement in myocardial function. During chronic ACE inhibitor therapy, renal blood flow increases and aldosterone secretion is suppressed; this may produce a natriuretic effect.[11] Reductions in other vasoconstrictors such as catecholamines, vasopressin or prostaglandins may also play a role.[12-14]

The magnitude of the hemodynamic changes produced by various ACE inhibitors is remarkably similar, although there are differences in dose, time of onset, and duration of action (Figure 2). Other types of vasodilators may produce hemodynamic changes similar to those seen with the ACE inhibitors. However, the hemodynamic effects of other vasodilators are not always sustained during chronic therapy.[15] In contrast the beneficial effects of the ACE inhibitors on hemodynamic parameters clearly are maintained during chronic therapy.[2,5]

Vasodilators that produce beneficial hemodynamic effects should also produce improvement in the patient's clinical status. However, the expected correlations between hemodynamic and clinical effects have not always been found.[16,17] As a class, the ACE inhibitors show the most consistent improvements in the patient's clinical status and exercise capacity in controlled

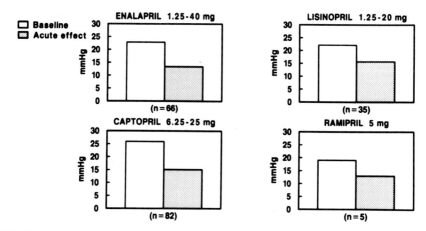

FIG. 2. Pulmonary capillary wedge pressure—acute effect. (Bottom left of figure adapted from Captopril Multicenter Research Group, *Am Heart J* 1985; **110**:439–447; bottom right of figure adapted from De Graeff et al, *Am J Cardiol* 1987; **59**:164D–170D).

double-blind studies. Improvement in exercise duration, signs and symptoms of heart failure and New York Heart Association (NYHA) classification improve fairly consistently with all of the ACE inhibitors tested.[2-8]

An extremely important property of certain vasodilators is the ability to improve survival in patients with heart failure. The Veterans Administration cooperative study showed that the combination of isosorbide dinitrate and hydralazine reduces mortality significantly compared to either placebo or prazosin.[18] The ACE inhibitor enalapril reduces mortality in patients with NYHA Class IV congestive heart failure.[4]

In view of their impressive efficacy, the risks of ACE inhibitor therapy in patients with heart failure are considered acceptable.[1,2,19] Patients with severe chronic congestive heart failure or the very old patient with congestive heart failure may be at added risk for developing adverse experiences with ACE inhibitors. Careful evaluation of patients prior to initiation of therapy with ACE inhibitors and careful observation during therapy can minimize the risks of ACE inhibitor therapy.

Hypotension is an expected effect of vasodilators, particularly in patients whose intravascular volume has been reduced by diuretic therapy. Hypotension is stated to be the most common adverse event attributable to converting-enzyme inhibition.[19,20,22] Risk factors for the development of hypotension have been defined in recent years. Severe heart failure is probably the most important risk factor. Aggressive use of diuretics and extremely low cardiac output cause a decrease in the arterial volume leading to heightened activation of the renin-angiotensin system. Hyponatremia may be observed in these patients.[23] Frequently, pre-renal azotemia is also present. High-dose diuretic therapy and a recent increase in diuretic dose are also risk factors. These patients can frequently be successfully begun on ACE inhibitor therapy by reducing the diuretic dose for several days prior to initiation of therapy. A patient in this situation should be observed in a medical setting following the administration of the first dose of any ACE inhibitor.[24] The risk of hypotension can be minimized by starting with low ACE inhibitor doses.[4]

The second most important risk of ACE inhibitor therapy is the development of renal dysfunction.[25] Possible explanations for this observation include the alteration in the balance of afferent and efferent vascular tone, systemic hypotension, and the reduction in renal blood flow and perfusion pressure due to withdrawal of sympathetic stimulation. Experience with enalapril, catopril and lisinopril have demonstrated that this is a class effect of all ACE inhibitors. The patients at greatest risk are the same patients at greatest risk for hypotension.

Table I presents the mean changes in serum creatinine for six major enalapril trials that involved a total of 498 enalapril-treated patients.

In most of the studies, the mean change was 0.2 mg/dl or less. The one exception was the 0.4 mg/dl increase seen in the captopril comparison study. The patient population in this study was primarily NYHA Class IV patients (86%); the remainder of the patients were NYHA Class III.[20] In addition, the diuretic dose was not adjusted during the course of this study, and we know now that these two factors predisposed the study patients to the development of functional renal insufficiency.[23,25] In addition, the enalapril dose used in this study (40 mg per day) was relatively high. Enalapril patients in the CONSENSUS mortality study, which included only NYHA Class IV patients, had a mean increase of only 0.2 mg/dl.[4] Dosage adjustments of diuretic and enalapril were permitted in the mortality study, which probably ac-

TABLE I. *Mean changes in serum creatinine (mg/dL)*

	Enalapril	Placebo	Captopril	Between Group Difference
Placebo — multinational (week 12)[3]	0.1	0.2	—	NS
Placebo — U.S. (week 12)	0.0	0.1	—	NS
Crossover (week 8)[11]	0.1*	0.0	—	p < 0.5
Mortality (week 6)[4]	0.2	0.0	—	p < 0.05
Open-label (week 16)				
b.i.d.	0.0	—	—	—
q.d.	0.2**	—	—	—
b.i.d. — open label	0.1	—	—	—
Vs. Captopril[20]	0.4**	—	0.1*	NS
	n = 498	n = 341	n = 21	

*, **Significantly diffferent from baseline: p < 0.05, p < 0.01, respectively.
NS = not significant.

TABLE II. *Mean changes in BUN (mg/dL)*

	Enalapril	Placebo	Captopril	Between Group Difference
Placebo — multinational (week 12)[3]	2.2	2.2	—	NS
Placebo — U.S. (week 12)	1.9	−0.9	—	p < 0.01
Crossover (week 8)[11]	4.2**	−0.6	—	p < 0.01
Mortality (week 6)[4]	—	—	—	—
Open-label (week 16)				
b.i.d.	3.0*	—	—	—
q.d.	5.0**	—	—	—
b.i.d. — open label	1.0	—	—	—
Vs. Captopril[20]	21.7**	—	10.1*	NS
	n = 371	n = 215	n = 21	

*, ** Significantly different from baseline: p < 0.05, p < 0.01, respectively.
NS = Not significant.

counted for the smaller increase in serum creatinine in this study compared to the captopril comparison study.

Mean changes in blood urea nitrogen (BUN) for five of the major enalapril trials are shown in Table II (BUN was not measured in the mortality trial). The mean increases of 1.0–5.0 mg/dl seen in the first four studies listed are less than the mean increase of 10.1 mg/dl observed in the captopril-treated patients from the captopril comparison study. This leads us to the conclusion that the most important factors governing the development of functional renal insufficiency in CHF patients treated with enalapril are the severity of the patient's heart failure and the volume status of the patient. Any differences between ACE inhibitors, if they exist, are secondary.

Patients with severe congestive heart failure (CHF) or those with low arterial volume are likely to be relatively dependent upon the renin-angiotensin system for the maintenance of glomerular filtration rate (GFR).[9,11,25] Markers for renin-angiotensin dependence in the CHF patient include hyponatremia, high-dose diuretic therapy or recent increase in diuretic dose, pretreatment elevation of BUN (which may indicate prerenal azotemia), and patients with a concomitant condition causing volume depletion, such as protracted diarrhea.

Patients who develop functional renal impairment while on an ACE inhibitor frequently respond to a reduction in the dose of concomitant diuretic, as shown in Figure 3. This patient, who was stabilized on digoxin and furosemide (40 mg) developed elevations in serum creatinine and BUN during the first month following the initiation of enalapril. The BUN and creatinine values returned to baseline when the furosemide dose was reduced to 20 mg. This patient's exercise duration continued to improve, despite the reduction

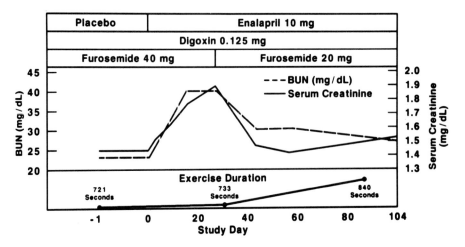

FIG. 3. Changes in BUN and serum creatinine for patient #2181.

of diuretic dose. This type of response is typical, although some patients may also require reduction or discontinuation of the ACE inhibitor.

EVOLVING CLINICAL ROLE OF THE ACE INHIBITORS IN HEART FAILURE

In recent years the use of the digitalis glycosides in patients with heart failure and sinus rhythm has been controversial. Studies have shown that some patients tolerate the withdrawal of digoxin without deterioration of their clinical status, and thus some clinicians believe that the benefits of digitalis therapy may not justify the risk in many patients with sinus rhythm.[26,27] Mechanistically there is no known reason why a patient with heart failure would need to be taking digoxin as well in order to benefit from ACE inhibitor therapy. Recently a large multicenter trial evaluated the beneficial effects of captopril, digoxin or placebo in patients receiving diuretic therapy.[28] Four hundred and sixty-four patients entered the washout/stabilization period; 164 discontinued during this phase of the study, 30 because of worsening heart failure. The remaining 300 patients were randomized, most of them classified as NYHA Class II. The study was a double-blind, parallel study. Captopril was used in doses of 25–50 mg t.i.d. and digoxin in doses of 0.125 to 0.375 mg once daily. Captopril or captopril placebo could be titrated based on patient response. Patients were treated for a period of 6 months. Without respect to exercise duration, only the captopril group had a significant change from baseline (Figure 4). The change was significantly better for captopril than for placebo, but there was no significantly difference between captopril and digoxin. On the other hand, digoxin produced a significant increase in

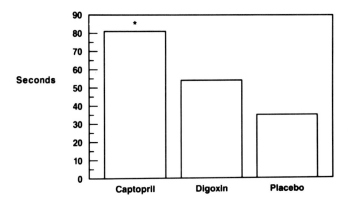

FIG. 4. Mean change in exercise duration in patients in the Captopril-Digoxin Multicenter Study. Asterisk indicates significantly greater change from baseline compared to placebo (p < 0.05). (Adapted from Captopril-Digoxin Research Group, *JAMA* 1988; **259**:539–544.)

ejection fraction, whereas captopril and placebo did not (Figure 5). This study did show however, that concomitant use of ACE inhibitors plus diuretics is useful in patients who cannot tolerate digoxin. The risk of digoxin toxicity is avoided, and the patients are likely to achieve a more favorable potassium balance. There is also a suggestion from this study that fewer ventricular arrhythmias occurred in the captopril group. The study results suggest that the effects of ACE inhibitors and digoxin are complimentary and that the ejection fractions were less in the group of patients who did not have the benefit of digoxin.

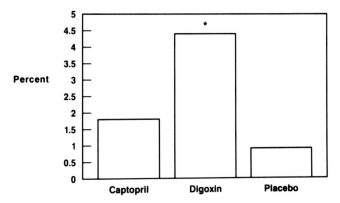

FIG. 5. Mean change in ejection fraction in patients in the Captopril-Digoxin Multicenter Study. Asterisk indicates greater change from baseline compared to placebo (p < 0.01) and captopril (p < 0.05). (Adapted from Captopril-Digoxin Research Group, *JAMA* 1988; **259**:539–544.)

ACE INHIBITORS AS MONOTHERAPY

A few small studies have evaluated the use of ACE inhibitors as initial therapy or monotherapy in patients with heart failure. The rationale of this approach is that, since ACE inhibitors reduce both preload and afterload, perhaps an ACE inhibitor alone would be sufficient for patients with mild heart failure. Richardson et al.[29] evaluated 14 patients with moderate CHF, despite therapy with furosemide (40 mg) and amiloride (5 mg) in a double-blind crossover study. One of the groups continued on its treatment with furosemide and amiloride, and the second group was switched to captopril 25 mg t.i.d. The treatment period was 8 weeks. Ten patients remained clinically stable when they were switched to captopril. Four patients, however, deteriorated while on captopril. All of these patients had a prior history of pulmonary edema, which indicates that it may be possible to define a subgroup of patients who are able to tolerate ACE inhibitors as monotherapy. There was no improvement in exercise tolerance in either of the treatment groups in this small study. We must conclude from this study that some patients with early heart failure controlled with diuretics cannot tolerate therapy with an ACE inhibitor alone.

Recently, the new ACE inhibitor, quinipril, has been evaluated as monotherapy.[30] The change in mean exercise time in patients in the quinipril group was comparable to those patients treated with diuretic alone.

The origin of sodium and water retention in heart failure probably is multifactorial.[31] Therefore, an intervention directed solely at the renin-angiotensin system may not be sufficient.

EFFECT ON PROGRESSION OF LEFT VENTRICULAR DYSFUNCTION AFTER ACUTE MYOCARDIAL INFARCTION

It is clear that increased afterload increases the work of the heart and hastens the deterioration of left ventricular dysfunction after acute myocardial infarction.[32] Sharpe et al. published the long-term effects of captopril in 60 asymptomatic patients with left ventricular dysfunction.[33] Patients were begun on therapy 1 week following the occurrence of a transmural myocardial infarction and were treated with either captopril 25 mg t.i.d., furosemide 40 mg q.d., or placebo. After 1 year asymptomatic left ventricular dysfunction improved with captopril; however further left ventricular dilatation occurred in the furosemide and the placebo groups (Figure 6).

More recently, Pfeffer et al. evaluated 59 patients with their first anterior myocardial infarction and ejection fractions of 45% or less.[34] These patients were randomly assigned to receive placebo or captopril 25–50 mg t.i.d. During 1 year of follow-up, the end diastolic volume increased in the placebo group, whereas the increase was not significant in the captopril group. In a

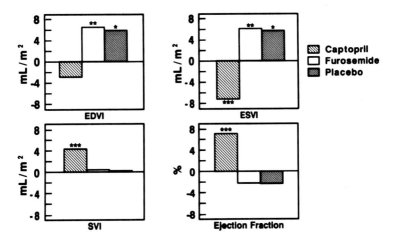

FIG. 6. Effect of ACE I on left ventricular dysfunction following myocardial infarction—change after 1 year. *, **, *** indicate significant change from baseline, p < 0.05, p < 0.01, p < 0.001, respectively. (Adapted from *Lancet* 1988; EDVI = end diastolic volume index; ESVI = end systolic volume index; SVI = stroke volume index.)

subset of 36 patients who were at highest risk for ventricular enlargement because of persistent occlusion of the left anterior descending coronary artery, captopril prevented further ventricular dilatation. Patients treated with captopril also had increased exercise capacity relative to placebo.

These important studies indicate that ACE inhibitors may be useful in patients with left ventricular dysfunction following myocardial infarction. Further studies are needed to clarify whether asymptomatic patients with left ventricular dysfunction not associated with a myocardial infarction would benefit from ACE inhibitor therapy.

EFFECT ON VENTRICULAR ARRHYTHMIAS

Several small studies have shown a reduction of ventricular arrhythmias in heart failure patients treated with ACE inhibitors.[35] There are a number of postulated mechanisms. First, ACE inhibitors reduce ventricular distention and wall stress. They also reduce the need for diuretic therapy, which will improve potassium and magnesium balance. Potassium balance may also improve through aldosterone suppression. The hemodynamic improvement that occurs with ACE inhibitors results in an improved balance of oxygen supply to the myocardium vs. demand. ACE inhibitors also produce a reduction in sympathetic outflow, which may influence ventricular arrhythmias. It is not known whether ANG II itself has any direct effects on the myocardium with respect to the production of arrhythmias. Webster *et al.* studied 20 NYHA Class II and III patients receiving digoxin and diuretics.[35] This was a double-blind parallel study of enalapril 5 mg b.i.d. vs. placebo. In the patients treated with enalapril, significant decreases were noted in ventricular premature beats, couplets and ventricular tachycardia. It is not known, however, whether the effect on ventricular arrhythmias is related to the increased survival in patients with severe heart failure. In the CONSENSUS study[4] there was no apparent reduction in the number of patients dying suddenly. A study currently being conducted by the National Heart Lung and Blood Institute [Studies of Left Ventricular Dysfunction (SOLVD)] is evaluating, in a subset of patients, whether the changes in ventricular arrhythmias produced by enalapril are correlated with mortality in a large group of patients randomized to enalapril or placebo.

CONCLUSION

The ACE inhibitors are effective when used as adjuvant therapy with diuretics, and this effect seems to be true whether or not digoxin is used concomitantly. The ACE inhibitors may be effective as monotherapy in certain subsets of patients, but these subsets have not yet been clearly defined. After acute myocardial infarction, patients with left ventricular dysfunction may benefit from the use of ACE inhibitors, which appear to slow the progression of left ventricular dysfunction. Preliminary studies indicate that ACE inhibitors reduce ventricular arrhythmias in heart failure patients.

In the 8 years since the identification of the ACE inhibitors, we have probably raised far more questions than we have answered. With respect to heart failure the most important questions may be as follows:

1. In what patient population, if any, can ACE inhibitors be used as monotherapy?

2. Are the positive effects of ACE inhibitors on survival confined to the severely ill patient or do they apply also to patients with NYHA Class II and III therapy?

3. Is digoxin required in order for the positive effects on survival to be manifest?

4. What are the mechanisms by which ACE inhibitors decrease ventricular arrhythmias?

5. Do ACE inhibitors reduce the incidence of sudden death in heart failure patients?

Most of the studies needed to answer these questions are already in progress. The next five years are likely to bring more changes in our medical management of patients with heart failure.

REFERENCES

1. Mulrow CD, Mulrow JP, Linn WD, Aguilar C, Ramirez G. Relative efficacy of vasodilator therapy in chronic digestive heart failure. *JAMA* 1988; **259**:3422–6.
2. Packer M. Vasodilator and inotropic drugs for the treatment of chronic heart failure: Distinguishing hype from hope. *J Am Coll Cardiol* 1988; **12**:1299–1317.

3. Enalapril congestive heart failure investigators. Long-term effects of enalapril in congestive heart failure: A multicenter placebo-controlled trial. *Heart Failure* 1987; 3:102–7.
4. Consensus Trial Study Group. Effects of enalapril on mortality in severe congestive heart failure: Results of the Cooperative North Scandinavian Enalapril Survival Study. *N Engl J Med* 1987; 316:1429–35.
5. Gomez HJ, Cirillo VJ, Davies RO, Bolognese JA, Walker JF. Enalapril in congestive heart failure: acute and chronic invasive hemodynamic evaluation. *Int J Cardiol* 1986; 11:37–48.
6. Captopril Multicenter Research Group. A placebo-controlled trial of captopril in congestive heart failure. *J Am Coll Cardiol* 1983; 2:755–63.
7. Uretsky BF, Shaver JA, Liang C, et al. Modulation of hemodynamic effects with a converting enzyme inhibitor: Acute hemodynamic dose-response relationship of a new angiotensin converting enzyme inhibitor, lisinopril, with observations on long-term clinical, functional, and biochemical responses. *Am Heart J* 1988; 116:480–88.
8. deGraeff PA, Kingma JH, Dunselman PHJM, Weisseling H, Lie KI. Acute hemodynamic and hormonal effects of ramipril in chronic congestive heart failure and comparison with captopril. *Am J Cardiol* 1987; 59:164D–70D.
9. Curtiss C, Cohn JN, Vrobel T, Franciosa JA. Role of the renin-angiotensin system in the systemic vasoconstriction of chronic congestive heart failure. *Circulation* 1978; 58:763–70.
10. LeJemtel T, Keung E, Frishman WH, Ribner HS, Sonnenblick EJ. Hemodynamic effects of captopril in patients with severe chronic heart failure. *Am J Cardiol* 1982; 49:1484–88.
11. Cleland JGF, Dargie HJ, Ball SG, et al. Effects of enalapril in heart failure: A double-blind study of the effects on exercise performance, renal function, hormones and metabolic state. *Br Heart J* 1985; 54:305–12.
12. Thomas JA, Marks BH. Plasma norepinephrine in congestive heart failure. *Am J Cardiol* 1978; 41:233–43.
13. Cohn JN, Levine TB, Francis GS, Goldsmith S. Neurohumoral control mechanisms in congestive heart failure. *Am Heart J* 1981; 102:509–14.
14. Goldsmith SR, Francis GS, Cowley AW, Levine TB, Cohn JN. Increased plasma arginine vasopressin in patients with congestive heart failure. *J Am Coll Cardiol* 1983; 1:1391–5.
15. Franciosa JA, Weber KT, Levine TB. Hydralazine in the long-term treatment of chronic heart failure: Lack of difference from placebo. *Am Heart J* 1982; 104:587–94.
16. Topic N, Kramer B, Massie B. Acute and long-term effects of captopril on exercise cardiac performance and exercise capacity in congestive heart failure. *Am Heart J* 1982; 104(5, Part 2):1172–1179.
17. Kirlin PC, Dansby C, Laird CK, Willis III PW. Discrepancy between first-dose converting enzyme inhibition at rest and subsequent inhibition during exercise in chronic heart failure. *Clin Pharmacol Ther* 1988; 43:616–622.
18. Cohn JN, Archibald DG, Ziesche S, et al: Effect of vasodilator therapy on mortality in chronic congestive heart failure: Results of a Veterans Administration Cooperative Study (V-HeFT). *N Engl J Med* 1986; 314:1547–52.
19. Warner NJ, Rush JE, Keegan ME. Tolerability of enalapril in congestive heart failure. *Am J Cardiol* 1989; 63:33D–37D.
20. Packer M, Lee WH, Yushak M, Medina N. Comparison of captopril and enalapril in patients with severe chronic heart failure. *N Engl J Med* 1986; 315:847–53.
21. O'Neill CJA, Bowes SG, Sullens CM, et al. Evaluation of the safety of enalapril in the treatment of heart failure in the very old. *Eur J Clin Pharmacol* 1988; 35:143–50.
22. Todd PA, Heel RC. Enalapril: A review of its pharmacodynamic and pharmacokinetic properties, and therapeutic use in hypertension and congestive heart failure. *Drugs* 1986; 31:198–248.
23. Packer M, Medina N, Yashak M. Relationship between serum sodium concentration and the hemodynamic and clinical responses to converting enzyme inhibition with captopril in severe heart failure. *J Am Coll Card* 1984; 3:1035–43.
24. Packer M, Kessler PD, Gottlieb SS. Adverse effects of converting-enzyme inhibition in patients with severe congestive heart failure: pathophysiology and management. *Postgrad Med J* 1986; 62(suppl 1):179–182.
25. Packer M, Medina N, Yushak M. Pathophysiologic factors underlying the development of worsening prerenal azotemia during captopril therapy for severe chronic heart failure. *Clin Res* 1983; 31:211A.
26. Gheorghiade M, Beller GA. Effects of discontinuing maintenance digoxin therapy in patients

with ischemic heart disease and congestive heart failure in sinus rhythm. *Am J Cardiol* 1983; **51**:1242–50.

27. Fleg JL, Gottlieb SH, Lakatta EG. Is digoxin really important in the treatment of compensated heart failure? A placebo-controlled crossover study in patients with sinus rhythm. *Am J Med* 1982; **73**:244–50.

28. The Captopril-Digoxin Multicenter Research Group. Comparative effects of therapy with captopril and digoxin in patients with mild to moderate heart failure. JAMA 1988; **259**:539–44.

29. Richardson A, Scriven A, Poole-Wilson PA, Bayliss J, Parameshwar J, Sutton GC. Double-blind comparison of captopril alone against furosemide plus amiloride in mild heart failure. Lancet 1987; ii:709–11.

30. Kromer EP, Riegger AJG, Medical University Clinic, Würzburg FRG. Effects of the ACE inhibitor quinapril as monotherapy in patients with congestive heart failure (CHF) NYHA Class II-III. European Heart Journal 1988; **9**(abs suppl 1):2.

31. Mettauer B, Rouleau JL, Bichet D, et al. Sodium and water excretion abnormalities in congestive heart failure: Determinant factors and clinical applications. Ann Intern Med 1986; **105**:161–7.

32. Pfeffer JM, Pfeffer MA, Braunwald E. Influence of chronic captopril therapy on the infarcted left ventricle of the rat. *Circ Res* 1985; **57**:84–95.

33. Sharpe N, Smith H, Murphy J, Hannan S. Treatment of patients with symptomless left ventricular dysfunction after myocardial infarction. Lancet 1988; i:255–9.

34. Pfeffer MA, Lamas CA, Vaughan DE, Parisia F, Braunwald E. Effect of captopril on progressive ventricular dilatation after anterior myocardial infarction. N Engl J Med 1988; **319**:80–5.

35. Webster MWI, Fitzpatrick A, Nicholls MG, Ikram H, Wells JE. Effect of enalapril on ventricular arrhythmias in congestive heart failure. *Am J Cardiol* 1985; **56**:566–9.

SUMMARY

Angiotensin converting enzyme (ACE) inhibitors have been shown to be highly efficacious in the treatment of patients with heart failure who remain symptomatic despite therapy with digoxin and diuretics. ACE inhibitors improve hemodynamic parameters, exercise duration, and the signs and symptoms of heart failure. In severe heart failure, enalapril improves survival. This review describes the efficacy and safety of ACE inhibitors used as adjunctive therapy to digoxin and diuretics. The evolving clinical role of ACE inhibitors in the treatment of heart failure is also discussed, and evidence is reviewed for the efficacy of ACE inhibitors used concomitantly with diuretics (in the absence of digoxin) and as monotherapy. The evidence that the use of ACE inhibitors prevents progression of left ventricular dysfunction in the setting of an acute myocardial infarction and their effect on ventricular arrhythmias in patients with heart failure are also discussed.

RÉSUMÉ

On a démontré que les inhibiteurs de l'enzyme de conversion de l'angiotensine (IEC) sont extrêment efficaces dans le traitement de patients atteints d'insuffisance cardiaque qui restent symptomatiques en dépit d'un traitement digitalique et diurétique. On a démontré que les inhibiteurs de l'enzyme de conversion de l'angiotensine (IEC) entraînent une amélioration des paramètres hémodynamiques, de la durée de la performance physique, et des signes et symtômes de l'insuffisance cardiaque. Dans le cas d'insuffisance cardiaque sévère, on a démontré que l'administration d'enalapril avait une action bénéfique sur la survie. Cette étude dêcrit l'efficacité et la sécurité de l'adjonction d'inhibiteurs de l'enzyme de conversion de l'angiotensine (IEC) à un traitement digitalique et diurétique. On discute aussi de l'évolution du rôle clinique que prennent les inhibiteurs de l'enzyme de conversion de l'angiotensine (IEC) dans le traitement des insuffisances cardiaques, et on décrit les preuves de l'efficacité des inhibiteurs de l'enzyme de conversion de l'angiotensine (IEC) lorqu'ils sont utilisés en association avec les diurétiques (en l'absence de digitaliques) et aussi lorsqu'ils sont utilisés en monothérapie. On met en évidence les avantages de l'utilisation des inhibiteurs de l'enzyme de conversion de l'angiotensine (IEC) pour éviter une détérioration progressive du ventricule gauche dans le cas d'un infarctus du myocarde et on discute aussi leur effet sur les arythmies ventriculaires chez les patients atteints d'insuffisance cardiaque.

ZUSAMMENFASSUNG

Inhibitoren des angiotensinkonvertierenden Enzyms ACE sind nach den Ergebnissen der Forschung hochwirksam in der Behandlung von Patienten mit Herzinsuffizienz, die trotz der Therapie mit Digoxin und Diuretika Symptome zurückbehalten. Es ist gezeigt worden, dass ACE-Inhibitoren die hämodynamischen Parameter, die Bewegungsdauer und die Anzeichen und Symptome der Herzinsuffizienz verbessern. Bei schwerem Herzversagen erhöht Enalapril nachweislich die Überlebenschancen. Die vorliegende Veröffentlichung bespricht die Wirksamkeit und Sicherheit von ACE-Inhibitoren in ihrer Verwendung als Beigabetherapie zu Digoxin und Diuretika. Auch diskutiert wird die wachsende klinische Rolle der ACE-Inhibitoren in der Behandlung von Herzinsuffizienz; und Beweise für die Wirksamkeit der ACE-Inhibitoren als Begleiter von Diuretika in der Abwesenheit von Digoxin und als Monotherapeutika werden besprochen. Es liegen auch Hinweise dafür vor, dass die Anwendung von ACE-Inhibitoren fortschreitende Dysfunktion der linken Herzkammer aufhält, wenn ein akuter myokardialer Infarkt vorliegt. Schliesslich wird auch der Effekt von ACE-Inhibitoren auf Herzkammer-Arrhythmie in Patienten mit Herzinsuffizienz besprochen.

RIASSUNTO

Gli inibitori dell'enzima isomerizzante dell'angiotensina (EIA) si sono dimostrati altamente efficaci nella cura di pazienti con insufficienza cardiaca che rimangono sintomatici malgrado terapia a base di digossina e diuretici. Gli inibitori dell'EIA si sono dimostrati capaci di migliorare i parametri emodinamici, la durata dell'esercizio fisico ed i segni e sintomi dell'insufficienza cardiaca. In casi di insufficienza cardiaca grave, è stato dimostrato che l'enalapril migliora le capacità di sopravvivenza. Questa rassegna descrive l'efficacia e la sicurezza degli inibitori dell'EIA usati come terapia aggiuntiva alla digossina ed ai diuretici. Viene anche discussa la continua evoluzione del ruolo clinico degli inibitori dell'EIA nella cura dell'insufficienza cardiaca e vengono esaminate le prove dell'efficacia degli inibitori dell'EIA usati in concomitanza ai diuretici (in assenza di digossina) e come monoterapia. Vengono anche discusse le prove evidenziali che l'uso di inibitori dell'EIA impedisce il progresso della disfunzione ventricolare sinistra nel caso di infarto miocardico acuto ed il loro effetto sulle aritmie ventricolari in pazienti con insufficienza cardiaca.

SUMÁRIO

Tem-se demonstrado que os inibidores da enzima convertidora da angiotensina (ACE) são muito eficazes no tratamento de pacientes com insuficiência cardíaca que ficam sintomáticos apesar da terapia com diogoxina e diuréticos. Tem-se demonstrado que os inibidores da ACE melhoram os parâmetros hemodinâmicos, duração dos exercícios, e os sinais e sintomas da insuficiência cardíaca. Tem-se demonstrado que o enalapril melhora a sobrevivência em casos de insuficiência cardíaca severa. Este trabalho descreve a eficacia e segurança dos inibidores la ACE utilizados como terapia adjuntiva à digoxina e aos diuréticos. Também discute-se a evolução do papel clínico dos inibidores da ACE no tratamento da insuficiência cardíaca, e revisa-se a evidência da eficácia dos inibidores da ACE utilizados concomitantemente com diuréticos (na ausência de digoxina) e como monoterapia. Também discute-se a evidência de que o uso dos inibidores da ACE evite a progressão da disfunção do ventrículo esquerdo em casos de infarto agudo miocárdico e seu efeito nas arritmias ventriculares em pacientes com insuficiência cardíaca.

RESUMEN

Se ha demostrado que los inhibidores de la enzima convertidora de la angiotensina (ACE) son muy eficaces en el tratamiento de pacientes con insuficiencia cardíca que permanecen sintomáticos a pesar de la terapia con digoxina y diuréticos. Se ha demostrado que los inhibidores de la ACE mejoran los parámetros hemodinámicos, duración de los ejercicios y los signos y síntomas de la insuficiencia cardíaca. Se ha demostrado que el enalapril mejora la supervivencia en casos de insuficiencia cardíaca severa. Este trabajo describe la eficacia y seguridad de los inhibidores de la ACE empleados concomitantemente con digoxina y diuréticos. También se discute la evolución del papel clínico de los inhibidores de la ACE en el tratamiento de la insuficiencia cardíaca, y se analizan las evidencias a favor de la eficacia de los inhibidores de la ACE empleados concomitantemente con diuréticos (en ausencia de digoxina) y como monoterapia. También se discute la evidencia de que el empleo de los inhibidores de la ACE previene la progresión de la disfunción del ventrículo izquierdo en casos de infarto agudo del miocardio y su efecto en las arritmias ventriculares en pacientes con insuficiencia cardíaca también se discute.

要約

ジゴキシンと利尿薬による治療にもかかわらず心不全の症状を示す心不全患者において，アンジオテンシン変換酵素（ACE）阻害薬は高い有効性を発揮することが示されている。ACE 阻害薬は，血行動態指標や運動持続時間，心不全の症状・症候のいずれをも改善することが明らかにされている。重症心不全において，エナラプリルは生存率を改善することが示された。

この総説では，ジゴキシンおよび利尿薬にさらに加えるべき治療法として用いた ACE 阻害薬の有効性と安全性について述べる。また，心不全治療における ACE 阻害薬のしだいに高まりつつある臨床的役割に関しても考察する。そして，利尿薬との併用療法（ジゴキシンなしで）および単独療法での ACE 阻害薬の有効性についても概説する。さらに，ACE 阻害薬の使用は急性心筋梗塞発症時の左室機能障害の進行を予防することや，心不全患者での心室性不整脈に対する効果についても考察する。

Cardiac and Renal Failure: An Expanding Role for ACE Inhibitors, edited by C. T. Dollery and L. M. Sherwood, Hanley & Belfus, Inc., Philadelphia.

Consensus Study and Beyond

John Kjekshus and Karl Swedberg

Thirty-five hospitals participated in the Consensus Trial[1]: 6 from Finland, 12 from Norway and 17 from Sweden. All patients were suffering from severe congestive heart failure (CHF). The primary objective of the trial was to look at mortality and mode of death following 6 months of treatment with the angiotensin converting enzyme (ACE) inhibitor, enalapril, compared with placebo. Mortality and mode of death at 12 months, tolerability, and clinical status and concurrent medication were also examined. We were particularly interested in survival rate according to risk factors such as neurohormonal activation.

PATIENTS AND METHODS

Enalapril Trial

Two hundred and fifty-three patients suffering from CHF were included in the trial. Inclusion criteria were as follows:

1. Patients should be in Functional Class IV (NYHA)—i.e., incapacitated at rest.

2. Heart should definitely be enlarged (male 600 ml, female 550 ml per square meter) on biplanar radiograph.

3. Patients should be above the lower legal age limit of 18 years, but there was no upper age limit.

4. All patients should be optimally treated with digitalis, diuretics, and vasodilators, excluding other ACE inhibitors.

The protocol recommended a starting dose of 5 mg twice daily, but hypotensive reactions occurred. The protocol was changed to a recommended starting dose of 2.5 mg once daily in patients considered to be at high risk—i.e., those with a low serum sodium, a raised serum creatinine, and other evidence of hypovolemia, especially among patients using diuretics. If enalapril was tolerated at this dosage, the dose could be stepped up to a maximum maintenance dose of 40 mg/day.

At the end of the study, we noticed that 4 out of 34 patients (12%) who had received enalapril, 5 mg bid, had been withdrawn because of symptomatic hypotension. By contrast, of 93 receiving 2.5 mg/once daily, 3% only (3 patients) had to be withdrawn.

At the point when patients had been entered, the Ethical Review Committee asked for termination of the trial. These patients were then randomized: 126 to placebo and 127 enalapril. The clinical characteristics of the two groups were comparable.[1] The final maintenance dose of enalapril was 18.4 mg and of matching placebo 27.3 mg (p<0.001).

RESULTS AND DISCUSSION

Enalapril versus Placebo Controlled Trial

As Figure 1 shows, soon after drug intervention had been started, the two curves representing the confidence limits for the Life Table Mortality Rates for placebo and enalapril started to diverge, and after 3 months there was virtually no overlap. By 6 months there was a 40% reduction in mortality in favor of enalapril. At 12 months, the reduction was 31%.

It has been suggested that because the two curves continue in parallel, there is a lack of continued effect. We should, however, be aware that once the trial had begun these two patient populations were no longer comparable. Since many more patients (the high-risk patients) died in the placebo-treated group, the remaining patients were good-risk patients, whereas those in the enala-

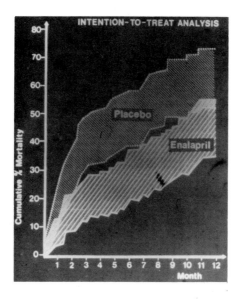

FIG. 1. Ninety-five percent confidence band for life-table mortality rates.

pril-treated group (of whom fewer had died) were consequently at much higher risk. The fact that the two curves continue in parallel may imply that the effect of enalapril was maintained over the months. More recently, after the termination of the study, we followed up these patients and the curves continued to run in parallel. This continued after we started to treat patients in an open fashion.

Mode of Death

By the end of the study, there were a total of 64 *cardiac* deaths in the placebo group and 44 in the enalapril-treated group (Table I). We defined sudden death as cardiac death within 24 hours or sudden cardiac death within 1 hour. There was no difference between the placebo- and enalapril-treated groups in the occurrence of sudden death, no matter how it was defined.

The beneficial effects of enalapril treatment were most clearly seen among those patients dying of progressive heart failure. In this group there were 44 deaths on placebo compared with 22 on enalapril — a reduction of 50%. For other modes of death, there was no difference between the enalapril- and placebo-treated groups. Except for one patient who died from a perforated ulcer, all patients died from cardiovascular causes; these included stroke and pulmonary embolism. In all, there were 68 deaths in the placebo group and 50 in the enalapril-treated group. This difference is statistically highly significant.

The mortality curves of placebo- and enalapril-treated patients dying from progressive heart failure showed a marked divergence, which continued up to the end of the trial, suggesting that there was a continued effect of enalapril treatment.

At the end of the study, the major cause of death from progression of CHF

TABLE I. *Mortality by mode of death*

	Placebo (N = 126) N	Enalapril (N = 127) N	p-Values Life-Table Analysis
• Any cardiac death	64	44	0.001
Cardiac death within 24 hours	19	20	<0.25
Sudden cardiac death within 1 hour	14	14	>0.25
Progression of CHF	44	22	0.001
Other cardiac death	1	2	
• Other cardiovascular death	4	5	>0.25
Stroke	2	1	
No stroke	2	4	>0.25
• Noncardiovascular death (perforated ulcer)	0	1	
Total mortality	68	50	0.003

was 65% in the placebo group. Interestingly, only a small number (21%) of patients died suddenly (within 1 hour). This is very surprising, since in most other studies of mild-to-moderate heart failure, the patients who died suddenly accounted for more than 50% of the deaths. It appears that sudden death is not a major cause of death among Class IV patients.

PREVENTION OF DEATH IN CONGESTIVE HEART FAILURE

The mechanism for death in severe CHF is as yet undefined. The three most likely approaches to preventing death in CHF are as follows:
Myocardial unloading
Antiarrhythmic treatment
Ischemic prophylaxis (the prevention of myocardial necrosis)

Myocardial Unloading

It could be argued that in the Consensus Trial many patients had a relatively high blood pressure (BP) at the start of the trial—the mean diastolic BP at baseline was 120 mmHg. Therefore, the data were analyzed relative to systolic blood pressure baseline (Figure 2). There was a tendency towards higher mortality with lower blood pressure, but among patients with a systolic BP above 135 mmHg, there was still a high (35%) mortality at 6 months. For any given blood pressure, high or low, at baseline, there was a reduction in mortality. Systolic BP was not an indicator of those patients who would benefit from treatment.

Figure 3 relates changes in systolic BP at 6 weeks of treatment to subsequent mortality at 6 months. In the placebo group, a fall in systolic BP of

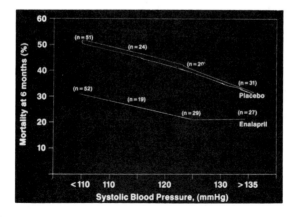

FIG. 2. Pretreatment systolic blood pressure and mortality.

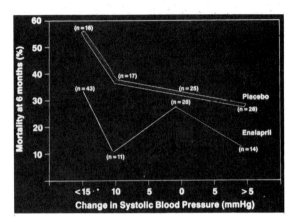

FIG. 3. Six-week change in systolic blood pressure from baseline.

more than 15 mmHg was associated with a high mortality. In the enalapril-treated group, many more patients had a fall in BP greater than 15 mmHg, but there was no clear evidence that this fall affected mortality. Interpretation of the curve is difficult, but it appears that the initial blood pressure or the reduction in pressure did not explain the effect in the enalapril-treated group.

This is in concert with the observed reduction in mortality among patients with mild heart failure[2] receiving combined treatment with hydralazine and isosorbide dinitrate. The favorable effect was obtained without reduction in blood pressure.

The unloading of the myocardium also implies a reduction of left ventricular filling pressure. This was not measured in the present study; however atrial natriuretic peptide (ANP) was determined. ANP is released during atrial distention, and blood levels relate to left ventricular filling pressure.[3] At 6 weeks ANP was reduced significantly by enalapril but not with placebo, suggesting a reduction of preload by treatment.[4]

Antiarrhythmic Prevention

It is intriguing that, so far, antiarrhythmic treatment in Class IV patients has not been very successful. In mild-to-moderate CHF, only beta-blockers have shown a reduction in sudden death. However, there are problems associated with the use of beta-blockers in heart failure.

Although enalapril has been shown to reduce ventricular arrhythmias among patients in mild heart failure,[5] no effect on sudden death was observed in the present study, although frequent ventricular arrhythmias were observed. However, the number of patients was small, and a positive effect might have been missed. Patients in severe CHF may behave differently from less sick patients, in that the myocardial stores of catecholamines are markedly depleted, which elevates the threshold for ventricular fibrillation.

Ischemic Prophylaxis

Heart rate determines myocardial oxygen consumption and is an indicator of subsequent mortality, as was also shown in the Consensus Study. Previous studies with beta blockers have shown that quantitative reduction of resting heart rate is associated with protection against death after myocardial infarction.[6] The average reduction in heart rate among patients receiving enalapril was 5 bpm, which was different from no change in the placebo group.[1]

In contrast to the placebo group, mortality in the enalapril-treated group was lower among patients with a baseline heart rate of 90 bpm or more. Among patients with a low heart rate, there was no clear difference in mortality between the enalapril- and placebo-treated groups.

The increase in heart rate during CHF is associated with marked activation of catecholamines. Since neurohormonal activation might increase myocardial oxygen consumption as well as induce coronary vasoconstriction, and thus cause ischemia and progressive damage of the myocardium, mortality was related to baseline neurohormonal activation.

Activation of Neurohormones

In the Consensus Trial, three different systems were analyzed[4]:
1. Renal system (ACE, angiotensin II [ANG II], aldosterone)
2. Neuroadrenal system (norepinephrine, epinephrine, dopamine)
3. Cardiac system (atrial naturetic peptide—ANP)

We analyzed mortality at 6 months relative to norepinephrine levels at baseline (Figure 4A). There was a clear relationship between the increase in norepinephrine and subsequent mortality at 6 months—from 30–35% at

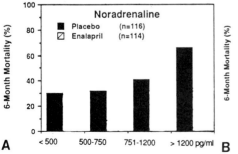 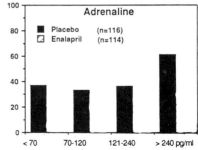

FIG. 4 A,B. Norepinephrine and epinephrine (in quartiles) at baseline vs. 6-month mortality.

baseline up to almost 70% among patients with the highest norepinephrine levels. This compares to previous findings.[7] Interestingly, in the enalapril-treated group, there was no such increase in mortality with increasing baseline levels of norepinephrine.[4] Among those patients with low norepinephrine levels, there was no change in mortality; the benefit was observed only among patients with elevated norepinephrine levels. A similar analysis was carried out for epinephrine. Although epinephrine was only slightly increased in these patients, a similar relationship was observed between low and high epinephrine levels with respect to 6-month mortality (Figure 4B).

Six-month mortality was also analyzed relative to ANG II and aldosterone levels (Figure 5A,B). Again, there was a strong relationship between hormone levels at baseline and 6-month mortality. The patients who benefited from treatment all had elevated hormone levels. For those patients whose hormone levels were not elevated at baseline, there was no difference between the enalapril- and placebo-treated groups.[4]

ANP activation was also found to be an index of subsequent mortality (Figure 6). There was a reduction in mortality at all levels of atrial natriuretic peptide (in the enalapril-treated group).

Thus, the greatest effect of enalapril was seen among those patients showing the greatest neurohormone activation. Low hormone activators did not respond to treatment.

We looked for comparability among patients with low and high levels of neuroendocrine activation. We could not discriminate between patients except for slightly lower serum sodium and slightly higher creatinine levels among the highest activators. Blood pressure and heart size were comparable. The demonstrated low activation of neurohormones in patients with severe heart failure may be similar to that observed by Dacker.[8] He demonstrated that patients who did not show reactive hyperreninemia following captopril did not respond hemodynamically to treatment. The nonresponders to treatment had no change in heart rates, whereas the responders had significantly reduced heart rate. This is in concert with findings in the present study.

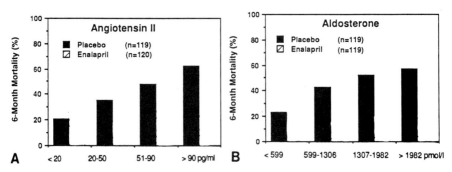

FIG. 5 A,B. Angiotensin II and aldosterone at baseline vs. 6-month mortality (in quartiles).

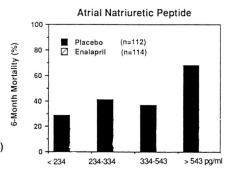

FIG. 6. Atrial natriuretic peptide (in quartiles) at baseline and 6-month mortality.

We also examined mode of death at low and high levels of hormones. Sudden death was distributed evenly among patients with low and high levels of neuroendocrine activation in both the placebo and enalapril-treated groups. Of the patients with progressive CHF, in the placebo group almost all those dying of progressive CHF were high activators. In the enalapril group, by contrast, the mortality was evenly distributed between high and low activators.

We also demonstrated a reduction in ACE, aldosterone, ANG II, ANP and norepinephrine by enalapril, although we found no such effect on epinephrine and dopamine.

The reason why some patients show low, and others high, levels of neurohormones is unclear. Since all patients were being treated concomitantly with diuretics, they would have all been equally activated by them. Individual variation in responsiveness of the neuroendocrine system to heart failure and diuretics seems to be a likely explanation.

CONCLUSION

The addition of enalapril to conventional therapy in severe congestive heart failure reduces mortality and improves symptoms. This effect appears to be due to a reduction in the number of deaths from progression of congestive heart failure among patients with marked activations of the neurohormonal system.

REFERENCES

1. The Consensus Trial Study Group. Effects of enalapril on mortality in severe congestive heart failure. *N Engl J Med* 1987; **316**:1429–1435.
2. Cohn JN, Archibald DG, Ziesche S, et al. Effect of vasodilator therapy on mortality in chronic congestive heart failure: results of a Veterans Administration Cooperative Study. *N Engl J Med* 1986; **314**:1547–52.
3. Richards AM, Cleland JGF, Tonolo G, McIntyre GD, Leckie BJ, Dargie HJ, Ball SG,

Robertson JIS. Plasma α natriuretic peptide in cardiac impairment. *Br Med J* 1986; **293**:409–412.

4. Swedberg K, Eneroth P, Kjekshus J, Wilhelmsen L. The Consensus Trial Study Group: Hormones regulating cardiovascular function in patients with severe congestive heart failure and the relation to mortality. (Submitted.)

5. Webster M, Fitzpatrick A, Nicholls G, Ikram H, Wells E. Effect of enalapril on ventricular arrhythmias in congestive heart failure.

6. Kjekshus J. Heart rate reduction—a mechanism of benefit? *Eur Heart J* 1987; **8(suppl L)**:115–122.

7. Cohn JN, Levine TB, Olivari MT et al, Plasma norepinephrine as a guide to prognosis in patients with chronic congestive heart failure. *N Engl J Med* 1984; **311**:819–823.

RÉSUMÉ

Nous rapportons, dans cette étude, les données de l'Essai de Consensus dans lequel 35 hôpitaux ont participé en Finlande, en Norvège et en Suède. Les 235 patients inclus dans l'essai souffraient d'insuffisance cardiaque congestive (progressive?) (Classification de New York: NYHA: Classe Fonctionnelle IV). Tous présentaient une cardiomégalie et étaient traités à fortes doses par des médicaments cardiovasculaires autres que les inhibiteurs de l'enzyme de conversion de l'angiotensine (IEC). L'essai avait pour objectif d'examiner la mortalité et les causes de décès à 6 mois et aussi à 12 mois chez les patients traités par l'inhibiteur de l'enzyme de conversion de l'angiotensine (IEC), l'énalapril. Le premier essai comprenait les patients traités uniquement par l'énalapril. Cet essai e été interrompu prématurément et un second essai entrepris avec des patients randomisés sous placebo ou enapril. Dans ce second essai, on a constaté la plus grande réduction de mortalité parmi les patients mourant d'insuffisance cardiaque progressive. Les chiffres de mortalité à 12 mois indiquent un effet continu du traitement par l'énalapril. Le niveau d'activation neuroendocrinienne varie énormément parmi les patients de la Classe IV atteints d'insuffisance cardiaque congestive sévère. On a observé une forte association entre les niveaux d'épinéphrine, d'angiotensine II, d'aldostcrone et de peptide natriurétique atrial (PNA) et de la mortalité qui s'ensuit dans les six mois. On a constaté que l'énalapril faisait baisser le risque accru de décès associé à de hauts niveaux de neurohormones.

ZUSAMMENFASSUNG

Die vorliegende Veröffentlichung befasst sich mit den Daten aus der CONSENSUS-Studie, an der 35 Krankenhäuser in Finnland, Norwegen und Schweden teilnahmen. Die 235 Patienten der Studie litten an hyperhämischer Herzinsuffizienz (progressiver Herzinsuffizienz?) der Funktionsklasse IV; NYHA. Alle hatten eine Cardiacusvergrösserung und wurden optimal behandelt mit Herz- und Kreislaufdrogen, die keine Inhibitoren des Angiotensinkonvertierenden Enzyms ACE enthielten. Das Ziel der Studie bestand darin, die Mortalitätsrate und die Todesart in Patienten zu bestimmen, die mit dem ACE-Inhibitor Enalapril behandelt wurden; und zwar nach 6 und nach 12 Monaten. Der erste Versuch beschäftigte sich mit Patienten, die nur mit Enalapril behandelt wurden. Dieser Versuch wurde vorzeitig abgebrochen und durch eine zweite Studie ersetzt, in der den Patienten willkürlich entweder Enalapril oder ein Placebo verschrieben wurde. Im Verlauf dieser zweiten Studie wurde die höchste Mortalitätsverringerung an den Patienten beobachtet, die an progressiver Herzinsuffizienz starben. Die Mortalitätsraten nach 12 Monaten zeigen einen kontinuierlichen Effekt in der Behandlung mit Enalapril. Das Ausmass der neuroendokrinen Aktivierung variiert stark in Patienten mit schwerer kongestiver Herzinsuffizienz der Klasse IV. Beobachtet wurde eine deutliche Korrelation zwischen den Mengen an Epinephrin, Norepinephrin, ANG II, Aldosteron und ANP und der Mortalitätsrate in den folgenden sechs Monaten. Die Ergebnisse zeigen, dass Enalapril in der Lage ist, das erhöhte Risiko des Todes durch grosse Mengen an Neurohormonen zu reduzieren.

RIASSUNTO

Questra tesi ripassa i dati dalla Prova Consensuale in cui hanno partecipato 35 ospedali nella Finlandia, nella Norvegia, e nella Svezia. I 235 pazienti inclusi nella prova soffrivano di arresto cardiaco congestivo (progessivo?) (Classe Funzionale IV; NYHA). Tutti avevano ingrossamento cardiaco e furono ottimamente trattati con droghe cardiovascolari oltre agli inibitori di enzima angiotensin-convertente (EAC). Lo scopo della prova era esaminare la mortalità e il modo della morte a sei e anche a dodici mesi nei pazienti trattati con l'inibitore EAC, enalapril. La prova iniziale incluse pazienti trattati solamente con enalapril. Questa prova fu terminata prematuramente e una seconda prova iniziò con pazienti trattati a casaccio con un rimedio fittizio o con enalapril. In questa seconda prova, la più grande riduzione nella mortalità fu vista tra quei pazienti morendo di arresto cardiaco progressivo. Le statistiche di mortalità a dodici mesi indicano un continuo effetto di un trattamento con enalapril. Il livello di attivazione neuroendocrina varia largamente tra i pazienti di Classe IV con grave arresto cardiaco congestivo. Un'associazione forte fu osservata tra i livelli di epinefrina, norepinefrina, ANG II, aldosterone e ANP e la mortalità susseguente a sei mesi. L'enalapril fu trovata a ridurre l'aumentato rischio di morte associata con alti livelli di neuroormoni.

SUMÁRIO

Revisam-se os dados do teste CONSENSUS, no qual participaram 35 hospitais na Finlândia, na Noruega e na Suécia. Os 235 pacientes incluídos no teste sofriam da insuficiência cardíaca congestiva (progressiva?) (Classe Funcional IV; NYHA). Todos tinham a hipertrofia cardíaca e foram otimamente tratados com drogas cardiovasculares distintas dos inibidores da enzima convertidora da angiotensina (ACE). A meta do teste foi de examinar a mortalidade e a modalidade da morte aos seis e também aos 12 meses nos pacientes tratados com o inhibidor ACE enalapril. O teste inicial envolveu pacientes tratados com enalapril só. Terminou-se prematuramente este teste e iniciou-se um segundo teste com os pacientes randomizados a um placebo ou ao enalapril. Neste segundo teste, viu-se a maior redução na mortalidade naqueles pacientes que estavam morrendo da insuficiência cardíaca progressiva. As cifras de mortalidade de 12 meses indicam um efeito contínuo do tratamento com enapril. O nível da ativação neuroendócrina varia consideravelmente entre os pacientes com a insuficiência cardíaca congestiva severa. Observou-se uma forte associação entre os níveis de epinefrina, norepinefrina, aldosterona, ANG II e ANP e a mortalidade posterior de seis meses. Determinou-se que o enalapril reduziu o risco aumentado de morte associado com níveis altos de neurohormônios.

RESUMEN

Este trabajo analiza los datos obtenidos en el Estudio de Consenso en el que participaron 35 hospitales de Finlandia, Noruega y Suecia. Los 235 pacientes incluidos en el estudio sufrían de insuficiencia cardíaca congestiva (progresiva?) (Clase funcional IV; NYHA). Todos presentaban agrandamiento del corazón y fueron óptimamente tratados con inhibidores de la enzima convertidora de la angiotensina (ACE). El propósito del estudio fue el examen de la mortalidad y el modo de muerte a los 6 y también a los 12 meses en pacientes tratados con el inhibitor de la ACE, enalapril. El estudio inicial incluyó tan solo pacientes tratados con el enalapril. Este estudio se terminó prematuramente y se empezó un segundo estudio, asignando pacientes aleatoriamente sea a un placebo o al enalapril. En este segundo estudio, la reducción más grande en la mortalidad se vio en aquellos pacientes que murieron a causa de insuficiencia cardíaca progresiva. Los datos de mortalidad de 12 meses indican un efecto continuo del tratamiento con el enalapril. El nivel de activación neuroendocrina varía ampliamente entre los pacientes de Clase IV con insuficiencia cardíaca congestiva severa. Se observó una fuerte asociación entre los niveles de epinefrina, norepinefrina, ANG II, aldosterona y ANP, y la mortalidad subsecuente a los 6 meses. Se determinó que el enalapril reduce el incremento en el riesgo de muerte asociado con niveles elevados de neurohormonas.

要約

　本論文は，フィンランド，ノルウェーおよびスウェーデンの 35 病院が参加した Consensus Trial の治験成績をまとめたものである。

　対象は 235 例のうっ血性心不全患者（NYHA 心機能分類 IV 度）で，すべて心拡大を呈し，アンジオテンシン変換酵素（ACE）阻害薬以外の心血管系薬剤の治療を適宜受けていた。本試験の目的は，ACE 阻害薬エナラプリル投与患者における治療後 6 カ月および 12 カ月目の死亡率と死亡状況を検討することであった。

　第一次試験では，エナラプリルのみを投与した。この予備試験の終了後，エナラプリルまたはプラセボ投与群に無作為に割り付ける第二次試験を開始した。

　第二次試験では，エナラプリル治療により，進行性の心不全で死亡の危険性のとくに高い患者において死亡率が著明に低下した。この死亡率低下効果は 12 カ月後にも継続してみられた。NYHA 心機能分類 IV 度の重症うっ血性心不全患者では，神経内分泌の活性レベルは非常に多様であった。エピネフリン，ノルエピネフリン，アンジオテンシン II，アルドステロンおよび心房性ナトリウム利尿ペプチドの測定値と，6 カ月目の死亡率との間に強い相関性が認められた。エナラプリルは，各種神経ホルモンの高レベルに伴う死亡の危険性の増大を抑制することが判明した。

Cardiac and Renal Failure: An Expanding Role for ACE Inhibitors, edited by C. T. Dollery and L. M. Sherwood, Hanley & Belfus, Inc., Philadelphia.

Roundtable 2: *Role of ACE Inhibitors in Heart Failure*

Chairman: Colin Dollery
Panelists: Jay N. Cohn, Paul Hugenholtz, John Kjekshus, John D. Irvin

THE PATIENT WITH CHRONIC SEVERE HEART FAILURE

"The advent of ACE inhibitors, and perhaps other vasodilators, has been a great advance in the treatment of severe heart failure," said Dr. Dollery, who continued ". . . this has to be put in context."

He asked the panel whether there are better ways of using existing drugs in the treatment of severe heart failure.

Are Diuretics Used Correctly?

Dr. Cohn underlined the fact that most patients are incorrectly treated, especially with respect to diuretics; they are either receiving too much or not enough. He suggested that patients should be given partial responsibility for their own therapy, in the way that diabetics monitor their own response to insulin therapy. Patients in heart failure, he suggested should be taught to adjust their diuretic dosage in accordance with their weight, calibrated against central venous pressure.

Dr. Kjekhus reported data from a Consensus study in which patients were initially receiving digitalis and diuretics. Patients who were given additional enalapril were able to reduce their use of other medications, whereas patients given placebo had an increased diuretic requirement. Nitrate therapy was also being administered to 50% of the patients in the study. This had no effect on the outcome. However, patients with an initially low blood pressure were unable to tolerate enalapril, and treatment was withdrawn.

223

When to Introduce ACE Inhibitors

Dr. Hugenholz pointed out that in many countries, physicians appear to prefer to use digitalis and diuretics. He suggested that initial treatment should include an ACE inhibitor. This was supported in part by Dr. Cohn, who emphasized that there are a great many people dying, "perhaps because we are intervening too late," and he stressed the need for combination treatment. Initial treatment should be a combination of a diuretic, an ACE inhibitor or other vasodilator, and digitalis. In his study, prazosin was not as effective as other vasodilators in improving mortality or exercise tolerance.

Dr. Rocha wanted to know how ACE inhibitors compare with the combination of hydralazine and isosorbide dinitrate—the cost and efficacy of the latter appear favorable. Dr. Cohn had no data on this comparison but suggested that it is possible to predict the effects of the two treatment regimens. ACE inhibitors reduce blood pressure, whereas the hydralazine/nitrate combination therapy does not. "The clear advantage of ACE inhibitors," said Dr. Cohn, "is the low incidence of side-effects. They have a favorable metabolic effect that one does not see with hydralazine and nitrate."

The Question of Diuretics With Vasodilators

The data from Professor Inman's Prescription Event Monitoring (PEM) study with enalapril was discussed. Among the patients who died from renal failure, a small number were judged to have had their death precipitated by treatment. Among the factors that were identified were excessive doses of loop diuretics, prolonged diarrhea, and concomitant use of nonsteroidal anti-inflammatory drugs. Two patients had died as a result of hyperkalemia from concomitant treatment with potassium-sparing diuretics.[1] Dr. Irvin emphasized that package inserts for ACE inhibitors warn against use with this type of diuretic.

Dr. Poole-Wilson raised the question of how clinicians judge the "optimal dose" of diuretics prior to the introduction of a vasodilator. Dr. Cohn answered that the diuretic needs to be titrated to achieve optimum filling pressure and stable body weight when a vasodilator is being given at an effective dose. He went on to describe how the central venous pressure should be measured when the ACE inhibitor is introduced and reviewed after 2–3 days. Only then should the diuretic dose be titrated. In contrast to this approach, Dr. Dollery was of the opinion that diuretic doses should be reduced substantially at the start of ACE inhibitor treatment. He was supported in this by Dr. Sonnenblick, who "would reduce or stop diuretics when I start an ACE inhibitor." He also suggested that fluctuations in the patient's weight are a good guide to the diuretic requirement.

Dr. Johnston pointed out the theoretical advantage of starting the ACE inhibitor before the diuretic: there is less chance of a profound hypotensive effect, and lower doses of the diuretic can be used from the outset.

HEART FAILURE DEVELOPING WITHIN A FEW DAYS OF ACUTE MYOCARDIAL INFARCTION

For and Against ACE Inhibitors

Dr. Hugenholz described the advent of thrombolytic therapy in acute myocardial infarction as "revolutionary;" however, he went on to say that "ACE inhibitors ought to be studied in the early phases of myocardial infarction." These drugs may be of use in patients who are unsuitable candidates for thrombolysis, for whatever reason. In these cases, ACE inhibitors should be used as early as possible. Dr. Kjekhus agreed with this, and his only question was "how long do you continue the therapy?" Dr. Poole-Wilson strongly disagreed with this point of view. His feeling was that "nitrates and other drugs should be used." Drawing on his interpretation of data from studies by Sharpe *et al.* and Pfeffer *et al.*, he declared himself "still unsure" and said that he would like to see stronger data before he used ACE inhibitors in this type of patient. Both views were qualified by Dr. Ledingham, who emphasized that the chance of a hypotensive response must be taken into account before an ACE inhibitor is used. If hypotension develops during ACE inhibitor treatment, dobutamine, dopamine or a phosphodiesterase III inhibitor can bring things back to normal, said Dr. Sonnenblick.

The Place of Other Drugs

Beta-blockers

Dr. Dollery opened this part of the discussion with the statement, "In most heart failure studies about half the patients have died suddenly under circumstances which suggest that arrhythmia may have played a part. What is the place of beta-blockers with or without partial agonist activity, such as xamoterol or pindolol?"

Dr. Kjekhus said that in all of the trials, high-risk patients do better if they are treated with beta-blockers. However, beta-blockers with agonist activity have not been shown to be particularly beneficial. In response, Dr. Dollery pointed out that the design of some of the trials involving the latter group of drugs had been criticized.

Studies from Sweden and the U.S. suggest that there is a subset of patients who have a favorable long-term response to beta-blockers.

Calcium Antagonists

Discussion then turned to the calcium antagonists. Dr. Sonnenblick was enthusiastic about data that suggest that verapamil is effective in preventing vascular spasm and preventing death of cardiac cells. However, Dr. Dollery was of the opinion that the results of secondary intervention studies with calcium antagonists after myocardial infarction have been discouraging. These two opposing views were in part reconciled by Dr. Hugenholz, who suggested that the clinical data are not encouraging because calcium antagonists are ineffective when ischemia has already occurred. They are effective, however, in the experimental situation, when they are given immediately before the induction of trauma.

Other Classes of Drugs

In response to a question on the usefulness of renin inhibitors and atrial natriuretic peptide (ANP), Dr. Irvin declared that neither of these types of compounds were likely to have therapeutic potential. ANP causes unpredictable symptomatic hypotension, often associated with bradycardia, and renin inhibitors are not likely to be clinically useful unless an orally active one can be developed.

In Japan, said Dr. Imura, i.v. infusion of ANP is being studied in acute and chronic heart failure. His study has found that the drop in blood pressure in these patients is not as marked as that seen in hypertensives or in normal volunteers. The size of the drop in blood pressure may relate to the amount of ANP given and its build-up in the body; Dr. Dollery suggested that the cumulative action of small doses may be beneficial and avoid the problem of acute hypotension. The use of neutral peptidase inhibitors to block the degradation of ANP, so increasing its concentration in the plasma, was briefly discussed. Dr. Brunner revealed that two such inhibitors will soon be going into clinical research, and Dr. Dollery thought that this approach might be beneficial in some heart failure patients.

THE PATIENT WITH A SMALL HEART

Many patients with heart failure have small hearts, which are fibrotic and have hypertrophy of the myocardial cells within the fibrous structure. What treatment should be used for this type of patient? Dr. Cohn felt that, since they have a better prognosis than patients with a dilated heart, they need less urgent therapy. He went on to question the effectiveness of the calcium antagonist and beta-blocker therapy that is often given. Dr. Sonnenblick felt that the existing therapy was adequate. He pointed out that one of the characteristics of a small hypertrophied heart with a normal ejection fraction is a prolongation of contraction and a marked delay in relaxation. Calcium blockers reduce the relaxation period. Diuretics will reduce pulmonary congestion, and drugs that help regression of hypertrophy are also beneficial. In response to Dr. Dollery's question about the prospects for new or existing inotropic drugs in this condition, Dr. Cohn said that trials with PDE inhibitors have been disappointing. There is a rationale for the use of calcium sensitizing agents, which appear to increase cell contractility without increasing cytosol calcium, and there are also other drugs that act on sodium and potassium channels. However, it has been difficult to design protocols to test their efficacy.

SUMMARY

There was a general consensus that the outlook for patients with severe heart failure is not good. Dr. Dollery expressed the opinion that ". . . the way we use existing drugs is not going to improve greatly the results for Grade III and IV heart failure. We must expect a mortality of 30–50% at 1 year." However, Dr. Kjekhus had found a decreased mortality of 36% in the enalapril group in the Consensus trial.

For patients with heart failure following acute myocardial infarction, there are a wide variety of treatments available. There was no real consensus about which therapeutic regimen is best, but it was evident that care must be taken in extrapolating data from animal studies to the human situation.

REFERENCE

1. Spiers CJ, et al. Post marketing surveillance of enalapril: Investigation of the potential role of enalapril in deaths from renal failure. *Br Med J* 1988; **297**:830–32.

*Cardiac and Renal Failure: An Expanding
Role for ACE Inhibitors,* edited by C. T.
Dollery and L. M. Sherwood, Hanley &
Belfus, Inc., Philadelphia.

The Formation of a
Glomerular Filtrate

Klaus Thurau

In the 16th and 17th century vitalism, divine revelation and other metaphysical notions were still considered as appropriate means of gaining insight into the processes of life. For the kidney and, in particular, for the function of the glomerulus, it was Carl Ludwig, a young scientist at the University of Marburg, who, in 1842, paved the way to a new concept based on materialist-mechanist views and physicochemical processes. The revolutionary element in the new philosophy is best documented by a paragraph from his famous textbook (1852):

> Concluded that all the phenomena of the animal body are the consequence of simple attractions and repulsions (between a limited number of chemical atoms) such as can be observed when these elementary components collide. This conclusion will be irrefutable, when it is proven, with mathematical precision, that the above mentioned elementary conditions are so ordered, with respect to direction, time and mass, in the animal body that all the accomplishments of the living or dead organism must, of necessity, follow from their interactions.

Carl Ludwig recognized the importance of the hydrostatic pressure in the glomerular filtration process that delivers extracellular fluid into Bowman's space and the tubules. He already made it clear that the transcapillary hydrostatic pressure forces across the capillary wall not only water but all other plasma constituents except proteins and cells. In 1924, the formation of an ultrafiltrate at the glomerular site was experimentally established by the work of Richards and Wearn, who were able to micropuncture Bowman's space and analyze the collected fluid. It was protein-free but contained considerable amounts of chloride and glucose.

FILTRATION EQUILIBRIUM AND DISEQUILIBRIUM

More recently, a major dispute arose from experiments designed to determine whether or not filtration equilibrium is reached at some point in the glomerular capillaries, ie., that the transcapillary hydrostatic pressure difference equals the oncotic pressure of plasma. If it does, fluid filtration becomes zero and filtration rate becomes highly plasma-flow dependent. Filtration equilibrium may occur in some experimental animals with low glomerular capillary pressure and high glomerular filtration coefficient. However, filtration equilibrium has not been universally observed, and depends on the species and strain of the animals, the degree of volume expansion, and differences in the physiological conditions under which the studies are performed. It appears that the filtration coefficient is not a fixed parameter and differs from species to species and even between strains of the same species. It remains to be shown whether differences in the filtration coefficient are the result of a different hydraulic conductivity or of different filtration surface areas. At present there is no information available concerning the occurrence of filtration equilibration or disequilibration in man. Since glomerular filtration rate (GFR) in man appears to be only loosely related to renal plasma flow under many functional conditions, it seems that filtration equilibrium may not exist.

COUPLING BETWEEN FILTRATION AND REABSORPTION, THE TUBULOGLOMERULAR FEEDBACK

The kidney, as the exacting guardian of our interior milieu, has been credited with discriminatory activity in the selection of filtered constituents for reabsorption or excretion. The large GFR is prerequisite for the kidney to serve its function as a reprocessing machine for the plasma. In this reprocessing, the entire circulating plasma volume is filtered and reabsorbed twice every hour.

The coupled events of filtration and reabsorption occur at the capillary end of all vascular beds and are accomplished in most organs by purely physical forces, the balance between hydrostatic and colloid oncotic pressure first described by Starling. By and large, the composition of filtrate and reabsorbate is the same and no discrimination is exercised. In the kidney, however, a layer of epithelial cells (the tubular wall) is interposed between the site of filtration and that of re-entry of the filtrate into the blood stream. This distinctive addition to the system refines the reabsorptive process and enables a degree of selectivity in solute excretion. Salt and water are reabsorbed in large quantities; creatinine and urea for the most part are excreted. Tubular cell activity defines the composition of both reabsorbate and final urine. Selectivity ends at the basal surface of tubular cells, and re-entry of the reabsorbate from the peritubular, interstitial space into the vascular compartment is accomplished, as in the peripheral circulation, by Starling forces, without further discrimination as to composition.

The energy source for glomerular filtration, the left ventricle, is distinct from the metabolic energy of reabsorption, generated locally by the tubular epithelial cells. It is this locally produced energy that brings to the blind force of filtration the refinement of differential selectivity in the reabsorptive process. Although the energies of these two basic renal operations are independently derived, they must be adaptively coupled to one another. The adaptive coupling is described phenomenologically as tubuloglomerular balance, a process by which the rate of tubular reabsorption (tubular reabsorptive capacity) sets the filtration rate. This setting is imperative, since failure of reabsorptive function in the presence of continued filtration would result in a devastating loss of body fluids.

In most systemic capillaries, filtration and reabsorption are intrinsically linked. The hydrostatic force that results in filtration at the arterial end of a capillary provides the energy for reabsorption by concentrating colloids. The opposing filtration pressure is dissipated by the resistance to blood flow of the capillaries, and colloid oncotic pressure becomes increasingly effective, favoring reabsorption.

What mechanism exists to adjust filtration rate to reabsorptive capacity in the nephron? To be effective it should comprise monitoring and reacting components by which some sensing device reads a signal reflecting the adequacy or inadequacy of reabsorption and initiates a response at the glomerular level. The structural basis for such a system has been found in every mammalian nephron examined and is embodied in the juxtaglomerular apparatus. The juxtaglomerular apparatus joins a late segment of each nephron to the vascular pole of its own glomerulus. At the end of the thick ascending limb of Henle's loop, where the nephron returns to its glomerulus, the cells of the tubular wall are differentiated into the macula densa cells and lie in intimate apposition to the walls of the glomerular arterioles. Here the cells of the media are transformed to large secretory-type cells filled with electron-dense granules (renin). This anatomic arrangement is ideally suited to monitor an intratubular event (reabsorption) and to initiate a response (filtration).

The signal that is read by the tubular component (macula densa) of the juxtaglomerular apparatus is the sodium chloride concentration of tubular fluid at that site. Present evidence more specifically favors chloride ion concentration as the definitive signal, and the concentration of this ion here is related to the reabsorptive activity of the entire nephron. The largest volume of filtrate is reabsorbed proximally, at a sodium chloride concentration close to the plasma value. Filtrate arriving at the site of the macula densa has, under normal conditions, lost over 80% of its original volume, and its sodium chloride concentration is, for the first time along the nephron, below plasma value — about one-seventh in fact. This low sodium chloride concentration is established by the thick ascending limb of Henle's loop, the cells of which actively transport sodium chloride without equivalent water.

An increased signal, reporting imbalance between filtration and reabsorption, can be induced experimentally in two ways: One is by augmenting the perfusion rate through the nephron, a condition simulating increased glomerular filtration rate. This leads to an increase in sodium chloride concentration at the macula densa, since tubular reabsorptive activity does not increase in proportion to the increased tubular flow rate. Another way is by reducing the tubular reabsorptive capacity. Here, the increased sodium chloride concentration at the macula densa reflects the failure of the tubular epithelium to reabsorb. Either maneuver causes an imbalance between solute load to the nephron and reabsorptive capacity of tubular cells.

The appropriate response to a signal-reporting reabsorptive failure is reduction in filtration rate; this has been found in experimental animals with induced acute renal failure (tubular insufficiency) and in the clinical condition of man. Filtration rate is reduced by vasoconstriction of the glomerular arterioles and, possibly by retraction of the glomerular tuft, activities that simultaneously reduce renal blood flow. Evidence is accumulating that the vasoactive material is angiotensin II, locally formed at the site of the juxtaglomerular apparatus and acting *in situ*. It has been shown that the juxtaglomerular apparatus is supplied with all the components necessary to manufacture and to degrade angiotensin II. Converting enzyme inhibitors reduce the intensity of the response as does depletion of renal renin.

Data have also been furnished to confirm the intrarenal formation of angiotensin II and its release primarily into the renal interstitium rather than into the blood. Experimentally, when tubular fluid sodium chloride concentration of a single nephron is increased at the macula densa, the renin activity of the attached juxtaglomerular apparatus increases proportionately and the filtration rate of the nephron decreases. These findings together demonstrate the existence of a tubuloglomerular feedback mechanism, whereby single nephron (and in the aggregate, whole kidney) glomerular filtration rate is regulated according to the efficiency of reabsorption.

The tubular-glomerular feedback described provides a means to maintain to a large extent a balance between the rate of filtrate delivered to the tubular epithelium for reprocessing and the capacity of the tubular epithelium to reabsorb selectively the filtrate. The feedback mechanism has been found to operate under physiological conditions, to possess the inherent capability for adjusting its effectiveness to the physiological needs (volume expansion vs. volume contraction) and to reduce glomerular filtration rate to conform to diminished reabsorptive capacity during acute tubular insufficiency. Under the latter condition, the glomerular shutdown shows that the glomeruli have taken over the volume conserving function normally exercised by the tubular epithelium. Volume conservation by glomerular shutdown is immediately effective and therefore life-saving. It has the disadvantage of being indiscriminate; consequently nitrogenous wastes and other constituents of the body regularly cleared by glomerular filtration are retained. The immediate threat by hypovolemia is averted at the expense of regulation of the body fluid composition, which allows the organism more time to repair structure and function of the tubular epithelium.

As glomerular shutdown is a logical response to tubular reabsorptive insufficiency in order to conserve body volume, it follows that any therapeutic attempt to increase glomerular filtration rate before tubular reabsorptive capacity has recovered must have deleterious effects upon the function of the organism as a whole.

SUMMARY

A large glomerular filtration rate (GFR) is a prerequisite for the kidney to function effectively as a reprocessing machine for the plasma. In the kidney, the coupled events of filtration and reabsorption are refined to allow selectivity in solute excretion at the basal surfaces of the tubular cells. A mechanism for adjusting filtration rate to the reabsorptive capacity of the nephron is essential if devastating loss of body fluids is to be avoided. The structural basis for such a system is found in the juxtaglomerular apparatus. The macula densa cells of the tubular wall are able to detect the sodium chloride concentration at that site and reflect the absorptive capacity of the entire nephron. The appropriate response to reabsorptive failure is a reduction in filtration rate, and the existence of a tubulo-glomerular feedback mechanism, which will achieve this, has been demonstrated. This feedback mechanism is affected by changes in renin activity in response to increases in the tubular fluid sodium chloride concentration. Tubulo-glomerular feedback allows the GFR to be reduced to conform to diminished absorptive capacity during acute tubular insufficiency. In such a situation, life-saving volume conservation can be achieved by glomerular shutdown. Any therapeutic attempt to increase GFR before the tubular reabsorptive capacity has recovered is likely to have adverse effects on the organism as a whole.

RÉSUMÉ

Pour que le rein fonctionne efficacement dans son rôle de redistribution du flux plasmatique, sanguin il est nécessaire que le taux de filtration glomérulaire soit important. Les phénomènes associés de filtration et de réabsorption, au niveau du rein, sont épurés de façon à permettre la sélectivité en excrétion dissoute aux surfaces basales des cellules tubulaires. Il est essentiel d'avoir un mécanisme apte à ajuster le taux de filtration à la capacité de réabsorption du néphron si l'on veut éviter une déshydradation importante. C'est dans l'appareil juxtaglomérulaire que l'on trouve la base de structure d'un tel système. Les cellules pigmentaires densa de la paroi tubulaire sont capables de détecter la concentration de chlorure de sodium à ce site et d'évoquer la capacité d'absorption du néphron entier. Lorsqu'il y a une insuffisance de réabsorption on note une diminution du taux de filtration, et l'existence du mécanisme d'autorégulation tubulo-glomérulaire a été démontrée. Ce mécanisme d'autorégulation intervient lorsqu'il y a des changements d'activité rénine en réponse aux augmentations de la concentration de chlorure de sodium tubulaire. L'autorégulation tubuloglomérulaire permet une réduction du taux de filtration glomérulaire en vue de s'adapter à la diminution de la capacité d'absorption au cours d'une insuffisance tubulaire aigue. Dans une telle situation on peut obtenir la conservation d'un volume vital par blocage glomérulaire. Toute tentative de traitement thérapeutique ayant pour objectif d'augmenter le taux de filtration glomérulaire avant d'avoir récupéré la capacité de réabsorption tubulaire risque d'avoir des effets délétères sur l'organisme dans son ensemble.

ZUSAMMENFASSUNG

Eine grosse glomeruläre Filtrationsrate ist eine notwendige Voraussetzung für die effektive Funktion der Niere als Wiederaufarbeitungsmaschine für das Plasma. In der Niere werden die gekoppelten Vorgänge der Filtration und der Reabsorption so verfeinert, dass Selektivität bei der Lösungabscheidung an den Basisflächen der tubulären Zellen möglich ist. Wichtig ist ein Mechanismus für die Anpassung der Filtrationsrate an die Reabsorptionskapazität des Nephrons, damit ein übermässiger Verlust an Körperflüssigkeit vermieden werden kann. Der juxtaglomeruläre Apparat stellt die strukturelle Basis für ein solches System dar. Die makulären Densa-Zellen der Tubulärwände sind in der Lage, die Konzentration an Natriumchlorid an eben diesem Ort festzustellen und so die Absorptionskapazität des ganzen Nephrons zu reflektieren. Die angemessene Antwort auf ein Versagen der Reabsorption besteht in einer Reduktion der Filtrationsrate; und die Existenz eines tubuloglomerulären Rückkopplungsmechanismus ist gezeigt worden, der genau dies erreicht. Dieser Rückkopplungsmechanismus arbeitet durch Veränderungen in der Reninaktivität als Reaktion auf Erhöhungen der Natriumchloridkonzentration in der tubulären Flüssigkeit. Tubulo-glomeruläre Rückkopplung erlaubt es der glomerulären Filtrationsrate, sich zu reduzieren als Anpassung an eine verringerte Absorptionskapazität im Verlauf einer akuten tubulären Insuffizienz. In einer solchen Situation kann eine lebensrettende Volumenerhaltung durch glomeruläre Schliessung erreicht werden. Therapeutische Versuche, die glomeruläre Filtrationsrate zu erhöhen, bevor die tubuläre Reabsorptionskapazität sich erhohlt hat, gehen das Risiko schädlicher Effekte auf den Restorganismus ein.

RIASSUNTO

Un alto tasso di filtrazione glomerulare è un prerequisito affinché il rene possa funzionare efficacemente come macchina di rielaborazione del plasma. Nel rene, gli eventi accoppiati di filtrazione e riassorbimento vengono raffinati per consentire la selettività nell'escrezione di soluto alle superfici basali delle cellule tubulari. Un meccanismo per adattare il tasso di filtrazione alla capacità di riassorbimento del nefrone è essenziale per evitare una catastrofica perdita di fluidi corporei. La base strutturale di tale sistema si trova nell'apparato juxtaglomerulare. Le cellule macula densa della parete tubulare sono in grado di riconoscere la concentrazione di cloruro di sodio in quel sito e riflettono la capacità di riassorbimento dell'intero nefrone. La reazione adeguata all'insufficienza di riassorbimento è una riduzione del tasso di filtrazione ed è strata clincostrata l'esistenza di un meccanismo di feedback tubuloglomerulare che los permette. Questo meccanismo di feedback viene attivato da cambiamenti nell'attività della renina come reazione ad aumenti della concentrazione di cloruro di sodio nel fluido tubulare. Il feedback tubuloglomerulare consente di ridurre il tasso di filtrazione glomerulare in modo da conformarsi alla diminuita capacità di riassorbimento durante l'insufficienza tubulare acuta. In tale situazione la conservazione del volume (e conseguente mantenimento in vita) può essere ottenuta mediante l'arresto glomerulare. Qualsiasi tentativo terapeutico di aumentare il tasso di filtrazione glomerulare prima della ripresa della capacità di riassorbimento tubulare avrà probabilmente effetti deleteri sull'insieme dell'organismo.

SUMÁRIO

Um elevado índice de filtração glomerular (GFR) é um prerequisito para que o rim funcione apropriadamente como máquina de reprocessamento do plasma. No rim, os eventos ligados da filtração são refinados para que permitam a seletividade na excreção de solutos nas superfícies basais das células tubulares. Para evitar a perda devastadora de fluidos corporais, precisa-se um mecanismo de ajuste do índice de filtração em relação com a capacidade de reabsorção do nefro. Encontra-se a base estrutural para tal sistema no aparelho justaglomerular. As células da mácula densa da parede tubular sáo capazes de detectar a concentração de cloreto de sódio neste síto e refletem a capacidade de absorção do nefro completo. A resposta apropriada à insuficiência cardíaca na reabsorção é uma redução do índice de filtração, e tem-se demonstrado a existência de um mecanismo de retroalimentação tubuloglomerular que possibilita isto. Este mecanismo de retroalimentação é efetuado mediante mudanças na atividade da renina em resposta a aumentos na concentração de cloreto de sódio no fluido tubular. A retroalimentação tubuloglomerular permite a redução do GFR para ajustar-se à capacidade reduzida de absorção durante a insuficiência tubular aguda. Em tal situação, uma concentração volumétrica que salve a vida pode conseguir-se mediante a paralisação da função glomerular. Qualquer intento terapêutico de aumentar o GFR antes de que se haja recuperado a capacidade de reabsorção tubular provavelmente cause efeitos nocivos no organismo como um todo.

RESUMEN

Un elevado índice de filtración glomerular (GFR) es un prerrequisito para que el riñón funcione apropiadamente como máquina de reprocesamiento del plasma. En el riñón, la filtración y reabsorción se han refinado para que permitan selectividad en la excreción de solutos en las superficies basales de las células tubulares. Para evitar la pérdida devastadora de fluidos corporales se necesita un mecanismo de ajuste del índice de filtración en relación a la capacidad de reabsorción del nefrón. La base estructural para tal sistema se encuentra en al aparato yuxtaglomerular. Las células de la mácula densa de la pared tubular son capaces de detectar la concentración de cloruro de sodio en ese sitio y reflejan la capacidad de absorción del nefrón completo. La respuesta apropiada a la insuficiencia en la reabsorción es una reducción del índice de filtración, y se ha demostrado la existencia de un mecanismo de retroalimentación tubuloglomerular que hace esto posible. Este mecanismo de retroalimentación tubuloglomerular tiene efecto debido a cambios en la actividad de la renina en respuesta a incrementos en la concentración de cloruro de sodio en el fluido tubular. La retroalimentación tubuloglomerular permite la reducción del GFR para ajustarse a la disminución en la capacidad de absorción durante la insuficiencia tubular aguda. En tal situación, una concentración volumétrica que salve la vida puede lograrse mediante la detención de la función glomerular. Cualquier intento terapéutico de incrementar el GFR antes de que se haya recuperado la capacidad le reabsorción tubular probablemente cause efectos nocivos en el organismo como un todo.

要約

腎が血漿の再生機構としての機能を効果的に発揮するためには，ある程度高い糸球体濾過値（GFR）が必要である。腎においては，互いに共役する濾過と再吸収とが，尿細管細胞の基底表層での溶質排出の選択性を精密に保っている。もし体液の甚大な損失を避ける必要がある場合には，GFR をネフロンの再吸収能に適合させる機序が不可欠である。このシステムの基本構造は，傍糸球体装置の中に

見出される。尿細管壁の密集斑細胞はその部位の NaCl 濃度を感知し，この情報を全ネフロンの再吸収能に反映させることができる。再吸収不全に対する適切な反応として，GFR が低下する。すなわち，尿細管‐糸球体フィードバック機構の存在が証明されている。

　このフィードバック機構は，尿細管の NaCl 濃度の増加に反応してレニン活性が変化することによって作動する。またこの機構は，急性尿細管機能不全時には失われた再吸収能に見合うように GFR を低下させる。このような一種の救命的な体液量の保持は，糸球体の閉鎖によってもたらされる。

　したがって，尿細管の再吸収能が回復する前に GFR を上昇させるいかなる治療も，生命体全体にとって有害であるといえる。

Cardiac and Renal Failure: An Expanding Role for ACE Inhibitors, edited by C. T. Dollery and L. M. Sherwood, Hanley & Belfus, Inc., Philadelphia.

Glomerular Microcirculatory Dynamics and Their Relationship to Progressive Renal Disease: Recent Concepts

William F. Keane
Michael P. O'Donnell
Bertram L. Kasiske

It is relatively well-established that, once a critical number of nephrons are destroyed by disease, renal function will progressively decline, even in clinical situations where the initial cause of the disease seems to have resolved.[1] Morphologically, the end-result of progressive renal injury is glomerulosclerosis. Frequently, focal glomerulosclerosis (FGS) is seen early in the course of progressive renal disease, and FGS is usually preceded by mesangial matrix expansion and by increased mesangial cellularity.[2] Glomerular epithelial cell vacuolization and focal detachment from the basement membrane have also been noted to precede the development of FGS.[2] However, it is not known what the relative contributions of each of these early morphological changes may be to the development of FGS.

The pathogenesis of progressive glomerular injury leading to FGS is still incompletely understood. It has been proposed that alterations in glomerular hemodynamics, particularly increased glomerular capillary pressure, play a pivotal role in the initiation and progression of renal disease.[3] Nonhemodynamic factors have also been considered important in glomerular injury leading to FGS.[4,5,6] Indeed, recent experimental data have suggested that some of these factors may have effects on glomerular injury that are independent of glomerular hemodynamics.[6,7,8] Clinically, the recognition that 30,000 new patients each year in the U.S. require dialysis or transplantation therapy and that the total cost of this program currently approximates 3.5 billion dollars have further underscored the importance of expanding our understanding of the pathogenesis of progressive renal disease.

237

GLOMERULAR HEMODYNAMIC ALTERATIONS AND THE PROGRESSION OF RENAL DISEASE: INFLUENCE OF DIETARY PROTEIN RESTRICTION AND ANTIHYPERTENSIVE THERAPY

Initial support for the notion that glomerular hemodynamic alterations are an important cause of glomerular injury comes from studies of rats with reduced renal mass. In these studies, surgical reduction of renal mass by 50–80% significantly accelerated the development of glomerular injury and protein-uria normally seen with aging.[3,9] The incidence and severity of glomerular injury paralleled the degree of nephron reduction. Renal ablation was uniformly followed by compensatory increases in single nephron glomerular filtration rate (SNGFR) and single nephron plasma flow (SNPF).[3,9] In rats with 80% ablation (remnant kidney model) induced by unilateral nephrectomy and segmental infarction of two-thirds of the remaining kidney, systemic hypertension and increased glomerular capillary pressure (P_{GC}) also occurred (Figure 1).[9] These studies suggested, therefore, that glomerular hyperfiltration, or some determinant thereof, was responsible for accelerated glomerular injury.

Further support for the contention that glomerular hemodynamic changes participated in progressive glomerular injury came from studies of dietary protein restriction,[10,11] as well as from studies in which pharmacologic interventions were used to treat systemic hypertension.[12] In rats with 80% renal ablation, dietary protein restriction, which limits the adaptive increases in

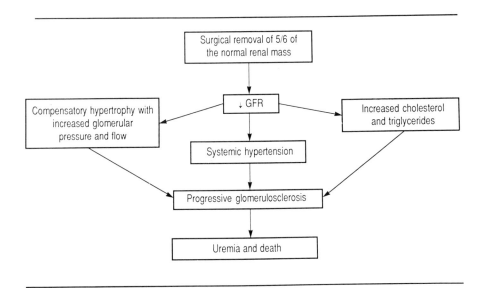

FIG. 1. Schematic outline of changes that occur after loss of functioning nephrons.

SNGFR, SNPF and P_{GC} without reducing systemic hypertension, resulted in amelioration of proteinuria and a lower frequency of FGS.[10] Moreover, when dietary protein restriction was started later in the course of glomerular disease, this intervention did not reduce SNGFR or SNPF, but did decrease P_{GC}, even though systemic hypertension persisted.[11] It should be noted, however, that the extent of protein restriction used in these studies was severe and was associated with retarded growth and potentially with other metabolic effects not evaluated.

Pharmacologic treatment of hypertension in the rat remnant kidney model has further suggested that glomerular hypertension is critical to the development of FGS. In these studies, two different therapeutic regimens were used for the treatment of hypertension, one a combination of hydrochlorothiazide, reserpine, and hydralazine, and the other the angiotensin-converting enzyme inhibitor, enalapril.[12] Although both regimens normalized systemic blood pressure, only enalapril reduced P_{GC}, and only enalapril therapy caused a reduction in proteinuria and a decrease in FGS.[12] Initiation of enalapril therapy after glomerular injury was established reduced systemic and glomerular pressures, and this was also associated with a reduction in the progression of glomerular injury.[13] Thus, persistent glomerular hypertension appeared important in the development of glomerular damage, whereas normalization of P_{GC} dramatically reduced glomerular injury.

ANGIOTENSIN-CONVERTING ENZYME INHIBITION: POTENTIAL NON-HEMODYNAMIC EFFECTS IN PROGRESSIVE RENAL DISEASE

Despite the evidence that hemodynamic factors can influence the development of FGS, the mechanism whereby glomerular hypertension causes glomerular injury is unclear. It is also unclear whether hemodynamic alterations are essential for the initiation of glomerular damage. In this regard, recent studies have been performed in the rat-remnant kidney model, in which serial micropuncture studies were performed in the same kidney. These investigations have questioned whether glomerular hypertension, present early in the course of this disease, is, in fact, predictive of which glomeruli will ultimately develop sclerosis.[14] It has also been demonstrated, in a model of progressive FGS induced by the aminonucleoside of puromycin, that amelioration of glomerular injury by an angiotensin converting enzyme (ACE) inhibitor occurred independently of any reduction in glomerular pressures.[15]

More recently, studies in obese Zucker rats have also suggested a nonhemodynamic beneficial effect of ACE inhibition.[16] This experimental model of chronic glomerular disease has been extensively investigated, and results to date have demonstrated that nonhemodynamic factors, specifically abnormal lipid metabolism, appear to be the predominant mechanism involved in the initiation of progressive renal insufficiency (see following discussion). Importantly, not only do these rats have normal glomerular hemodynamics, but they also have low circulating renin concentrations.[16] Therapy with enalapril over approximately an 8-month time interval resulted in a significant reduction in albuminuria in obese rats, prevention of a progressive increase in serum cholesterol, and, ultimately, a five-fold reduction in the extent of glomerular injury (Table I). Blood pressures, although within the normal range, were slightly lower in the enalapril treatment group.

Kidney size was significantly less in obese Zucker rats treated with enalapril (Table I). In addition, the degree of mesangial cellularity and matrix expansion was reduced in enalapril-treated rats. In this regard, ACE therapy also limits the degree of compensatory glomerular hypertrophy in the remnant kidney model.[12] Evidence that ACE inhibitors have a direct effect on glomerular cell growth and proliferation can also be derived from experiments that have demonstrated attenuation of maturational growth independent of changes in glomerular pressures.[17] Based on these recent results, it is reasonable to postulate that the beneficial effects of ACE inhibition may be more a result of their effect on cell proliferation and growth than on glomerular hemodynamic changes.

NONHEMODYNAMIC MECHANISMS AND THE PROGRESSION OF RENAL DISEASE

The possibility that nonhemodynamic mechanisms participate in the pathogenesis of progressive renal disease was initially suggested by studies using anticoagulants.[18] Specifically, heparin was shown to reduce the incidence of FGS in the renal ablation model without affecting glomerular hemodynamics.[18,19] This effect was probably not a result of heparin's anticoagulant properties, because low-molecular-weight heparin, which is devoid of anticoagulant effects, also reduced glomerular injury in rats with renal ablation.[19] The precise mechanism whereby heparin exerted these salutary effects is not understood. However, heparin molecules have cell growth inhibitory properties in a variety of *in vitro* settings. Specifically, heparin has been shown to inhibit mesangial cell growth in a dose dependent fashion.[20]

More recently, experimental results have suggested that abnormalities of lipid metabolism also may be an important factor in the progression of glomerular injury.[21] In these studies, two chemically different lipid lowering agents, clofibric acid, the pharmacologically-active form of clofibrate, and the 3-hydroxy-3-methylglutaryl (HMG) coenzyme-A reductase inhibitor, lovastatin, were used.[21] In the obese Zucker rat, progressive, glomerular injury, resulting in renal insufficiency, occurred over a period of one year.[22,23] In addition, hyperlipidemia was evident at an early age and this became more pronounced as proteinuria increases. Since neither glomerular hyperfiltration

TABLE I.   *Effect of angiotensin enzyme converting enzyme inhibition in Zucker rats.*

Group	PRA (ng AI · ml⁻¹ · hr⁻¹)	BP (mmHg)	CHOL (mg/dL)	$U_{alb}V$ (mg/24h)	Kidney Wt (g)	FGS (%)
Obese Zucker	9.0[a]	144[a]	149[a]	98[a]	2.92[a]	8.3[a]
(n = 9)	± 1.9	18	29	29	0.06	2.5
Obese Zucker	19.2[b]	125[b]	105[b]	25[b]	2.50[b]	1.4[b]
+ enalapril (n = 7)	± 4.5	9	9	8	0.07	0.8
Lean Zuckers	22.8[b]	124[b]	75[b]	3[c]	2.47[b]	0.5[b]
(n = 8)	± 3.0	4	5	1	0.04	0.5

Male obese Zucker rats were treated from 8–38 weeks of age with enalapril (50 mg/L) in their drinking water. Results (mean ± SE) are at 38 weeks of age. Different superscripts (a, b, c) indicate $p < 0.05$ by ANOVA.

Abbreviations: PRA, plasma renin activity; BP, tail cuff awake blood pressure; CHOL, fasting serum cholesterol; $U_{alb}V$, urinary albumin excretion; Wt, weight; FGS, focal glomerulosclerosis.

nor glomerular hypertension anteceded the development of FGS, it was hypothesized that the hyperlipidemia observed in this model participated in the development of FGS.[21,24] Indeed, therapy with the lipid-lowering agents clofibric acid or lovastatin dramatically reduced albuminuria and FGS.[21] Interestingly, reduction in glomerular mesangial matrix expansion as well as mesangial cellularity were conspicuous findings in these studies. These beneficial effects were independent of changes in systemic or glomerular pressures.[21]

Therapy with lipid-lowering agents also appears to have a significant impact on the progression of renal diseases in hyperlipidemic models in which systemic and glomerular hypertension are present. In the rat-remnant kidney model, therapy with clofibric acid or lovastatin effectively decreased hyperlipidemia. In addition, therapy with these agents dramatically reduced proteinuria and the incidence of FGS independent of changes in systemic blood pressure or glomerular hemodynamics.[7] Recently, studies have also shown that the Dahl-salt-sensitive ("S") rat exhibits multiple risk factors for glomerular injury. Hyperlipidemia, for example, occurs at an early age in Dahl "S" rats.[25] In this model, development of systemic hypertension is also associated with increased glomerular pressures.[26] Ultimately, marked albuminuria and extensive FGS developed in hypertensive "S" rats. Thus, in this model, glomerular hypertension and hyperlipidemia coexist and are associated with the development of severe glomerular injury, reminiscent of findings seen after removal of 80% of renal mass. Importantly, lovastatin therapy abrogated the progressive hyperlipidemia seen in hypertensive Dahl "S" rats, and this was associated with amelioration of glomerular injury, despite the presence of severe systemic hypertension (Figure 2). Thus, in two models of systemic hypertension in which glomerular hypertension occurs, the remnant-kidney model and the Dahl "S" rat, reduction in circulating lipids by pharmacologi-

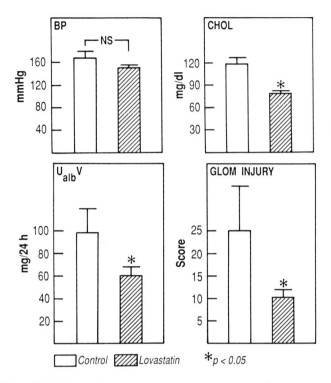

FIG. 2. Effect of daily lovastatin therapy in hypertensive Dahl salt-sensitive rats fed 4% NaCl diet since 6 weeks of age. Data (mean ± SE) are those obtained at 28 weeks of age.

cal agents dramatically reduced the extent and severity of glomerular injury. Collectively, these experimental data indicate that nonhemodynamic factors involving lipid metabolism are important modulators of progressive renal injury. These effects are also independent of glomerular hemodynamic changes. Whether an interaction between abnormal lipid metabolism and glomerular hypertension exists in progressive renal injury is unknown.

The mechanisms whereby abnormal lipid metabolism may initiate and/or participate in the development of FGS are unknown. A number of important effects of hyperlipidemia on cell function have been defined. Hyperlipidemia appears to alter renal structure and may be associated with altered renal tissue lipid composition.[27] Experimental results have suggested that changes in mesangial matrix and cellularity are dramatically reduced by therapy with lipid-lowering agents, suggesting a possible mechanism of lipid-mediated glomerular injury. An increased number of macrophage-derived cells, e.g., foam cells, is evident in glomeruli of rats with hyperlipidemia.[7,21] Macrophages have been implicated as important cellular mediators of glomerular injury in immune-mediated diseases.[28] In addition, hyperlipidemia has been shown to affect a number of monocyte functions.[29] Thus, it is possible that monocytes contribute to injury in the setting of hyperlipidemia, possibly in a manner analogous to that postulated in atherosclerosis.[29]

In addition, abnormalities of fatty acid metabolism have been identified as an important renal lipid alteration that correlates with glomerular injury.[27] Specifically, relative deficiencies in polyunsaturated fatty acids of the omega-6 series, e.g., linoleic and arachidonic acids, have been described.[27] In this regard, dietary supplementation with linoleic acid has been shown to ameliorate glomerular injury in the rat remnant kidney model.[30,31] These omega-6 fatty acids are intimately involved in the production of various eicosanoids that may modulate mesangial cell proliferation and matrix production, attracting circulating monocytes as well as influencing the production of other cytokines.[32,33]

ACKNOWLEDGEMENTS

This work was supported by grants R01-AM37396, R23-AM37112 and DK01628-01A from the National Institutes of Health.

REFERENCES

1. Mitch WE, Walser M, Buffington GA, Leman NJ. A simple method of estimating progression of chronic renal failure. *Lancet* 1976; **ii**:1326–1328.
2. Rennke HG. Structural alterations associated with glomerular hyperfiltration. In Mitch WE, Brenner BM, Stein JM (eds). *The Progressive Nature of Renal Disease.* New York: Churchill Livingstone, 1986, pp 111–131.
3. Brenner BM. Nephron adaption to renal injury or ablation. *Am J Physiol* 1985; **249**: F324–F337.
4. Klahr S, Schreiner G, Ichikawa I. The progression of renal disease. *N Engl J Med* 1988; **318**:1657–1666.
5. Keane WF, Kasiske BL, O'Donnell MP. Hyperlipidemia and the progression of renal disease. *Am J Clin Nutr* 1988; **47**:157–160.
6. Ichikawa I, Yoshida Y, Purkerson ML, Klahr S. The effect of heparin administration on the glomerular structure and function of remnant nephrons. *J Hypertens* 1986; **4**:S566.
7. Kasiske BL, O'Donnell MP, Garvis WJ, Keane WF. Pharmacological treatment of hyperlipidemia reduces glomerular injury in rat 5/6 nephrectomy model of chronic renal failure. *Circ Res* 1988; **62**:367–374.
8. Purkerson ML, Joist JH, Yates SJ, Valdes A, Morrison A, Klahr S. Inhibition of thromboxane synthesis ameliorates the progressive kidney disease of rats with subtotal renal ablation. *Proc Natl Acad Sci* (USA) 1985; **82**:193–197.
9. Hostetter TH, Olson JL, Rennke HG, Venkatachalam MA, Brenner BM. Hyperfiltration in remnant nephrons: a potentially adverse response to renal ablation. *Am J Physiol* 1981; **241**:F85–F93.
10. Hostetter TH, Meyer TW, Rennke HG, Brenner BM. Chronic effects of dietary protein on renal structure and function in the rat with intact and reduced renal mass. *Kidney Int* 1986; **30**:509–517.

11. Nath KA, Kren SM, Hostetter TH. Dietary protein restriction and established renal injury in the rat. Selective role of glomerular capillary pressure and progressive glomerular dysfunction. *J Clin Invest* 1986; **78**:1199–1205.

12. Anderson S, Rennke HG, Brenner BM. Therapeutic advantage of converting enzyme inhibitors in arresting progressive renal disease associated with systemic hypertension in the rat. *J Clin Invest* 1986; **77**:1993–2000.

13. Meyer TW, Anderson S, Rennke HG, Brenner BM. Reversing glomerular hypertension stabilizes established injury. *Kidney Int* 1987; **31**:752–759.

14. Yoshida Y, Fogo A, Shiraga H, Glick AD, Ichikawa I. Serial micropuncture analysis of single nephron function in subtotal renal ablation. *Kidney Int* 1988; **33**:855–867.

15. Fogo A, Yoshia Y, Glick AD, Homma T, Ichikawa I. Serial micropuncture analysis of glomerular function in two rat models of glomerulosclerosis. *J Clin Invest* 1988; **82**:322–330.

16. O'Donnell MP, Kasiske BL, Katz SA, Schmitz PG, Keane WF. Enalapril reduces glomerular injury in obese Zucker rats. *Abstracts of the American Society of Nephrology* 1988; **21**.

17. Yoshida Y, Fogo A, Ichikawa I. Glomerular hypertrophy has a greater impact on glomerular sclerosis than the adaptive hyperfunction in remnant nephrons. *Kidney Int* 1988; **33**:327 (abstract).

18. Klahr S, Heifets M, Purkerson ML. The influence of anticoagulation on the progression of experimental renal disease. In Mitch WE, Brenner BM, Stein JH (eds). *The Progressive Nature of Renal Disease.* New York: Churchill Livingstone, 1986, pp 45–64.

19. Purkerson ML, Tollefsen BM, Klahr S. N-desulfated-acetylated heparin ameliorates the progression of renal disease in rats with subtotal renal ablation. *J Clin Invest* 1988; **81**:69–74.

20. Castellanot JJ, Hoover RL, Harper RA, Karnovsky MJ. Heparin and glomerular epithelial cell-secreted heparin-like species inhibit mesangial cell proliferation. *Am J Pathol* 1985; **120**:427–435.

21. Kasiske BL, O'Donnell MP, Cleary MP, Keane WF. Treatment of hyperlipidemia reduces glomerular injury in obese Zucker rats. *Kidney Int* 1988; **33**:667–672.

22. Kasiske BL, Cleary MP, O'Donnell MP, Keane WF. Effects of genetic obesity on renal structure and function in the Zucker rat. *J Lab Clin Med* 1985; **106**:598–604.

23. O'Donnell MP, Kasiske BL, Cleary MP, Keane WF. Effects of genetic obesity on renal structure and function in the Zucker rat. II. Micropuncture studies. *J Lab Clin Med* 1985; **106**:605–610.

24. Kasiske BL, O'Donnell MP, Keane WF. The obese Zucker rat model of glomerular injury in type II diabetes. *J Diabetic Complications* 1987; **1**:26–29.

25. O'Donnell MP, Kasiske BL, Keane WF. Factors underlying differences in glomerular injury between Dahl salt-sensitive rats and spontaneously hypertensive rats. *Am J Hypertens* 1988; **2**:9–13.

26. Raij L, Azar S, Keane WF. Mesangial immune injury, hypertension and progressive glomerular damage in Dahl rats. *Kidney Int* 1984; **26**:137–143.

27. Kasiske BL, O'Donnell MP, Cleary MP, Keane WF. The effects of reduced renal mass on tissue lipids and renal injury in hyperlipidemic obese Zucker rats. *Kidney Int* 1989; **35**:40–47.

28. Schreiner GF, Cotran RS, Unanue ER. Macrophages and cellular immunity in experimental glomerulonephritis. *Sem Immunopath* 1982; **5**:251–267.

29. Mitchison MJ, Ball RY. Macrophages and atherogenesis. *Lancet* 1987; **ii**:146–149.

30. Barcelli UO, Weiss M, Pollak BE. Effects of a dietary prostaglandin precursor on the progression of experimentally induced chronic renal failure. *J Lab Clin Med* 1982; **100**:786–797.

31. Heifets M, Morrissey JJ, Purkerson ML, Morrison AR, Klahr S. Effect of dietary lipids on renal function in rats with subtotal nephrectomy. *Kidney Int* 1987; **32**:335–341.

32. Parker CW. Lipid mediators produced through lipoxygenase pathway. *Ann Rev Immunol* 1987; **5**:65–84.

33. Lefkowith JB, Schreiner G. Essential fatty acid deficiency depletes rat glomeruli of resident macrophages and inhibits angiotensin II-induced eicosanoid synthesis. *J Clin Invest* 1987; **80**:947–956.

SUMMARY

At present, the role that lipid abnormalities and cellular changes play in progressive renal injury remains to be determined. It is intriguing to speculate that both ACE inhibitors and lipid-lowering agents may have a common mechanism of action in the pathogenesis of progressive renal disease by affecting cell growth/proliferation. It is increasingly evident that the pathogenesis of progressive renal disease involves multiple factors. The availability of new pharmacological agents, such as ACE inhibitors and lipid-lowering agents, has allowed the development of important new concepts as they pertain to mechanisms of renal injury.

RÉSUMÉ

Actuellement, le rôle que les anomalies lipidiques et les changements cellulaires jouent dans l'insuffisance rénale progressive n'a pas encore été déterminé. Il est intéressant de spéculer qu'à la fois les inhibiteurs de l'enzyme de conversion de l'angiotensine et les agents qui entraînent une baisse lipidique ont un mécanisme commun d'action dans la pathogenèse de l'insuffisance rénale progressive: ils affectent la croissance/prolifération des cellules. Il apparaît de plus en plus évident que la pathogenèse de l'insuffisance rénale progressive implique de multiples facteurs. L'apparition de nouveaux agents pharmacologiques, tels les inhibiteurs de l'enzyme de conversion de l'angiotensine et les agents qui entraînent une baisse des lipides ont permis le développement de nouveaux concepts importants étant donné que leur impact le plus remarquable touche aux mécanismes de dégradation de la fonction rénale.

ZUSAMMENFASSUNG

Die Rolle, die lipide Abnormalitäten und Zellveränderungen bei fortschreitender Nierenverletzung spielen, ist gegenwärtig noch nicht geklärt. Eine interessante Spekulation stützt sich auf die Annahme, dass sowohl Inhibitoren des angiotensinkonvertierenden Enzyms als auch lipidverringernde Mittel einen gemeinsamen Aktionsmechanismus in der Pathogenese fortschreitender Nierenkrankheit aufweisen, indem sie das Zellenwachstum/Proliferation beeinflussen. Es gibt mehr und mehr Hinweise dafür, dass die Pathogenese der progressiven Nierenkrankheit von diversen Faktoren abhängig ist. Der Zugang zu neuen pharmakologischen Mitteln, wie Inhibitoren des angiotensinkonvertierenden Enzyms und lipidverringernden

Mitteln, hat die Entwicklung wichtiger neuer Konzepte möglich gemacht, die die Mechanismen der Nierenverletzung aufdecken.

RIASSUNTO

Attualmente il ruolo svolto dalle anormalitá dei lipidi e le mutazioni cellulari nelle lesioni renali progressive è ancora da determinare. E' interessante pensare che sia gli inibitori dell'enzima isomerizzante dell'angiotensina che gli agenti di abbassamento dei lipidi possano avere un meccanismo d'azione in commune nella patogenesi del morbo renale progressivo, influendo sulla crescita/proliferazione delle cellule. E' sempre più evidente che la patogenesi del morbo renale progressivo implica molteplici fattori. La disponibilità di nuovi agenti farmacologici quali gli inibitori dell'enzima isomerizzante dell'angiotensina e gli agenti di abbassamento dei lipidi ha permesso lo sviluppo di importanti nuovi concetti quanto ai meccanismi della lesione renale.

SUMÁRIO

Atualmente, o papel que jogam as anormalidades dos lípidos e as mudanças celulares nas lesões renais progressivas ainda está por ser determinado. É intrigante especular que tanto os inibidores da enzima convertidora da angiotensina como os agentes que diminuem o conteúdo de lípidos podem ter un mecanismo de ação comum na patogênese da doença renal progressiva pelo seu efeito sobre o crescimento/proliferação celular. Resulta cada vez mais evidente que a patogênese da doença renal progressiva envolve muitos fatores. A disponibilidade de novos agentes farmacológicos, tais como os inibidores da enzima convertidora da angiotensina e agentes que diminuem o conteúdo de lípidos, tem permitido o desenvolvimento de importantes novos conceitos no que respeita aos mecanismos de lesões renais.

RESUMEN

Todavía hace falta determinar el papel que las anormalidades de los lípidos y cambios celulares tienen en las lesiones renales progresivas. Es intrigante especular que tanto los inhibidores de la enzima convertidora de la angiotensina como los agentes que disminuyen el contenido lípido peuden tener un mecanismo de acción común en la patogénesis de la enfermedad renal progresiva por su efecto sobre el crecimiento/proliferación celular. Resulta cada vez más evidente que la patogénesis de la enfermedad renal progresiva incluye muchos factores. La disponibilidad de nuevos agentes farmacológicos, tales como los inhibidores de la enzima convertidora de la angiotensina y agentes que disminuyen el contenido lípido, han permitido el desarrollo de importantes nuevos conceptos en lo que respecta a los mecanismos causantes de lesiones renales.

要約

現在，進行性腎障害における脂質異常と細胞変化の果たす役割については，明らかではない。興味深いことに，アンジオテンシン変換酵素（ACE）阻害薬や脂質低下薬は，ともに細胞の成長・増殖に作用することによって，進行性の腎疾患の発症における共通の作用機序を有していると考えられている。

進行性の腎疾患の発症には，多くの因子が関与することが次第に明らかにされている。ACE阻害薬や脂質低下薬などの新しい薬剤の使用が可能になり，腎障害の発生機序に関する重要な新しい考え方が生まれつつある。

Cardiac and Renal Failure: An Expanding Role for ACE Inhibitors, edited by C. T. Dollery and L. M. Sherwood, Hanley & Belfus, Inc., Philadelphia.

The Role of Eicosanoids in Chronic Glomerular Disease

Carlo Patrono and Alessandro Pierucci

Eicosanoid is the generic term that refers to lipoxygenase and cyclooxygenase products of arachidonate metabolism. Prostaglandins (PG) and the other eicosanoids are autacoids that do not have a circulating endocrine function but rather act in a paracrine or autocrine manner, affecting cells close to or at the site of PG synthesis.[1] Nonsteroidal anti-inflammatory drugs (NSAIDs) inhibit either irreversibly (aspirin) or reversibly the cyclooxygenase enzyme that converts arachidonate to the PG-endoperoxides. Presently, no similar inhibitory agents are clinically available that inhibit the lipoxygenase enzymes converting arachidonate to leukotrienes and monohydroxy fatty acids. Although glucocorticoids can limit substrate availability through the induction of a recently characterized phospholipase A_2-inhibitory protein (named lipocortin), their *in vivo* effects on endogenous PG production are rather inconsistent.

LOCALIZATION OF RENAL PROSTAGLANDIN SYNTHESIS

Eicosanoid synthesis in the kidney is localized to specific sites and is not uniformly present throughout the nephron.[1] Since the initial discovery of PG synthesis in the renal medulla, it has been recognized that the medullary tissue synthesizes greater amounts of PGs than the cortex. It is generally accepted that the regional heterogeneity of arachidonate metabolism, as well as the lack of vascular communications between the medulla and the cortex, dictate that PGs synthesized in the cortex (glomeruli and vasculature) regulate cortical function, and PGs synthesized in the medulla (collecting tubule and medullary interstitial cells) regulate medullary function.[1] Table I summarizes the principal sites of PG synthesis in the kidney, the major PGs produced at each site, and their principal actions. Assessment of PG synthesis by different components of the nephron is based on immunofluorescent microscopy,

TABLE I. *Principal renal sites of prostaglandin synthesis and major actions.*

Site	Eicosanoid	Action
Vasculature	PGI_2	Vasodilation
Glomerulus	PGI_2, PGE_2	Maintain GFR
	TXA_2	Reduce GFR*
Collecting tubule	PGE_2, $PGF_{2\alpha}$	Enhance excretion of NaCl and water
Medullary interstitial cells	PGE_2	Vasodilation and natriuresis-diuresis

*TXA_2 reduces GFR in pathophysiologic situations such as glomerulonephritis, transplant rejection, and ureteral obstruction.
Reproduced from Patrono C, Dunn MJ. *Kidney Int* 1987; **32**:1–12, with permission.[18]

separation of glomeruli and nephron segments with measurement of PG synthesis, or by cell cultures of specific components of the nephron with measurements of eicosanoid turnover.[1,2] Some species variation exists, and the majority of data are based on studies of rat, rabbit, and human kidney. In the cortex, the major sites of PG synthesis include arteries, arterioles and the glomerulus. The proximal tubule and the loop of Henle show little cyclooxygenase activity but may convert arachidonate to several epoxygenase derivatives.[2] The large amounts of PGE_2 produced by the renal medulla primarily derive from the substantial biosynthetic activity of collecting tubule and interstitial cells. Eicosanoids synthesized within the kidney are either degraded in the kidney, by enzymes acting on the $\Delta 13,14$ double bond and on the hydroxyl group at C-15, or are removed from the kidney in the lymphatic and venous drainage or by excretion into the urine.[1] As discussed below, measurement of urinary unmetabolized PGs or their stable hydrolysis products provides the best clinical assessment of the state of renal PG production.

MEASUREMENTS OF URINARY PROSTAGLANDINS AND THROMBOXANE B_2 AS A REFLECTION OF RENAL CYCLOOXYGENASE ACTIVITY

Because detection of primary PGs in renal venous plasma has major limitations, measurement of PGE_2 and $PGF_{2\alpha}$ in urine has gained general acceptance following the original report by Frolich *et al.*[3] suggesting their renal origin in healthy women. Urine, besides having a PG concentration that is two orders of magnitude greater than that of renal venous plasma, has the additional advantage of being virtually free of platelet eicosanoids and of providing a noninvasive and continuous, rather than episodic, measure of renal PG synthesis. In addition to PGE_2 and $PGF_{2\alpha}$, human urine contains measurable amounts of 6-keto-$PGF_{1\alpha}$[4] and thromboxane $(TX)B_2$,[5] chemically stable hydration products of PGI_2 and TXA_2, respectively. In a number of pathophysiologic conditions examined thus far, the urinary excretion of 6-

keto-PGF$_{1\alpha}$ and TXB$_2$ is largely a reflection of the renal synthesis of the unstable parent compounds.[6,7] The evidence supporting this statement is summarized in Table II. No information of similar nature is available in animal studies, even though measurements of urinary TXB$_2$ have been used extensively in rat and murine models of glomerular disease. Although no clear-cut evidence exists for a differential origin of any given urinary eicosanoid from a well-defined nephron segment, a working hypothesis can be proposed as outlined in Table III.

Radioimmunoassay and gas chromatography-mass spectrometry have been employed to quantitate urinary PG and TXB$_2$ excretion. Although the latter method can provide definitive identification of a given eicosanoid, with adequate sensitivity particularly in the negative-ion chemical ionization mode,[8] the former represents a highly sophisticated form of bioassay, substituting the classic smooth-muscle strip with a soluble antibody as the biological reactant. Consequently, the biologic readout (i.e., variably reduced binding of the labeled eicosanoid to a presumably "specific" anti-eicosanoid serum as a function of increasing concentrations of the unlabeled homologous as well as heterologous ligands) is liable to all forms of artifacts possibly affecting bioassay. In particular, the presence in urine of a large number (up to 20 in the case of TXB$_2$) of potentially cross-reacting enzymatic derivatives of PGs and TXB$_2$ excreted in up to a ten-fold excess vis-à-vis unmetabolized eicosanoids represents a serious potential limitation to the specificity of such measurements. Unfortunately, immunologic characterization of anti-eicosanoid sera is often limited to primary PGs and TXB$_2$, with limited information, if any, on the cross-reactivity of major urinary metabolites such as the 2,3-dinor-derivatives of PGI$_2$ and TXB$_2$. Moreover, reduction of the measured urinary PG-like immunoreactivity by cyclooxygenase inhibitors is often presented as evidence of the "specificity" of such measurements. This is

TABLE II. *Drug-induced or disease-associated changes in urinary 6-Keto-PGF$_{1\alpha}$ and thromboxane B$_2$ and corresponding 2,3-dinor derivatives*

Drug or Disease	6-Keto-PGF$_{1\alpha}$	2,3-Dinor-6-keto-PGF$_{1\alpha}$	Thromboxane B$_2$	2,3-Dinor-thromboxane B$_2$
Loop diuretics	↑	⇆	↑	ND*
Sulindac	⇆	↓	⇆	↓
Low-dose aspirin	⇆	↓	⇆	↓
Systemic lupus erythematosus	↓	ND	↑	⇆
Bartter's syndrome	↑	⇆	↑	ND

*ND = not determined.

6-keto-PGF$_{1\alpha}$ and thromboxane B$_2$ excretions are considered to reflect the renal synthesis of PGI$_2$ and thromboxane A$_2$, respectively, whereas 2,3-dinor-6-keto-PGF$_{1\alpha}$ and 2,3-dinor-thromboxane B$_2$ represent major urinary metabolites of exogenously infused PGI$_2$ and thromboxane B$_2$, presumably reflecting a systemic extrarenal origin (reviewed in ref. 6).

TABLE III.   *Sites of synthesis and action, and stable urinary derivatives of the major cyclooxygenase products identified in the human kidney*[*]

Biologically Active Eicosanoids	Sites of Synthesis	Sites of Action	Stable Urinary Derivatives
PGI_2	Glomerulus; arterioles	Mesangium Vascular smooth muscle Juxtaglomerular apparatus	6-Keto-$PGF_{1\alpha}$
Thromboxane A_2	Glomerulus	Mesangium Vascular smooth muscle	Thromboxane B_2
PGE_2	Medullary interstitium; tubules	Vascular smooth muscle Loop of Henle Collecting tubule	PGE_2
$PGF_{2\alpha}$	Medullary interstitium; tubules	Vascular smooth muscle? Collecting tubule?	$PGF_{2\alpha}$

[*]These data provide a working hypothesis as to the origin and functional correlates of urinary eicosanoids.

misleading, inasmuch as the renal and extrarenal synthesis of all eicosanoids will be suppressed by nonselective cyclooxygenase inhibitors (e.g., indomethacin), thereby causing a simultaneous reduction in the urinary excretion of both primary unmetabolized PGs (presumably reflecting a renal origin) and potentially cross-reacting systemic metabolites. On the other hand, such methodologic problems will obscure the effects of selective cyclooxygenase inhibitors on the kidney (e.g., sulindac, low-dose aspirin, sulphinpyrazone) by virtue of the reduced excretion of cross-reacting systemic metabolites masking the continued synthesis and excretion of renal PGs.

Validation criteria allowing the assessment of the specificity of urinary PG measurements by radioimmunoassay include: (1) characterization of the thin-layer or high-pressure liquid chromatographic pattern of distribution of the extracted PG-like immunoreactivity; (2) use of multiple antisera; and (3) comparison with gas chromatography-mass spectrometry determinations.[4,7] Such an integrated approach can provide meaningful information on renal PG and TXA_2 synthesis in health and disease.

URINARY PROSTAGLANDIN AND THROMBOXANE B_2 EXCRETION IN CHRONIC GLOMERULAR DISEASE

A number of studies have addressed the issue of urinary PGE_2 excretion in chronic renal disease (reviewed in ref. 9). With the exception of patients with severe renal failure (inulin clearance less than 25 ml per minute) in whom the excretion rate of PGE_2 was profoundly diminished,[9] and patients with systemic lupus erythematosus (SLE) in whom urinary PGE_2 excretion was moderately increased,[10] most patients with mild to moderate renal failure were described as having normal excretory rates.[9] The inclusion of male patients in some of these studies is a potentially confounding factor, in view of the highly variable and unpredictable origin (i.e., renal versus seminal) of PGE_2 in male urine.[11] In a study of 20 healthy women and 16 female patients with biopsy-diagnosed chronic glomerulonephritis (creatinine clearance: 110 ± 5 and 91 ± 19 ml/minute/1.73 m^2, respectively; mean $\pm$ SD), we found that control subjects and patients excreted PGE_2 at almost identical rates, i.e., 7.6 ± 2.7 versus 7.4 ± 2.4 ng per hour.[12] Although urinary PGE_2 excretion was significantly increased in a group of 23 female patients with SLE nephritis, only eight patients (six with active renal lesions) had urinary PGE_2 excretion in excess of two standard deviations of the normal mean.[7] In most of these studies, the urinary excretion of PGE_2 did not correlate with any of the measured parameters of cortical or medullary function to a statistically significant extent, in either patients or control subjects. An entirely novel finding of our group was the demonstration of a significantly reduced excretion of 6-keto-$PGF_{1\alpha}$ in female patients with chronic glomerular disease, (Table IV) including SLE nephropathy.[12] In SLE patients with active renal lesions, the reduction was greater than 50%,[7] i.e., similar to that which is inducible by the administration of a relatively high dose of aspirin in healthy women.[13] In these patients, the urinary excretion of 6-keto-$PGF_{1\alpha}$ showed a statistically significant positive correlation with both the glomerular filtration rate and renal blood flow.[7] That such a biochemical change is not a consequence of a chronic immune disease process is indicated by the finding of a normal excretion rate of 6-keto-$PGF_{1\alpha}$ in a group of 25 age-matched female patients with rheumatoid arthritis (Ciabattoni, Caruso, and Patrono, unpublished observations). Although the reduced excretion of the PGI_2 hydration product in chronic glomerular disease may have reflected a reduced glomerular mass

TABLE IV. *Urinary eicosanoids in healthy women (n = 20) and female patients with chronic glomerular disease (n = 16)*

Eicosanoid	Patients	Control Subjects	p Value
PGE_2	$7.4 \pm 2.4*$	7.6 ± 2.7	NS
$PGF_{2\alpha}$	15.7 ± 7.1	18.1 ± 6.8	NS
6-keto-$PGF_{1\alpha}$	2.3 ± 1.0	4.1 ± 0.9	<0.001
Thromboxane B_2	1.9 ± 0.4	2.0 ± 0.6	NS

*Mean $\pm$ SD
NS = not significant
All values are expressed as ng per hour.
Data are from Patrono et al.[7] and Ciabattoni et al.[12]

available for PGI_2 synthesis, this appears to be unlikely inasmuch as TXB_2, the second most abundant cyclooxygenase product in human glomeruli, was excreted at a normal rate or at an accelerated rate under the same circumstances.[7]

At least two distinct mechanisms may account for the reduction in the glomerular synthesis of PGI_2: inhibition of PGI_2 synthase by hydroperoxy-derivatives of arachidonate;[14] or feedback regulation of PGI_2 synthesis by the hemodynamic changes associated with progressive glomerular sclerosis.[15] To the extent that PGI_2 is a major determinant of glomerular hemodynamics because of its effects on glomerular capillary plasma flow rate and on glomerular ultrafiltration coefficient,[16] our findings clearly establish that the adaptive increases in glomerular capillary pressures and flow that characterize progressive glomerular sclerosis are not mediated by increased PGI_2 production. PGI_2 synthesis appears to be switched off by such hemodynamic changes, as would be expected in homeostatic terms.

Urinary TXB_2 excretion is markedly enhanced in SLE patients but not in patients with other forms of chronic glomerular disease.[7] Moreover, patients with active renal lesions differ significantly from those with inactive lesions by having a two-fold higher TXB_2 excretion rate (Table V). A non-platelet intrarenal source of enhanced TXA_2 production was suggested by the unaltered *ex vivo* and *in vivo* indices of platelet TXB_2 production.[7] Interestingly, the *ex vivo* renal synthesis of TXB_2 is also increased in the MRL-lpr and NZBxW mice with spontaneous lupus nephritis.[17] As in the human disease, a platelet source of increased intrarenal TXB_2 production could be excluded on the basis of inhibitor studies.[17] Glomerular mesangial cells and monocytes were indicated as the most likely sources of TXA_2 synthesis.[17] A cellular source allowing the interaction of TXA_2 with mesangial receptors is consistent with our finding of a significant inverse correlation between urinary TXB_2 and glomerular filtration rate.[7] The mechanism(s) responsible for enhanced glomerular TXA_2 production in lupus nephritis remain entirely spec-

TABLE V. *Urinary eicosanoids in patients with systemic lupus erythematosus and active (SLE-A; n = 13) or inactive (SLE-I; n = 10) renal lesions*

Eicosanoid	SLE-A	SLE-I	p Value
PGE_2	15.0 ± 10.2*	10.9 ± 4.7	NS
$PGF_{2\alpha}$	16.4 ± 6.2	15.9 ± 4.2	NS
6-keto-$PGF_{1\alpha}$	2.0 ± 1.0	3.0 ± 0.4	<0.001
Thromboxane B_2	9.4 ± 4.5	4.6 ± 1.6	<0.001

*Mean ± SD
NS = not significant
All values are expressed as ng per hour
Data are from Patrono et al.[7]

ulative.[7,17] Although such biochemical alteration might contribute to deteriorating renal function in SLE nephropathy, the precise role of enhanced intrarenal TXA_2 production remains to be assessed by specific receptor antagonists or tissue-selective synthesis inhibitors (see below).

RENAL PROSTAGLANDIN-SYNTHESIS INHIBITION IN MAN

Pharmacologic inhibition of renal PG synthesis is thought to be reflected by a variably reduced excretion of primary unmetabolized PGs. Most, if not all, widely used NSAIDs have been tested for their acute and/or chronic effects on urinary PG excretion. These include indomethacin, ibuprofen, naproxen, aspirin, fenoprofen, diclofenac, sulindac, piroxicam and flurbiprofen.[18] Their effects have been characterized in healthy subjects as well as in patients with renal, hepatic, rheumatic and cardiovascular disease. Some generalizations can be drawn from the results of such studies:[18]

1. With the possible exception of sulindac (see below), all of these NSAIDs have been shown to reduce urinary PG excretion by at least 50% when used at full antiinflammatory dosage; a maximal reduction in the range of 60 to 80% has been described with the vast majority of these agents, although no detailed dose-response studies have been carried out to allow a quantitative assessment of relative potencies;

2. Such a maximal suppression of renal PG synthesis can be shown to occur within 24 to 48 hours of treatment, and is fully reversible within 48 to 72 hours after drug withdrawal, depending upon pharmacokinetics of the individual agent;

3. The apparent reduction in urinary PG excretion following a given cyclooxygenase inhibitor is not substantially modified by disease processes affecting renal or hepatic function, although the latter can obviously alter the pharmacokinetics of some NSAIDs;

4. Despite early reports of partial attenuation of NSAID-induced biochemical and functional changes during continued drug administration, such a phenomenon has not been confirmed in controlled studies.

Eighteen studies of sulindac administration in health and disease have been reviewed recently.[18] The following points have emerged from such a critical overview:

1. When given to human subjects at the recommended therapeutic dose of 400 mg/day, sulindac does not appear to influence cortical sites of renal cyclooxygenase activity,[12,19,20] as reflected by urinary 6-keto-$PGF_{1\alpha}$, with the possible exception of patients with cirrhosis and ascites;

2. Under the same circumstances, the drug may affect medullary sites of cyclooxygenase activity,[21] as reflected by urinary PGE_2, in approximately one third of the cases thus far evaluated;

3. The drug does appear to blunt i.v. furosemide-induced PGE_2 release;[22]

4. The mechanism(s) underlying these peculiar features of sulindac is largely unknown, although it is likely to be related to its redox pro-drug nature.[18]

A different mechanism is responsible for the selective sparing of renal cyclooxygenase activity by low-dose aspirin.[23] The mechanism underlying this selectivity is probably related to a different rate of recovery of cyclooxygenase activity in glomeruli versus platelets, following irreversible acetylation of the enzyme, and possibly to a different aspirin "sensitivity" of glomerular cyclooxygenase. The finding of a normal pattern of furosemide-induced renin release and urinary 6-keto-$PGF_{1\alpha}$ excretion after three to four weeks of low-dose (0.45 mg/kg/day) aspirin treatment in healthy subjects indicates that renal PGI_2-producing cells are readily activatable at a time of virtually complete suppression of platelet cyclooxygenase activity. Thus, low-dose aspirin represents an ideal pharmacologic tool to investigate the role of intraglomerular platelet activation in the progression of chronic glomerular disease without the risk inherent in higher conventional dosage that might compromise PG-dependent renal function.

THE EFFECTS OF PROSTAGLANDINS AND CYCLOOXYGENASE INHIBITORS ON RENAL FUNCTION

Renal function is not critically dependent upon the integrity of PG synthesis, at least under normal circumstances.[1,24] Inhibition of PG synthesis in healthy animals and humans does not induce a significant decline of renal function. It is probable that basal, endogenous PG synthesis does contribute to control of renal vascular resistance, glomerular filtration, and salt excretion in healthy subjects, but administration of an NSAID does not alter renal function, since other regulatory mechanisms (adrenergic tone, renin secretion, dopamine, adenosine) are uncompromised and can compensate for the inhibition of PG-synthesis.[18] In animals under anesthesia, especially after laparotomy, acute inhibition of PG synthesis reduces renal blood flow substantially, although GFR is largely unaffected. Different responses of anesthetized surgically-stressed dogs and conscious animals to the acute inhibition of PG synthesis are partially attributable to the effects of anesthesia and surgery on major vasoconstrictor hormones, especially angiotensin II, vasopressin, and catecholamines. In experimental and clinical circumstances, in which the vasoconstrictor hormones are increased, renal PG synthesis is augmented and renal function becomes "PG-dependent."[24] Infusion of angiotensin II, vasopressin, or norepinephrine into the renal artery stimulates renal PG synthesis measured either as secretion into renal venous blood or excretion into the urine. In vitro studies have confirmed that angiotensin and vasopressin stimulate vasodilatory PG release in glomerular mesangial and epithelial cells, and renal medullary interstitial cells.[18] Pretreatment with an NSAID potentiated the renal vasoconstriction induced by angiotensin II, α-adrenergic nerve stimulation, and norepinephrine or α-adrenergic drugs. These experiments reinforce the belief that the vasoconstrictor substances stimulate cortical PGE_2 and PGI_2 which modulate the constrictor action of angiotensin or norepinephrine.[18] The major clinical circumstances in which vasoconstrictor hormones increase to maintain cardiovascular homeostasis include extracellular volume depletion, congestive heart failure, nephrotic syndrome and hepatic disease.[18]

Diseases such as atherosclerotic cardiovascular disease and chronic glomerular disease (including lupus nephritis) may reduce renal PGE_2 or PGI_2 and thereby enhance the susceptibility to NSAIDs, despite normal levels of constrictor hormones.[12] Figure 1 summarizes the hypothesis[18] about the modulating effect of renal PGE_2 and PGI_2 on the intrarenal constrictor action of angiotensin II, vasopressin, and norepinephrine. According to this hypothesis, drug- and/or disease-induced suppression of cortical PG synthesis is associated with a lower threshold for the contractile response of the glomerular mesangium and arterioles to a variety of agonists. This simplified scheme

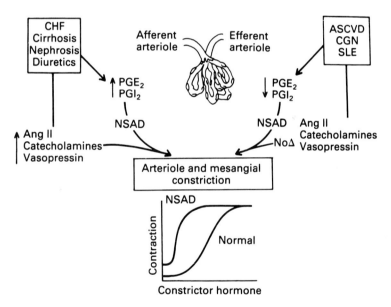

FIG. 1. Scheme depicting the balance between vasoconstriction and vasodilation existing in the pre- and post-glomerular circulation, and the glomerular mesangium. Abbreviations include: arteriosclerotic cardiovascular disease (ASCVD); chronic glomerulonephritis (CGN); systemic lupus erythematosus (SLE); congestive heart failure (CHF); angiotensin II (ANG II); nonsteroidal antiinflammatory drugs (NSAD). The graph schematically depicts the enhanced arteriolar and mesangial contraction to constrictor hormones after inhibition of prostaglandin synthesis. Reproduced from Patrono C, Dunn MJ. *Kidney Int* 1987; **32**:1–12, with permission.

does not include the important possibility that glomerular and vascular PGE_2 and PGI_2 may antagonize the renal effects of diverse contractile compounds, such as platelet-activating factor, TXA_2, leukotriene C_4-D_4, and other vaso-constrictor agents.

CYCLOOXYGENASE INHIBITORS IN ANIMAL MODELS OF RENAL DISEASE

The effects of cyclooxygenase inhibitors have been studied in several animal models of immune and nonimmune renal disease. Nephrotoxic serum nephritis, produced by the administration of heterologous antiglomerular basement membrane antibody, is a well-established model of immune glomerulonephritis. Stork and Dunn[25] have studied the effects of meclofena-mate and indomethacin in a rat model of nephrotoxic serum nephritis. Short-term treatment with either cyclooxygenase inhibitor on day 14 of the autologous phase resulted in a 50% decrease in both renal plasma flow and GFR, suggesting that vasodilator PGE_2 is of greater relative significance than is vasoconstrictor TXA_2 with respect to renal function in the rat model of nephrotoxic serum nephritis.[25] The long-term consequences of selective versus nonselective cyclooxygenase inhibition have been studied by Bertani et al.[26] in a rabbit model of nephrotoxic serum nephritis. Aspirin, at a dose (100 mg/kg per day during the autologous phase of the disease) that almost com-pletely suppressed cyclooxygenase activity in both circulating cells and the kidney, worsened the morphologic expression of nephrotoxic serum nephritis and negatively influenced the clinical course of the disease.[26] In contrast, sulindac, at a dose (60 mg/kg per day) that suppressed circulating platelet cyclooxygenase activity by 90% but substantially spared renal PGE_2 and PGI_2 production, prevented extracapillary proliferation and reduced proteinuria without creating a negative influence on glomerular hemodynamics.[26] The beneficial effect of sulindac was interpreted as being related to suppression of eicosanoid synthesis in blood-derived infiltrating cells, a potential source of inflammatory mediators contributing to glomerular damage. Kelley et al.[17] administered ibuprofen (8 to 9 mg/kg per day) for one week to two different strains of mice with autoimmune lupus nephritis. The drug did not alter TXB_2 or PGE_2 levels in the renal cortex or medulla, although it suppressed platelet TXB_2 production by 90%. Long-term treatment with ibuprofen, begun at 2 months of age, did not modify development of renal disease or 12-month survival in NZBxW mice.[27] However, ibuprofen did change the site of immune complex localization from the subepithelial to the subendothelial aspect of the glomerular basement membrane, a shift not associated with alterations in renal function.[27] Nath et al.[28] studied the effect of a short-term indomethacin infusion (5 mg/kg I.V.) on glomerular hemodynamics in euvo-lemic subtotally nephrectomized rats. Indomethacin reduced the single-nephron GFR by 23% by decreasing glomerular plasma flow rate and the ultrafiltration coefficient. These investigators also found that urinary excretions per nephron of PGE and 6-keto-PGF$_{1\alpha}$ were strikingly increased in nephrectomized compared with control rats.[28] These data were interpreted to suggest that adaptive increments in vasodilatory PG synthesis per nephron attend and sustain, at least in part, hyperfiltration in the remnant nephron due to their effects on intrarenal vascular resistances and the ultrafiltration coefficient. Since extrapolation of these experimental findings to the clinical situation might be taken to suggest beneficial effects from the use of cyclooxygenase inhibitors, a note of caution appears appropriate. Thus, the large increase in glomerular plasma flow rate, which occurred in the adapted remnant nephron (416 versus 140 nl per minute), was only moderately blunted (416 to 321 nl per minute) by such a large dose of indomethacin.[28] This would imply that approximately two-thirds of such an adaptive increase is mediated by mechanism(s) independent of cyclooxygenase activity. Moreover, the observed hemodynamic changes, i.e., increased afferent and efferent vascular resistances, might be related to the inherent vasoconstrictor effect of indomethacin, also observed in humans[29] independently of reduced PG synthesis.

A role of the renal PG system in the maintenance of the adaptive changes to a diminished nephron population has also been suggested by Kirschenbaum and Serros[30] in a rabbit model and by Rubinger et al.[31] in a rat model. The latter study involved a comparative evaluation of the effects of indomethacin (33.3 mg/kg in 48 hours) and sulindac (30 mg/kg in 48 hours) in five-sixths nephrectomized rats. Indomethacin reduced the 24-hour urinary sodium excretion and the fractional excretion of sodium, independently of changes in GFR, possibly as the result of direct tubular transport mechanisms. In contrast, sulindac had no effect on renal function or electrolyte excretion in rats with reduced renal mass. Indomethacin suppressed urinary PGE$_2$ and TXB$_2$ excretion in these animals, whereas sulindac had no effect.[31] It seems worth mentioning in this context that eicosapentaenoic acid, a potential substrate for both cyclooxygenase and 5-lipoxygenase, delays progression of immune-mediated renal disease,[32] although it accelerates the rate of glomerular sclerosis in renoprival nephropathy.[33] However, the relevance of intrarenal changes in eicosanoid production, induced by this dietary manipulation to such strikingly different patterns of evolution, remains to be established.

PLATELET AND/OR GLOMERULAR EICOSANOID INHIBITION IN CHRONIC GLOMERULAR DISEASE

In many renal diseases, loss of renal function correlates with evidence on biopsy of the deposition of fibrin and, less obviously, platelets in glomerular arteries and arterioles.[34] It has been argued by Kincaid-Smith[34] that in many

glomerular diseases progression is the result of thrombosis and the hyaliniza-
tion of glomerular thrombi or their organization by myointimal proliferation
in arteries. A critical viewpoint has been put forth by Border,[35] suggesting that
activation of the coagulation system is merely an epiphenomenon of glomerular injury. As the value of anticoagulants in the treatment of renal disease[34,35]
is beyond the scope of this article, we restrict ourselves to a brief discussion of
the independent role of platelets and antiplatelet drugs in chronic glomerular
disease.

Platelets are potential sources of a number of mediators possibly affecting
immune-complex deposition, capillary permeability, mesangial function, and
glomerular hemodynamics. Moreover, platelets contain at least two mitogens
—epidermal growth factor and platelet-derived growth factor—and a number of potentially chemotactic factors (reviewed in ref. 36). In a manner
similar to their proposed contribution to atherosclerotic lesions,[36] platelets
might contribute to glomerular lesions, e.g., by inducing proliferation of
mesangial cells with an increase of the mesangium as is seen in membranoproliferative glomerulonephritis.[37] The experimental and clinical evidence
supporting the involvement of platelets in mediating or amplifying glomerular injury has been reviewed by Cameron.[38] Platelets and/or platelet-related
antigens can be found within the glomeruli of patients with glomerulonephritis.[38] Moreover, platelet survival can be shortened and the intraplatelet concentration of serotonin can be reduced.[38]

With the notable exception of platelets from nephrotic patients, which
synthesize more TXB_2 when challenged *ex vivo,* possibly as a result of hy-
poalbuminemia,[39] platelets obtained from patients with different forms of
chronic glomerular disease do not differ from normal platelets in terms of
maximal capacity to produce TXB_2 in response to thrombin.[7] However, no
information is available on *in vivo* platelet TXB_2 production except for SLE
patients, in whom we have recently 'described[7] a normal excretion rate of
2,3-dinor-TXB_2. Interestingly, glomerular thrombi occur frequently in SLE
(in 50% of biopsies with diffuse and focal proliferative glomerulonephritis)
and appear to represent a singularly important factor in predicting whether
glomerulosclerosis subsequently develops.[40]

To test the hypothesis that the vasoconstrictor and mesangial contractile
actions of TXA_2 might influence glomerular hemodynamics in lupus
nephritis, we examined the short-term functional effects of a selective thromboxane receptor antagonist, BM 13,177, and of low-dose aspirin in two
separate randomized, placebo-controlled studies.[41] Forty-eight hour continuous infusion of BM 13,177 in 10 patients was associated with a statistically
significant increase of inulin and para-aminohippurate clearances by 24 ± 12
and $26 \pm 13\%$, respectively, and with a doubling of bleeding time.[42] These
hemodynamic changes were associated with a significant increase in sodium
excretion, with no change in arterial blood pressure. Single oral doses of

aspirin in the range 25 to 200 mg caused a dose-dependent irreversible inhibition of platelet TXB_2 production, with a pattern substantially similar to that previously described in healthy subjects.[23] Repeated b.i.d. dosing with 20 mg aspirin for 4 weeks caused a selective, cumulative inhibition of platelet cyclooxygenase activity and a doubling of bleeding time. Neither time- nor treatment-related differences were detected in urinary TXB_2 and 6-keto-$PGF_{1\alpha}$ excretion and inulin clearance in ten patients.[43]

These findings would suggest that, in lupus nephritis, impairment of renal function is, at least in part, hemodynamically mediated and reversible. Moreover, platelets do not represent a major source of intraglomerular TXA_2 synthesis and action. Whether the short-term changes in renal function associated with thromboxane antagonism can translate into long-term benefits in terms of progression of lupus nephritis remains to be determined.

In contrast to other areas of human disease, such as coronary artery disease, where a role for local platelet activation can be strongly argued for on the basis of inhibitor trials,[44] the case for glomerular thrombosis playing an important role in the development of glomerular sclerosis and progressive renal disease remains to be proved in humans. The results of trials employing a combination of anticoagulants, steroids, cytotoxic drugs, and dipyridamole[35,37] are difficult to interpret in trying to understand the contribution, if any, of each individual agent. In a recent prospective, randomized, double-blind trial,[45] 40 patients with type I membranoproliferative glomerulonephritis were treated with dipyridamole (75 mg three times daily) and aspirin (325 mg three times daily) or with placebo for as long as 84 months, with the masked conditions of the trial ending after 1 year of treatment. Efficacy analysis revealed that aspirin and dipyridamole significantly decreased the rate of decline of renal function and the development of end-stage renal failure. However, if in addition to loss of renal function, complications of treatment were also designated as failures, then the difference between the two groups was not statistically significant. Moreover, no difference between the groups was noted with regard to proteinuria. Perhaps the most impressive results are related to the follow-up of these patients. Thus, nine of the 19 patients who were originally assigned to the placebo group acquired end-stage renal disease, on average 33 months after entry into the study. In the active treatment group, only three of the 21 patients acquired end-stage renal disease, on average 62 months after entry into the study. It should be pointed out that data from 20% of the patients entered into the trial were not analysed for various reasons,[45] thus preventing an intention-to-treat analysis. The mechanism(s) underlying the apparent beneficial effect of this combined treatment is probably related to suppression of TXA_2-related platelet function by aspirin. Any effect on glomerular cyclooxygenase activity is likely to have influenced glomerular eicosanoid production only partially and non-selectively with negative consequences, if any, on glomerular hemodynamics. The contribution of dipyridamole to the observed effects of the combination cannot be derived from this study. In a recent prospective trial, 47 patients with type I membranoproliferative glomerulonephritis were randomly assigned to treatment with a combination of cyclophosphamide, coumadin, and dipyridamole (100 mg four times daily), or to no specific therapy[46] for 18 months. Actuarial survival, progression of the renal disease, and proteinuria did not differ between the two groups to any statistically significant extent.[46]

That platelet activation and intraglomerular thrombosis may have a broader role in the development of glomerulosclerosis is suggested by the study of Purkerson et al.[47] in rats with subtotal renal ablation. Long-term oral administration of OKY 1581, a selective TX-synthase inhibitor, in rats with a remnant kidney increased renal blood flow and GFR, decreased protein excretion, lowered blood pressure, and improved renal histology.[47] Unfortunately, the use of a rather large dose of the inhibitor (20 mg/kg twice daily) precludes the possibility of distinguishing the effects resulting from inhibition of platelet TX-synthase from those resulting from inhibition of the glomerular enzyme. Of particular interest was the finding that despite the increase in hyperfiltration and hyperperfusion seen with the administration of OKY 1581, there was amelioration of the renal disease in this model.[47]

It should also be mentioned that in the studies of Purkerson et al.,[47,48] most of the maneuvers designed to decrease the progressive glomerulosclerosis also resulted in marked decreases in arterial blood pressure. These included OKY-1581, aspirin when given alone in low doses (5 mg/kg) or in combination with dipyridamole (50 and 10 mg/kg, respectively), heparin, coumadin and a combination of antihypertensive drugs. The following sequence of events has been suggested by these investigators:[48] Reduced renal mass causing vasodilation of arterioles in residual glomeruli would lead to hyperperfusion and intraglomerular hypertension. The latter will result in mechanical damage of the endothelium of glomerular capillaries followed by platelet aggregation, intraglomerular thrombosis, and release of factors that may produce hyperplasia and hypertrophy of medium and small arterioles and subsequent sclerosis of the tissue (Figure 2). Conflicting results have been obtained by Zoja et al.,[49] showing that selective inhibition of platelet TXB_2 generation by low-dose aspirin (a loading dose of 100 mg/kg followed by 15 mg/kg daily) failed to protect rats with reduced renal mass from the development of progressive glomerular sclerosis. These investigators have argued that the beneficial results obtained by Purkerson et al.[47] with a selective TX-synthase inhibitor might be attributed to an effect on TXA_2 synthesis by resident glomerular cells (not inhibited by low-dose aspirin) or to lowering of systemic blood pressure.[49] The Milan normotensive rat strain (MNS) is characterized by a genetically determined, age-related glomerular sclerosis accompanied by heavy proteinuria and deterioration of renal function.[50] Increased glomerular production of TXB_2 has been described in this model of spontaneous glomerular damage not associated with systemic hypertension.[51] Long-

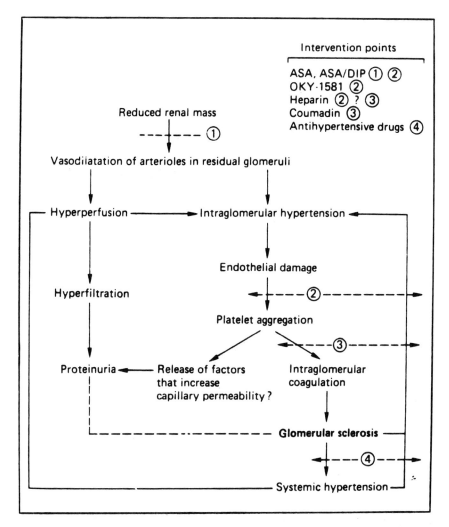

FIG. 2.   Proposed scheme for pathogenesis of the progressive glomerulosclerosis that occurs in rats with subtotal renal ablation and postulated sites of different interventions known to ameliorate the progression of the renal disease. Reproduced from Purkerson ML, et al. *Mineral Electrolyte Metab* 13: **370;** 1987, by copyright permission from S. Karger AG, Basel.

term administration of FCE 22178, a selective TX-synthase inhibitor, reduced proteinuria, preserved renal function, and improved renal histology with no significant change in systemic blood pressure.[52] These results would support the contention that selective inhibition of intraglomerular TXA_2 production *per se* is responsible for the prevention of progressive glomerular damage irrespective of changes in arterial blood pressure.

Whether intraglomerular platelet activation and/or enhanced TXA_2 production by glomerular mesangial and epithelial cells is the primary target of FCE 22178 remains to be determined. This drug inhibits TXB_2 production in isolated MNS glomeruli at significantly lower concentrations than in whole blood from the same animals,[53] a finding at variance with previous results obtained with dazoxiben[54] and other imidazole-analogue TX-synthase inhibitors. Thus, "tissue-selective" inhibitors, such as FCE 22178, may help to clarify the relative contribution of glomerular vis-a-vis platelet TX-synthase in the progression of glomerulosclerosis and may provide new therapeutic strategies in TXA_2-dependent loss of renal function.

ACKNOWLEDGEMENT

We wish to thank Maria Luisa Bonanomi for expert editorial assistance.

REFERENCES

1. Dunn MJ. Renal prostaglandins. In Dunn MJ, ed. Renal Endocrinology. Baltimore, Williams and Wilkins, 1983; 1–74.
2. Schlondorff D. Renal prostaglandin synthesis: sites of production and specific actions of prostaglandins. *Am J Med* 1986; **81**:1–11.
3. Frolich JC, Wilson FW, Sweetman BJ, et al. Urinary prostaglandins: identification and origin. *J Clin Invest* 1975; **55**:763–70.
4. Patrono C, Pugliese F, Ciabattoni G, et al. Evidence for a direct stimulatory effect of prostacyclin on renin release in man. *J Clin Invest* 1982; **69**:231–9.
5. Ciabattoni G, Pugliese F, Cinotti GA, et al. Characterisation of furosemide-induced activation of the renal prostaglandin system. *Eur J Pharmacol* 1979; **60**:181–7.
6. FitzGerald GA, Pedersen AK, Patrono C. Analysis of prostacyclin and thromboxane biosynthesis in cardiovascular disease. *Circulation* 1983; **67**:1174–7.
7. Patrono C, Ciabattoni G, Remuzzi G, et al. Functional significance of renal prostacyclin and thromboxane A_2 production in patients with systemic lupus erythematosus. *J Clin Invest* 1985; **76**:1011–8.
8. Lawson JA, Brash AR, Doran J, FitzGerald GA. Measurements of urinary 2,3-dinor-thromboxane B_2 and thromboxane B_2 using bonded phase phenylboronic acid columns and capillary gas chromatography negative ion chemical ionization mass spectrometry. *Anal Biochem* 1985; **150**:463–70.
9. Lebel M, Grose JH. Abnormal renal prostaglandin production during the evolution of chronic nephropathy. *Am J Nephrol* 1986; **6**:96–100.
10. Kimberly RP, Gill JR Jr, Bowden RE, Keiser HR, Plotz PH. Elevated urinary prostaglandins and the effects of aspirin on renal function in lupus erythematosus. *Ann Intern Med* 1978; **89**:336–41.
11. Patrono C, Wennmalm A, Ciabattoni G, Nowak J, Pugliese F, Cinotti GA. Evidence for an extrarenal origin of urinary prostaglandin E_2 in healthy men. *Prostaglandins* 1979; **18**:623–9.
12. Ciabattoni G, Cinotti GA, Pierucci A, et al. Effects of sulindac and ibuprofen in patients with chronic glomerular disease. Evidence for the dependence of renal function on prostacyclin. *N Engl J Med* 1984; **310**:279–83.
13. Reimann IW, Golbs E, Fischer C, Frolich JC. Influence of intravenous acetylsalicylic acid and sodium salicylate on human renal function and lithium clearance. *Eur J Clin Pharmacol* 1985; **29**:435–41.

14. Gryglewski RJ, Bunting S, Moncada S, Flower RJ, Vane JR. Arterial walls are protected against deposition of platelet thrombi by a substance (prostaglandin X) which they make from prostaglandin endoperoxides. *Prostaglandins* 1976; **12**:685–713.
15. Brenner BM, Meyer TW, Hostetter TH. Dietary protein intake and the progressive nature of kidney disease: the role of hemodynamically mediated glomerular injury in the pathogenesis of progressive glomerular sclerosis in aging, renal ablation, and intrinsic renal disease. *N Engl J Med* 1982; **307**:652–9.
16. Brenner BM, Schor N. Studies of prostaglandin action on the glomerular microcirculation. In Dunn MJ, Patrono C, Cinotti GA, eds. *Prostaglandins and the Kidney:* Biochemistry, Physiology, Pharmacology, and Clinical Applications. New York, Plenum Press, 1983; 125–32.
17. Kelley VE, Sneve S, Musinski S. Increased renal thromboxane production in murine lupus nephritis. *J Clin Invest* 1986; **77**:252–9.
18. Patrono C, Dunn MJ. The clinical significance of inhibition of renal prostaglandin synthesis. *Kidney Int* 1987; **32**:1–12.
19. Ciabattoni G, Boss AH, Patrignani P, et al. Effects of sulindac on renal and extrarenal eicosanoid synthesis. *Clin Pharmacol Ther* 1987; **41**:380–3.
20. Sedor JR, Williams SL, Chremos AN, Johnson CL, Dunn MJ. Effects of sulindac and indomethacin on renal prostaglandin synthesis. *Clin Pharmacol Ther* 1984; **36**:85–91.
21. Roberts DG, Gerber JG, Barnes JS, Zerbe GO, Nies AS. Sulindac is not renal-sparing in man. *Clin Pharmacol Ther* 1985; **38**:258–65.
22. Brater DC, Anderson S, Baird B, Campbell WB. Effects of ibuprofen, naproxen, and sulindac on prostaglandins in men. *Kidney Int* 1985; **27**:66–73.
23. Patrignani P, Filabozzi P, Patrono C. Selective cumulative inhibition of platelet thromboxane production by low-dose aspirin in healthy subjects. *J Clin Invest* 1982; **69**:1366–72.
24. Dunn MJ. Nonsteroidal antiinflammatory drugs and renal function. *Ann Rev Med* 1984; **35**:411–28.
25. Stork JE, Dunn MJ. Hemodynamic roles of thromboxane A_2 and prostaglandin E_2 in glomerulonephritis. *J Pharmacol Exp Ther* 1985; **37**:298–300.
26. Bertani T, Benigni A, Cutillo F, et al. Effect of aspirin and sulindac in rabbit nephrotoxic nephritis. *J Lab Clin Med* 1986; **107**:261–8.
27. Kelley VE, Izui S, Halushka PV. Effect of ibuprofen, a fatty acid cyclooxygenase inhibitor, on murine lupus. *Clin Immunol Immunopathol* 1982; **25**:223–31.
28. Nath KA, Chmielewski D, Hostetter TH. Regulatory role of prostanoids in glomerular microcirculation of remnant nephrons. *Am. J. Physiol.* 1987; **252**:F829–F837.
29. Edlund A, Berglund B, Van Dorne D, et al. Coronary flow regulation in patients with ischemic heart disease: release of purines and prostacyclin and the effect of inhibitors of prostaglandin formation. *Circulation* 1985; **71**:1113–20.
30. Kirschenbaum MA, Serros ER. Effect of prostaglandin inhibition on glomerular filtration rate in normal and uremic rabbits. *Prostaglandins* 1981; **22**:245–54.
31. Rubinger D, Frishberg Y, Eldor A, Popovtzer MM. The effect of suppression of prostaglandin synthesis on renal function in rats with intact and reduced renal mass. *Prostaglandins* 1985; **30**:651–68.
32. Kelley VE, Ferretti A, Izui S, Strom TB. A fish oil diet rich in eicosapentaenoic acid reduces cyclooxygenase metabolites, and suppresses lupus in MRL-lpr mice. *J Immunol* 1985; **134**:1914–9.
33. Scharschmidt LA, Gibbons NB, McGarry L, et al. Effects of dietary fish oil on renal insufficiency in rats with subtotal nephrectomy. *Kidney Int.* 1987; **32**:700–709.
34. Kincaid-Smith P. Anticoagulants are of value in the treatment of renal disease. *Am J Kidney Dis* 1984; **3**:299–307.
35. Border WA. Anticoagulants are of little value in the treatment of renal disease. *Am J Kidney Dis* 1984; **3**:308–12.
36. Ross R. The pathogenesis of atherosclerosis. An update. *N Engl J Med* 1986; **314**:488–500.
37. Hayslett JP. Role of platelets in glomerulonephritis. *N Engl J Med* 1984; **310**:1457–8.
38. Cameron JS. Platelets in glomerular disease. *Ann Rev Med* 1984; **35**:175–80.
39. Remuzzi G, Mecca G, Marchesi D, et al. Platelet hyperaggregability and the nephrotic syndrome. *Thromb Res* 1979; **16**:345–54.
40. Kant KS, Pollak VE, Weiss MA, Glueck HI, Miller MA, Hesse EV. Glomerular thrombosis

in systemic lupus erythematosus: prevalence and significance. *Medicine* (Baltimore) 1981; **60**:71–86.

41. Pierucci A, Simonetti BM, Pecci G, et al. Thromboxane antagonism improves renal function in lupus nephritis. *N Engl J Med* 1989; **320**:421.

42. Pierucci A, Simonetti BM, Pecci G, et al. Acute effects of a thromboxane receptor antagonist on real function in patients with lupus nephritis [abstract]. *Kidney Int* 1987; **31**:283.

43. Pierucci A, Simonetti BM, Pecci G, et al. Low dose aspirin in patients with lupus nephritis [abstract]. *Kidney Int* 1988; **33**:281.

44. Patrono C. Aspirin for the prevention of coronary thrombosis: current facts and perspectives. *Eur Heart J* 1986; **7**:454–9.

45. Donadio JV, Anderson CF, Mitchell JC, et al. Membranoproliferative glomerulonephritis. A prospective clinical trial of platelet-inhibitor therapy. *N Engl J Med* 1984; **310**:1421–6.

46. Cattran DC, Cardella CJ, Roscoe JM, et al. Results of a controlled drug trial in membrano-proliferative glomerulonephritis. *Kidney Int* 1985; **27**:436–441.

47. Purkerson ML, Joist JH, Yates J, Valdes A, Morrison A, Klahr S. Inhibition of thromboxane synthesis ameliorates the progressive kidney disease of rats with subtotal renal ablation. *Proc Natl Acad Sci USA* 1985; **82**:193–7.

48. Purkerson ML, Joist JH, Yates J, Klahr S. Role of hypertension and coagulation in the progressive glomerulopathy of rats with subtotal renal ablation. *Mineral Electrolyte Metab* 1987; **13**:370–6.

49. Zoja C, Benigni A, Livio M, et al. Selective inhibition of platelet thromboxane generation with low-dose aspirin does not protect rats with reduced renal mass from the development of progressive disease. (Submitted for publication.)

50. Brandis A, Bianchi G, Reale E, Helmechen U, Kunn K. Age-dependent glomerulosclerosis and proteinuria occurring in rats of the Milan normotensive strain and not in rats of the Milan hypertensive strain. *J Lab Invest* 1986; **55**:234–43.

51. Pugliese F, Menè P, Cinotti GA. Glomerular prostaglandin and thromboxane synthesis in normotensive and hypertensive rats of the Milan strain before and after development of hypertension. *J Hypertens* 1984; **4(suppl 3)**:S391–3.

52. Salvati P, Ferti C, Duzzi L, et al. Effect of thromboxane synthase inhibitor on age-dependent glomerulosclerosis in Milan normotensive rats [abstract]. London, 10th International Congress of Nephrology, 1987.

53. Salvati P, Pugliese F, Ferti C, et al. Selective inhibition of glomerular thromboxane-synthase in rat models of progressive glomerulosclerosis [abstract]. *Kidney Int* 1989; **35**:296.

54. Patrignani P, Filabozzi P, Catella F, Pugliese F, Patrono C. Differential effects of dazoxiben, a selective thromboxane-synthase inhibitor, on platelet and renal prostaglandin endoperoxide metabolism. *J Pharmacol Exp Ther* 1984; **228**:472–7.

SUMMARY

This paper provides an extensive review of the literature concerning the role of eicosanoids in chronic glomerular disease. In particular, the localisation of renal prostaglandin (PG) synthesis, measurement of its activity, and its inhibition are discussed. The effects of prostaglandins and cyclooxygenase inhibitors on renal function are examined and data from animal model studies are presented. Platelet and glomerular eicosanoid inhibition in chronic glomerular disease are also discussed.

Eicosanoids, which include prostaglandins, are the lipoxygenase and cyclooxygenase products of arachidonate metabolism. PG synthesis has been demonstrated in the renal medulla and cortex, but in greater amounts in the former. The measurement of urinary unmetabolized PGs (and also thromboxane B_2 (TXB_2)) provides the best clinical assessment of the state of renal

PG production and hence cyclooxygenase activity. Urinary excretion of PGE_2 does not appear to be altered in chronic renal failure, but 6-keto-$PGF_{1\alpha}$ is significantly reduced in patients with chronic glomerular disease, including systemic lupus erythematosus nephropathy. PGI_2 synthesis is reduced under these circumstances, and the mechanisms thought to be involved are outlined. Pharmacologic inhibition of renal PG synthesis (as demonstrated by reduced urinary PG excretion) can be effected by a number of compounds, including aspirin and the nonsteroidal anti-inflammatory drugs (NSAIDs). In healthy individuals, inhibition of PG synthesis does not induce a significant decline in renal function, but diseases such as chronic glomerular disease may reduce PGE_2 or PGI_2 and thereby enhance the susceptibility to NSAIDs, despite normal levels of constrictor hormones. A hypothesis of the modulating effect of renal PGE_2 and PGI_2 on the intrarenal constrictor action of angiotensin II, vasopressin, and norepinephrine is outlined.

The role of intrarenal TXA_2 production in the progression of chronic glomerular disease is also reviewed, with emphasis on human studies of lupus nephritis and animal models of progressive glomerulosclerosis. The protective effects of TX-synthase inhibitors and TXA_2 receptor antagonists are discussed vis-à-vis the potential cellular sources of enhanced TXA_2 biosynthesis.

RÉSUMÉ

Cette étude fait le recensement des publications consacrées au rôle des eicosanoides dans les maladies glomérulaires chroniques. On discute, en particulier, de la localisation de la synthèse de la prostaglandine rénale, de la mesure de son activité et de son inhibition. On examine les effets des inhibiteurs de la cyclooxygénase et de la prostaglandine sur la fonction rénale et on présente les données d'études faites chez l'animal. On discute aussi de l'inhibition de l'eicosanoide glomérulaire et des platelettes dans les maladies glomérulaires chroniques.

Les eicosanoides, qui comprennent les prostaglandines, sont les produits de cyclooxygénase et de lipooxygénase du métabolisme arachidonique. On a démontré la synthèse des prostaglandines dans la medulla rénale et dans la substance corticale, mais en quantité plus importante dans la première. La mesure des prostaglandines urinaires que ne sont pas métabolisées (et aussi de la thromboxane B2 (TXB2)) fournit la meilleure évaluation clinique de l'état de la production de prostaglandine rénale et de là de l'activité de la cyclooxygénase.

L'excrétion urinaire des prostaglandines (PGE2) ne semble pas être modifiée dans l'insuffisance rénale chronique, mais la prostaglandine (6-keto PGF1α) est réduite significativement chez les patients atteints d'une maladie glomérulaire chronique, y compris la néphropathie systémique de lupus érythémateux. Dans ces circonstances la synthèse de la prostaglandine (PGI2) est réduite, et l'on décrit les mécanismes que l'on pense être impliqués. Un certain nombre de médicaments (NSAIDs), y compris l'aspirine et les médicaments stéroïdiens antiinflammatoires peuvent déclencher l'inhibition pharmacologique de la synthèse rénale de la prostaglandine (comme il est démontré par l'excrétion urinaire réduite de la prostaglandine). Chez les personnes en bonne santé, l'inhibition de la synthèse de la prostaglandine ne provoque pas une diminution significative de la fonction rénale, mais des maladies telle que l'insuffisance glomérulaire chronique peuvent réduire la prostaglandine (PGE2 ou PGI1α) et de ce fait accroître la susceptibilité aux médicaments stéroïdiens antiinflammatoires, en dépit des taux normaux d'hormones constrictives. On présente une hypothèse de l'effet modulateur de la prostaglandine rénale (PGE2 et PGI2) sur l'action constrictive intrarénale de l'angiotensine II, de la vasopressine et de la norépinéphrine.

On examine aussi le rôle de la production de TXA2 dans la progression de la maladie glomérulaire chronique, en mettant l'accent sur des études de néphrite de lupus chez l'homme et de glomérulosclérose progressive chez les animaux. On discute des effets protecteurs des inhibiteurs de la synthèse TX et des antagonistes du récepteur TXA2 vis-à-vis des sources cellulaires potentielles d'une meilleure biosynthèse de TXA2.

ZUSAMMENFASSUNG

Diese Veröffentlichung bietet eine gründliche Übersicht über die Literatur, die sich mit der Rolle von Eicosanoiden bei chronischer glomerulärer Krankheit befasst. Speziell werden die Lokalisierung der Synthese des Nierenprostaglandins (PG) und die Messung seiner Aktivität und seiner Inhibition diskutiert. Die Effekte der Prostaglandin- und Cyclooxygenase- Inhibitoren auf die Nierenfunktion werden untersucht, und Daten, die aus Tier-Modellversuchen stammen, werden vorgestellt. Schliesslich präsentiert der Autor die Plättchen- und glomeruläre Eicosanoid-Inhibition bei chronischer glomerulärer Krankheit.

Eicosanoide, einschliesslich der Prostaglandine (PGs), bilden die Lipooxygenase- und Cyclooxygenaseprodukte des Arachidonatmetabolismus. Die Prostaglandinsynthese in der Nierenmedulla und der Rinde ist nachgewiesen worden; jedoch tritt sie in der ersteren in grösseren Mengen auf. Die beste klinische Auswertung des Zustandes der Nierenprostaglandinproduktion und damit auch der Cyclooxygenaseaktivität wird erreicht durch die Messung der unmetabolisierten Prostaglandine im Urin (und auch Thromboxan B_2(TXB$_2$)). Die Urinausscheidung des PGE_2 scheint sich bei chronischem Nierenversagen nicht zu verändern; jedoch wird 6-keto-PGF_2 deutlich reduziert in Patienten mit chronischer glomerulärer Krankheit, einschliesslich systemischer Erythematodes-Nephropathie. Unter diesen Umständen wird die PGI$_2$-Synthese unterdrückt, und der Autor beschreibt die Mechanismen, die diesem Vorgang wahrscheinlich zugrundeliegen. Die pharmakologische Inhibition der Prostaglandinsynthese in den Nieren (wie demonstriert durch die reduzierte Prostaglandinausscheidung im Urin) kann durch eine Reihe von Verbindungen hervorgerufen werden, einschliesslich Aspirin und die nonsteroiden anti-entzündlichen Drogen (NSAIDs). In gesunden Individuen ruft die Inhibition der Prostaglandinsynthese keine signifikante Reduktion der Nierenfunktion hervor; aber Krankheiten wie die chronische glomeruläre Krankheit können das PGE$_2$ oder das PGI$_2$ reduzieren und damit die Anfälligkeit gegenüber NSAIDs erhöhen, obwohl normale Mengen von Konstriktor-Hormomen vorliegen. Der Text beschreibt eine Hypothese für den modulierenden Effekt des PG$_2$ und des PGI$_2$ in der Niere auf die intrarenale Konstriktoraktivität des Angiotensin II, des Vasopressin und des Norepinephrin.

Die Besprechung beinhaltet die Rolle der intrarenalen TXA$_2$-Produktion im Verlauf der chronischen glomerulären Krankheit, mit Betonung auf menschlichen Studien des Lupus Nephritis und Tiermodellen für progressive Glomerulosklerose. Diskutiert werden die Schutzeffekte der TX-Synthase-Inhibitoren und der TXA$_2$-Rezeptor-Antagonisten vis-à-vis der potentiellen zellulären Quellen für verbesserte TXA$_2$-Biosynthese.

RIASSUNTO

Questo articolo fornisce un'estesa rassegna della letteratura sul ruolo degli eicosanoidi nel morbo glomerulare cronico. In particolare vengono discusse l'individuazione della sintesi della prostaglandina (PB) renale, la misurazione della sua attività e la sua inibizione. Vengono esaminati gli effetti delle prostaglandine e degli inibitori della cicloossigenasi sulla funzione renale e presentati dati da studi su modelli animali. Viene anche discussa l'inibizione di piastrine e eicosanoidi glomerulari nel morbo glomerulare cronico.

Gli eicosanoidi, che includono le prostaglandine (PG), sono i prodotti di lipoossigenasi e cicloossigenasi del metabolismo arachidonato. La sintesi delle PG è stata dimostrata nel midollo e nella corteccia renali, ma in maggiori quantità nella prima. La misurazione delle PG urinarie non metabolizzate (ed anche trombossane B2 (TXB2) fornisce la migliore valutazione clinica dello stato della produzione di PG e quindi di attività di cicloossigenasi.

L'escrezione urinaria di PGE2 non sembra venire alterata nell'insufficienza renale cronica ma la 6-keto-PGF1a è significativamente ridotta in pazienti con morbo glomerulare cronico, nefropatia di lupus eritematoso sistemico compresa. In queste circostanze la sintesi della PGI2 è ridotta e vengono delineati i meccanismi che si pensa siano coinvolti.

L'inibizione farmacologica della sintesi della PG renale (dimostrata dalla ridotta escrezione della PG urinaria) può essere effettuata da un certo numero di composti, aspirina e farmaci antiinflammatori non steroidali (FAINS). Negli individui sani, l'inibizione sintesi della PG non induce un significativo degrado della funzione renale ma malattie quali il morbo glomerulare cronico possono ridurre la PGE2 o la PGI2 e quindi aumentare la suscettibilità ai FAINS, malgrado livelli normali di ormoni costrittori. Viene delineata un'ipotesi dell'effetto modulatorio della PGE2 e della PGI2 sull'azione costrittrice intrarenale di angiotensina II, vasopressina e norepinefrina.

Viene anche passato in rassegna il ruolo della produzione di TXA2 nel progresso del morbo glomerulare cronico, con enfasi sugli studi umani del lupus nefritico e su modelli animali di glomerulosclerosi progressiva. Vengono discussi gli effetti protettivi degli inibitori della sintesi di TX e gli antagonisti dei recettori TXA2 in confronto alle fonti potenziali di biosintesi TXA2 ottimizzata.

SUMÁRIO

Este trabalho proporciona uma revisão extensa da literatura sobre o papel dos eicosanóides na doença glomerular crônica. Em particular, discutem-se a localização da síntese das prostaglandinas renais (PG), a medição de sua atividade e sua inibição. Examinam-se os efeitos das prostaglandinas e os inibidores da ciclooxigenasa sobre a função renal e presentam-se dados obtidos em estudos com animais modelo. Também discute-se a inibição de plaquetas e eicosanóides glomerulares na doença glomerular crônica. Os eicosanóides, que incluem as prostaglandinas (PG), são os produtos lipooxyigenasa e ciclooxigenasa do metabolismo araquidonato. Tem-se demonstrado a síntese de PG na medula e no córtex renais, mas em maior quantidade na primeira. A medição de PG urinárias não metabolizadas (e também tromboxano B_2 [TXB_2]) proporciona a melhor avaliação clínica do estado da produção renal de PG e por isso da atividade da ciclooxigenasa. A excreção urinária de PGE_2 não parece ser modificada na insuficiência renal crônica, mas a 6-ceto-$PGF_{1\alpha}$ é significativamente reduzida em pacientes com doença glomerular crônica, inclusive a nefropatia sistémica lúpus eritematoso. A síntese de PGI_2 é reduzida nestas circunstâncias, e esboçam-se os mecanismos que se pensam ser implicados. A inibição farmacológica da síntese de PG no rim (conforme demonstrada pela reduzida excreção urinária de PG) pode ser efetuada mediante uma série de compostos, inclusive a aspirina e as drogas antiinflamatórias não esteroidais (NSAID). Nos indivíduos sadios, a inibição da síntese de PG não induz um decremento significativo na função renal, mas doenças tais como a doença glomerular crônica poderiam reduzir os níveis de PGE_2 ou PGI_2, assim aumentando a suscetibilidade aos NSAID, apesar dos níveis normais de hormônios constritores. Esboçase uma hipótese acerca do efeito modulator dos níveis renais de PGE_2 e PGI_2 na ação constritora intrarrenal da angiotensina II, a vasopressina e a norepinefrina. Tambêm revisase o papel da produção intrarrenal de TXA_2 na progressão da doença glomerular crônica, com ênfase em estudos humanos de lúpus nefrite e modelos animais da glomeruloesclerose progressiva. Discutem-se os efeitos protetores dos inibidores de TX-sintasa e os antagonistas do receptor de TXA_2 em frente das fontes celulares potenciais de aumento da biosíntese de TXA_2.

RESUMEN

Este trabajo proporciona un repaso extenso de la literature en cuanto al papel de los eicosanoides en la enfermedad glomerular crónica. En particular se discute la localización de la síntesis de prostaglandinas (PG) en el riñón, la medida de su actividad y su inhibición. Se examinan los efectos de las prostaglandinas y los inhibidores de la ciclooxigenasa sobre la función renal y se presentan datos obtenidos en estudios con animales modelo. También se discute la inhibición de plaquetas y eicosanoides glomerulares en la enfermedad glomerular crónica. Los eicosanoides, que incluyen las prostaglandinas, son los productos lipooxigenasa y ciclooxigenasa del metabolismo del araquidonato. Se ha demostrado que existe síntesis de PG en la médula y corteza renales, pero en mayor cantidad en la primera. La medida de PG no metabolizadas en la orina (y también tromboxano B_2 [TXB_2]) proporciona la mejor evaluación clínica del estado de la producción renal de PG y de allí de la actividad de la ciclooxigenasa. La excreción urinaria de PGE_2 no parece verse alterada en la insuficiencia renal crónica, pero la 6-ceto-$PGF_{1\alpha}$ se ve significativamente reducida en pacientes con enfermedad glomerular crónica, incluyendo la nefropatía sistémica lupus eritematoso. La síntesis de PGI_2 se ve reducida en estas circunstancias, y se bosquejan los mecanismos que se piensa se hallan involucrados. La inhibición farmacológica de la síntesis de PG en el riñón (según demuestra la reducida excreción urinaria de PG) puede presentarse debido a un número de compuestos, incluyendo la aspirina y los fármacos antiinflamatorios no esteroides (FAINE). En individuos saludables, la inhibición de la síntesis de PG no induce un decremento significativo en la función renal, pero enfermedades tales como la enfermedad glomerular crónica podrían reducir los niveles de PGE_2 o PGI_2 causando así un incremento en la susceptibilidad a los FAINE, a pesar de los niveles normales de hormonas constrictoras. Se bosqueja una hipótesis acerca del efecto modulador de los niveles renales de PGE_2 y PGI_2 en la acción constrictoria intrarrenal de la angiotensina II, la vasopresina y la norepinefrina. También se analiza el papel de la producción intrarrenal de TXA_2 en la progresión de la enfermedad glomerular crónica, poniendo énfasis en estudios humanos de lupus nefritis y animales modelos de glomeruloesclerosis progresiva. Se discuten los efectos protectores de los inhibidores de TX-sintasa y los antagonistas del receptor de

TXA$_2$ en comparación con fuentes celulares potenciales de incremento de al biosíntesis de TXA$_2$.

要約

　本論文では，慢性糸球体疾患におけるエイコサノイドの役割に関して，広範な概説を試みる。とくに，腎プロスタグランジン（PG）合成の局在部位，その活性測定およびその抑制について考察する。腎機能に対するPGおよびシクロオキシゲナーゼ抑制薬の効果について検討し，動物実験のデータを紹介する。また，慢性糸球体疾患における血小板と糸球体エイコサノイド抑制の問題についても考察する。

　PGを含むエイコサノイドはリポキシゲナーゼおよびシクロオキシゲナーゼによるアラキドン酸代謝産物である。PG合成は腎髄質と皮質の両方で認められるが，前者が圧倒的に多い。尿中の未変化体PG［およびトロンボキサンB$_2$（TXB$_2$）］の測定は，腎PG産生の状態，すなわちシクロオキシゲナーゼ活性を臨床的に評価するのに最もよい方法である。慢性腎不全ではPGE$_2$の尿中排泄量は変化を示さないが，全身性エリテマトーデス腎症を含む慢性糸球体疾患患者では，6-ケト-PGF$_1\alpha$が有意に減少している。PGI$_2$合成はこのような状態では低下し，これに関与すると考えられる機序の概略を呈示する。

　腎PG合成の薬理学的抑制（尿中PG排泄量の減少で証明される）は，アスピリンや各種非ステロイド性抗炎症薬（NSAID）などを含むいくつかの化合物によってもたらされる。健常者ではPG合成抑制は腎機能の有意な低下をひき起こさない。しかし，慢性糸球体疾患のような病態では，PGE$_2$あるいはPGI$_2$が減少し，収縮ホルモンは正常レベルにあってもNSAIDに対する感受性が亢進する。ここでは，アンジオテンシンII，バソプレシンおよびノルエピネフリンの腎内収縮作用に及ぼす腎PGE$_2$およびPGI$_2$の調節作用の仮説について概説する。

　慢性糸球体疾患の進展における腎内TXA$_2$産生の役割についても，とくにループス腎炎の臨床研究および進行性糸球体硬化症の動物モデルでの研究に重点をおいて総括する。また，TX合成酵素阻害薬およびTXA$_2$受容体拮抗薬の防御効果について，TXA$_2$生合成亢進の細胞源と考えられるものと対比しながら考察する。

Cardiac and Renal Failure: An Expanding Role for ACE Inhibitors, edited by C. T. Dollery and L. M. Sherwood, Hanley & Belfus, Inc., Philadelphia.

Angiotensin-Converting Enzyme Inhibition in Renal Disease

Paul E. de Jong, Gerjan Navis, Jan E. Heeg, Dick de Zeeuw

BLOOD PRESSURE

From the early days of their introduction angiotensin I-converting enzyme (ACE) inhibitors have been successfully used as antihypertensive drugs in patients with renal hypertension. The use of ACE inhibitors in this specific population was not only the logical consequence of the efficacy of this class of antihypertensives, but, more importantly, a consequence of the specific mechanism of action of these drugs. Since a stimulated renin-angiotensin-aldosterone system (RAAS) frequently contributes to the hypertension in patients with renal artery stenosis and renal parenchymal disease, a drug that interferes with the production of the vasoconstrictor angiotensin II (ANG II) would particularly be efficacious in lowering the blood pressure in these patients. At least two RAAS-related factors contribute to the antihypertensive effect of ACE inhibitors in this specific population. First of all, the reduction of the usually stimulated circulating ANG II will result in systemic vasodilatation. The degree of vasodilation of any vascular bed is dependent on the initial vascular tone. This could well explain why the initial blood pressure response to ACE inhibition is correlated with the pre-treatment plasma renin activity.[1-4] Another factor that can contribute to the antihypertensive effect in patients with essential hypertension is the diuretic effect of these drugs. ACE inhibitors have been found to promote sodium excretion.[5-9] It has, moreover, been shown that such a natriuresis, occurring both during a low and a high salt intake,[10] results in a negative sodium and volume balance with a fall in body weight (Figure 1).[10,11] This net loss of sodium seems to be due to an effect on both the proximal and distal tubule.[6,9] Thus far, no data are available that show that ACE inhibitors also induce a natriuresis in patients with renal parenchymal disease or renal artery stenosis. It could be expected that such

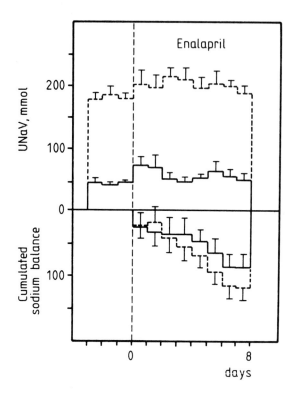

FIG. 1. Effects of enalapril (10 mg bid) on sodium excretion (top panel) and sodium balance (lower panel) in patients with essential hypertension (n = 9). Data on low sodium intake are depicted by continuous lines, data on liberal sodium intake by broken lines. Data are presented as mean ± SEM. From Navis, et al. Kidney Int 1987; **31**:815–819, with permission of the publisher.

tubular effects only are present if glomerular filtration rate (GFR) does not change (see subsequent discussion). Although such a natriuresis has not yet been documented in these patients, both in renal parenchymal disease[12,13] and in renal artery stenosis ACE inhibitors have been found to be effective antihypertensive agents.[14,15] However, despite their proven efficacy in both these conditions, caution is needed when using ACE inhibitors in patients with impaired renal function. Firstly, because ACE inhibition in these patients could result in a decrease in GFR (see below), and secondly, because ACE inhibitors are, at least partly, excreted via the kidney[16] and thus dose adjustment is required in case of impaired renal function.[17,18] We recently showed in patients with renal parenchymatous disease and a GFR of 30–60 ml/min that a dose of 28 ± 13 mg lisinopril gave a good antihypertensive effect, whereas patients with a GFR of 10–30 ml/min only needed 16 ± 16 mg.[18] In patients on chronic hemodialysis, lisinopril can induce an adequate antihypertensive effect in doses of 1–2.5 mg two or three times a week. A further gradual fall in blood pressure may occur after the initial titration period, and it is frequently possible to lower the dose of the drug during longer follow-up.[18]

RENAL HEMODYNAMICS

Apart from their antihypertensive effects, ACE inhibitors have profound effects on renal hemodynamics. These effects also result from inhibition of ANG II production, since this vasoactive peptide is of prime importance in the regulation of renal hemodynamics. Angiotensin II increases postglomerular capillary resistance[19] and thus induces a rise in intraglomerular capillary pressure. At low levels of perfusion pressure, adequate renal autoregulation (the capacity to maintain glomerular filtration during a fall in systemic pressure) is in fact dependent on the capacity to constrict the postglomerular arteriole, and thus on (local) ANG II.[20] This is particularly true in the case of renal artery stenosis and intrinsic renal parenchymal disease, especially in the presence of a concomitant volume depletion.

In patients with normal renal function, ACE inhibition results in a rise in effective renal plasma flow (ERPF) with a stable or elevated GFR.[8,9,21-24] Consequently, filtration fraction, which with some restrictions can be used as an index of postglomerular resistance, is decreased. Interestingly, the extent to which GFR may rise has been found to be dependent upon pre-existing volume depletion.[25] Only in patients on a low sodium diet did GFR increase after treatment with enalapril. GFR remained stable after enalapril treatment when the same patients were on a high sodium diet (Figure 2). As Figure 2

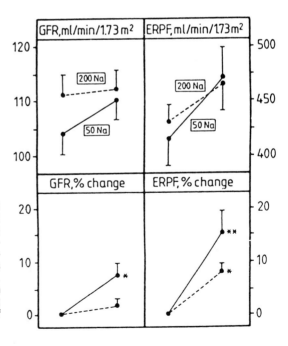

FIG. 2. Effects of enalapril (10 mg bid during one week) on GFR and ERPF on liberal (broken lines) and on low (continuous lines) sodium intake. Data are given as absolute values (upper panel) and as percentage change (lower panel). Mean ± SEM. *p < 0.01. From Navis, et al. Kidney Int 1987; 31:815–819, with permission of the publisher.

shows, this difference in response to ACE inhibition on a low versus a high sodium diet is explained by the differing pretreatment GFRs. Glomerular filtration rate is lower during low salt intake, probably as a consequence of the increased ANG II level under these circumstances. This demonstrates the intricate balance between the RAAS and the state of volume balance in interpreting the renal effects of ACE inhibitors. Moreover it shows that, as had been demonstrated for the antihypertensive effects,[10] the net renal hemo-dynamic effects of the ACE inhibitor are enhanced during sodium depletion.

The observed effects of ACE inhibitors on GFR in patients with impaired renal function due to renal parenchymatous disease are more conflicting. Whereas ERPF in these patients has generally been found to increase after ACE inhibition, both a rise[26-28] and a fall[13,29-32] in GFR have been described. We found that lisinopril induced a 21 ± 10% fall in GFR in patients with hypertension and renal function impairment (GFR 10–60 ml/min)[13] and a 9 ± 7% fall in GFR in patients with the nephrotic syndrome (generally without hypertension) with a pretreatment GFR of 78 ± 29 ml/min.[33] In both

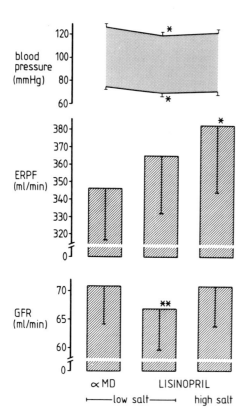

FIG. 3. The influence of changes in salt intake on the effects of lisinopril on blood pressure, ERPF, and GFR compared to a period with alpha-methyldopa (α-MD) in nine patients with the nephrotic syndrome. Low salt indicates 50 mmol sodium, high salt 200 mmol sodium per day. Mean ± SEM. *p < 0.05, **p < 0.01. From Heeg, et al. *Current Opinion in Cardiology* (in press), with permission of the publisher.

studies patients adhered to a low sodium diet. We recently showed, however, that the lisinopril-induced fall in GFR in sodium-depleted patients with the nephrotic syndrome was nearly totally abolished when the patients switched from the low sodium (50 mmol) to a high sodium (200 mmol) diet.[34] On the high sodium diet GFR was comparable to the level observed during similar blood pressure lowering with alpha-methyldopa (Figure 3). This highlights the importance of closely monitoring sodium balance when interpreting the renal effects of ACE inhibitors. These findings are in contrast with the data on ACE inhibition in patients with normal renal function in whom GFR is increased on a low sodium diet. The data in patients with renal function impairment indicate an increased dependency of GFR on ANG II-mediated efferent vasoconstriction unmasked by sodium depletion. This suggests an impairment of the vasodilator capacity of the afferent arteriole (the normal response to a fall in blood pressure), either because the vasodilation is already maximal or because of an intrinsic defect.

Special attention should be paid to the data on the effects of ACE inhibitors in patients with renal artery stenosis. Several reports mentioned a fall in GFR in patients with a bilateral renal artery stenosis or a renal artery stenosis in a solitary kidney.[35-38] Even complete cessation of GFR has been described. In the case of severely impaired renal blood flow behind a stenosis, glomerular filtration is fully dependent on ANG II-mediated postglomerular vasoconstriction. In these circumstances, if ANG II production is blocked, the fall in intraglomerular pressure due to the postglomerular vasodilation causes the already restricted blood flow to bypass the glomerulus. This interpretation is in agreement with the reversible character of the fall in glomerular filtration after withdrawal of the drug and after volume repletion.[39] These effects of ACE inhibitors have consequences for clinical practice; in patients with a bilateral renal artery stenosis, or a renal artery stenosis in a solitary kidney, ACE inhibition can result in a rise in serum creatinine. In such cases, serum creatinine will usually have been somewhat elevated prior to ACE inhibition. We therefore recommend that serum creatinine is measured before administration of an ACE inhibitor to a patient in whom the possibility of a renal artery stenosis has not been excluded. In the case of abnormal results, further investigations are needed to establish the underlying cause of that renal function disturbance. In the case of normal results before treatment, serum creatinine should still be checked within a week after starting the ACE inhibitor. If a rise should have occurred, further diagnostic procedures are necessary. Used in this way, ACE inhibitors may be of value since they may help to unmask treatable causes of the elevated blood pressure. Recent studies describe the use of renal isotope scanning (either with 131-I-hippuran or Tc-DTPA) before and after ACE inhibition as a diagnostic aid in the detection of a renal artery stenosis, and also in the case of a unilateral renal artery stenosis with a contralateral normal kidney.[40,41] The same pathophysiological mechanism probably applies in both cases.

PROTEINURIA AND NEPHROTIC SYNDROME

Proteinuria frequently occurs in patients with renal parenchymal disease, and it has also been described in some patients with renal artery stenosis. The number of drugs that are effective in the treatment of proteinuria in cases of a non-steroid-sensitive nephrotic syndrome is rather limited. Until recently, non-steroidal anti-inflammatory drugs like indomethacin have been the most successful in the treatment of proteinuria in nephrotic syndrome.[42-44] Since 1985, however, a number of reports show the efficacy of ACE inhibition in this context.[13,28,45-49] Some of these studies are restricted to patients with diabetic nephropathy.[45,46] However, ACE inhibitors also reduce proteinuria in patients with renal disease of different etiology.[13,28,47-49] We showed a fall in proteinuria from 4.2 ± 3.2 to 2.3 ± 3.4 g/day after 3 months of treatment with lisinopril, whereas previous conventional antihypertensive therapy did not influence urinary protein loss (Figure 4).[13] More interestingly, the anti-proteinuric effect occurred, although was not maximal, at quite low doses of the drug. The antiproteinuric effect, however, appeared to vary considerably between individuals. In a subsequent study, the response was found not to be dependent on initial blood pressure or GFR.[50] However, we have shown that

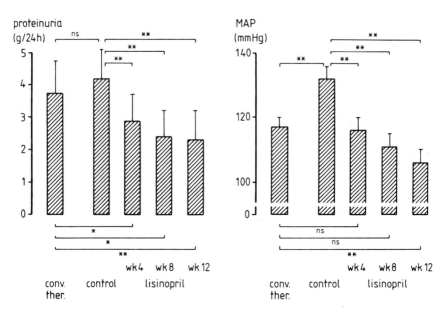

FIG. 4. The effect of lisinopril (in increasing doses during a 12-week treatment period) on proteinuria (left panel) and mean arterial pressure (right panel) as compared to a period on conventional antihypertensive therapy and a 2-week period without antihypertensives (control) in 13 patients with renal functional impairment. Mean ± SEM. *p < 0.05, **p < 0.01. From Heeg, et al. Kidney Int 1987; **32**:78–83, with permission of the publisher.

the response is markedly dependent on volume balance. Although lisinopril induced a $52 \pm 14\%$ fall in proteinuria in patients on a low sodium diet (from 6.4 ± 2.0 to 3.1 ± 1.4 g/day), this antiproteinuric effect disappeared when the patients switched to a high sodium diet (24-hour protein excretion being 5.9 ± 3.0 g).[50] Thus, as shown before for the effects on GFR, the effect of ACE inhibition on urinary protein excretion is also enhanced during a low sodium intake. We further showed that the antiproteinuric effect was related to the effect on filtration fraction: the more the filtration fraction fell, the more proteinuria decreased.[13] This argues in favor of a hemodynamically mediated mechanism and suggests that the fall in proteinuria is due to a lowering of intraglomerular capillary pressure.

In this respect the data on the occurrence of proteinuria in renal artery stenosis are of interest. Proteinuria in these patients has been reported to be related to increased ANG II production[51-57] and to improve either after nephrectomy of the post-stenotic kidney,[51-53] after renal angioplasty[56,57] or after ACE inhibition.[54,55]

PREVENTION OF PROGRESSIVE DECLINE IN RENAL FUNCTION

In cases of loss of GFR (through whatever cause), the natural course will be a steady progression in loss of renal function. This is thought to be the result of ongoing glomerular damage caused by an increased glomerular pressure in the remaining stressed filter units. Indeed, it has been demonstrated in different animal models that ACE inhibitors (that lower intraglomerular capillary pressure) are able to prevent progressive renal function decline, whereas conventional antihypertensive agents have little or no protective effect.[58-61] So far, human data to substantiate these findings are limited. No prospective studies — except for diabetic nephropathy[62] — are available. One retrospective study,[63] however, indicates that the findings may also be applicable to human renal insufficiency. The authors showed that ACE inhibition in hypertensive patients with a moderate degree of renal function impairment resulted in a stable serum creatinine over a period of more than 1 year, whereas a comparable control group treated with conventional antihypertensives (producing a comparable fall in blood pressure) showed a steady rise in serum creatinine levels.

CONCLUSIONS

It can be concluded that ACE inhibitors are effective antihypertensive drugs in patients with renal artery stenosis and renal parenchymal disease. When renal function is compromised, dose adjustments are warranted and often quite low doses of the drug will be sufficient to maintain adequate blood pressure control, particularly when the patient is on a sodium-restricted diet.

ERPF generally rises during ACE inhibition in patients with renal parenchymal disease. The short-term effects on GFR are variable and are affected by the initial sodium balance. GFR may decrease after treatment with ACE inhibitors in patients with renal parenchymal disease and renal artery stenosis, particularly in case of a low sodium diet. The resulting fall in filtration fraction indicates a postglomerular vasodilation with a concomitant fall in intraglomerular capillary pressure. This also explains the antiproteinuric effect of the ACE inhibitors, which again is particularly evident when sodium intake is low. Whether this fall in glomerular capillary pressure will also contribute to the prevention of progressive loss of renal function in these patients has still to be proven.

REFERENCES

1. Case DB, Wallace JM, Keim HJ, Weber MA, Sealey JE, Laragh JH. Possible role of renin in hypertension as suggested by renin-sodium profiling and inhibition of converting enzyme. *N Engl J Med* 1977; **296**:641–646.
2. Bravo EL, Tarazi RC. Converting enzyme inhibition with an orally active compound in hypertensive man. *Hypertension* 1979; **1**:39–46.
3. Brunner HR, Gavras H, Waeber B, Textor SC, Turini GA, Wauters JP. Clinical use of an orally active converting enzyme inhibitor captopril. *Hypertension* 1980; **2**:558–566.
4. Navis GJ, de Jong PE, Donker AJM, van der Hem GK, de Zeeuw D. Blood pressure response to enalaprilic acid; dose-response and effect of pre-treatment with furosemide. *Eur J Clin Pharmacol* 1985; **29**:9–15.
5. McCaa RE, Hall JE, McCaa CS. The effect of angiotensin I converting enzyme inhibition on arterial blood pressure and urinary sodium excretion. Role of the renal renin angiotensin and kallikrein-kinin system. *Circ Res* 1978; **43(suppl 1)**:32–39.
6. Atlas SA, Case DB, Sealey JE, Laragh JH, McKinstry DN. Interruption of the renin-angiotensin system in hypertensive patients by captopril induces sustained reduction in aldosterone excretion, potassium retention and natriuresis. *Hypertension* 1979; **1**:274–280.
7. Zimmerman BG, Wong PC. Alterations in renal function produced by angiotensin converting enzyme inhibitors. In Horowitz ZP, ed. *Angiotensin Converting Enzyme Inhibitors. Mechanisms of Action and Therapeutic Implications.* Baltimore and Munich, Urban & Schwartzenberg, 1981; 239–255.
8. de Zeeuw D, Navis GJ, Donker AJM, de Jong PE. The angiotensin converting enzyme inhibitor enalapril and its effects on renal function. *J Hypertens* 1983; **I(suppl)**:93–97.
9. Navis GJ, de Jong PE, Donker AJM, van der Hem GK, de Zeeuw D. Effects of enalaprilic acid on sodium excretion and renal hemodynamics in essential hypertension. *J Clin Hypertens* 1985; **1**:228–238.
10. Navis GJ, de Jong PE, Donker AJM, van der Hem GK, de Zeeuw D. Diuretic effects of ACE-inhibition; comparison of low and liberal sodium diet in hypertensive patients. *J Cardiovasc Pharmacol* 1987; **9**:743–748.
11. MacGregor GA, Markandu ND, Roulston JE, Jones JC, Morton JJ. Maintenance of blood pressure by the renin angiotensin system in normal man. *Nature* 1981; **291**:329–331.
12. Bauer JH. Role of angiotensin converting enzyme inhibitors in essential and renal hypertension. Effects of captopril and enalapril on renin-angiotensin-aldosterone, renal function and hemodynamics, salt and water excretion, and body fluid composition. *Am J Med* 1984; **77(suppl 2a)**:43–51.
13. Heeg JE, de Jong PE, van der Hem GK, de Zeeuw D. Reduction of proteinuria by angiotensin converting enzyme inhibition. *Kidney Int* 1987; **32**:78–83.
14. Case DB, Atlas SA, Marion RM, Laragh JH. Long-term efficacy of captopril in renovascular and essential hypertension. *Am J Cardiol* 1982; **49**:1440–1445.
15. Hodsman GP, Brown JJ, Cumming AMM, Davies DL, East BW, Lever AF, Morton JJ,

Murray GD, Robertson JI. Enalapril in treatment of hypertension with renal artery stenosis. Changes in blood pressure, renin, angiotensin I and II, renal function, and body composition. *Am J Med* 1984; **77(suppl 2a)**:52–60.

16. Ulm EH, Hichens M, Gomez HJ, Till EA, Hand EL, Vassil TC, Biollaz J, Brunner HR, Schelling JL. Enalapril maleate and a lysine analogue: disposition in man. *Br J Clin Pharmacol* 1982; **14**:357–362.

17. van Schaik BAM, Geyskes GG, Boer P. Lisinopril in hypertensive patients with and without renal failure. *Eur J Clin Pharmacol* 1987; **32**:11–16.

18. de Jong PE, Apperloo AJ, Heeg JE, de Zeeuw D. Lisinopril in hypertensive patients with renal function impairment. *Nephron* (in press).

19. Edwards RM. Segmental effects of norepinephrine and angiotensin on isolated renal microvessels. *Am J Physiol* 1983; **244**:F526–534.

20. Hall JE, Guyton AC, Jackson TE, Coleman TG, Lohmeier TE, Trippodo NC. Control of glomerular filtration rate by renin-angiotensin system. *Am J Physiol* 1972; **233**:366–372.

21. Hollenberg NK, Meggs LG, Williams GH, Katz J, Garnic JD, Harrington DP. Sodium intake and renal responses to captopril in normal man and in essential hypertension. *Kidney Int* 1981; **20**:240–245.

22. Navis GJ, de Jong PE, Donker AJM, de Zeeuw D. Effects of enalapril on blood pressure and renal hemodynamics in essential hypertension. *Proc EDTA* 1983; **20**:577–581.

23. Bauer JH, Reams G, Gaddy P. Renal function and hemodynamics during treatment with enalapril in primary hypertension. *Nephron* 1986; **44 (suppl 1)**:83–86.

24. Navis GJ, de Jong PE, Donker AJM, van der Hem GK, de Zeeuw D. Enalapril and the kidney: renal vasodilation and natriuresis due to the inhibition of angiotensin II information. *J Cardiovasc Pharmacol* 1985; **8(suppl 1)**:30–34.

25. Navis GJ, de Jong PE, Donker AJM, van der Hem GK, de Zeeuw D. Renal response to moderate sodium restriction in essential hypertension; effects of ACE-inhibition. *Kidney Int* 1987; **31**:815–819.

26. Rasmussen S, Ibsen H, Giese J. Contrasting effects of the renin-angiotensin system on renal function disclosed during converting enzyme inhibition in patients with renal hypertension. *Scand J Urol Nephrol* 1984; **79(suppl)**:49–52.

27. Delink K, Aurell M, Herlitz H. Captopril in the treatment of hypertension in predialytic end-stage renal disease. *Contr Nephrol* 1984; **41**:299–303.

28. Herlitz H, Edeno C, Mulec H, Westberg G, Aurell M. Captopril treatment of hypertension and renal failure in systemic lupus erythematosus. *Nephron* 1984; **38**:253–256.

29. Beroniade V. Severe side-effects of captopril in advanced chronic kidney insufficiency. *Kidney Int* 1983; **24**:423.

30. Bjork S, Herlitz H, Nijberg G, Granerus G, Aurell M. Effect of captopril on renal hemodynamics in the treatment of resistant renal hypertension. *Hypertension* 1983; **5(suppl III)**:152–153.

31. Verbeelen DL, de Boel S. Reversible acute on chronic renal failure during captopril treatment. *Br Med J* 1984; **289**:20–21.

32. Brivet F, Roulot D, Poitrine A, Dormont J. Reversible acute renal failure during enalapril treatment in patient with chronic glomerulonephritis without renal artery stenosis. *Lancet* 1985; **i**:1512.

33. Heeg JE, de Jong PE, van der Hem GK, de Zeeuw D. Antiproteinuric effect of the ACE-inhibitor lisinopril in comparison with the NSAID indomethacin. *Nephr Dial Transpl* 1988; **3**:510–511(A).

34. Heeg JE, de Zeeuw D, de Jong PE. The effects of lisinopril on renal hemodynamics in patients with renal disease. *Curr Opinion in Cardiology* 1988 (in press).

35. Collste P, Haglund K, Lundgren G, Magnussen G, Ostman J. Reversible renal failure during treatment with captopril. *Br Med J* 1979; **2**:612–613.

36. Farrow PR, Wilkinson R. Reversible renal failure during treatment with captopril. *Br Med J* 1979; **1**:1680.

37. Hricik DE, Browning PJ, Kopelman R, Goorno WE, Madias NE, Dzau VJ. Captopril-induced functional renal insufficiency in patients with bilateral renal artery stenosis or renal artery stenosis in a solitary kidney. *N Engl J Med* 1983; **308**:373–376.

38. van der Woude FJ, van Son WJ, Tegzess AM, Donker AJM, Slooff MJH, van der Slikke LB, Hoorntje SJ. Effect of captopril on blood pressure and renal function in patients with transplant renal artery stenosis. *Nephron* 1985; **39**:134–188.

39. Watson ML, Bell GM, Muir AL, Buist TAS, Kellett RJ, Padfield PL. Captopril/diuretic combinations in severe renovascular disease: a cautionary note. *Lancet* 1983; **i**:44–45.
40. Geyskes GG, Oei HY, Puylaert CBAJ, Dorhout Mees EJ. Renovascular hypertension identified by captopril-induced changes in the renogram. *Hypertension* 1987; **9**:451–458.
41. Sfakianakis GN, Bourgoignie JJ, Jaffe D, Kyriakides G, Perez-Stable E, Duncan RC. Single-dose captopril scintigraphy in the diagnosis of renovascular hypertension. *J Nucl Med* 1987; **28**:1383–1392.
42. Arisz L, Donker AJM, Brentjens JRH, van der Hem GK. The effect of indomethacin on proteinuria and kidney function in the nephrotic syndrome. *Acta Med Scand* 1976; **199**:122–125.
43. Donker AJM, Brentjens JRH, van der Hem GK, Arisz L. Treatment of the nephrotic syndrome with indomethacin. *Nephron* 1978; **22**:374–381.
44. Vriesendorp R, Donker AJM, de Zeeuw D, de Jong PE, van der Hem GK, Brentjens JRH. Effects of nonsteroidal anti-inflammatory drugs on proteinuria. *Am J Med* 1986; **81(2B)**:84–94.
45. Taguma Y, Kitamoto Y, Futaki G, Ueda H, Monma H, Ishazaki M, Takahashi H, Sekino H, Saski Y. Effect of captopril on heavy proteinuria in azotemic diabetics. *N Engl J Med* 1985; **313**:1617–1620.
46. Hommel E, Parving HH, Mathiesen E, Edsberg B, Nielsen MD, Giese J. Effect of captopril on kidney function in insulin-dependent diabetic patients with nephropathy. *Br Med J* 1986; **293**:446–470.
47. Reams GP, Bauer JH. Effect of enalapril in subjects with hypertension associated with moderate to severe renal dysfunction. *Arch Intern Med* 1986; **146**:2145–2148.
48. Lagrue G, Robeva R, Laurent J. Antiproteinuric effect of captopril in primary glomerular disease. *Nephron* 1987; **46**:99–100.
49. Trachtman H, Gauthier B. Effects of ACE inhibitor therapy on proteinuria in children with renal disease. *J Pediatr* 1988; **112**:255–298.
50. Heeg JE, de Jong PE, van der Hem GK, de Zeeuw D. Efficacy and variability of the antiproteinuric effect of ACE-inhibition by lisinopril—a comparison with indomethacin. *Kidney Int* 1989 (in press).
51. Montoliu J, Botey A, Torras A, Darnell A, Revert L. Renin-induced massive proteinuria in man. *Clin Nephrol* 1979; **11**:267–271.
52. Kumar A, Shapiro AP. Proteinuria and nephrotic syndrome induced by renin in patients with renal artery stenosis. *Arch Intern Med* 1980; **140**:1631–1634.
53. Eiser AR, Katz SM, Swartz C. Reversible nephrotic range proteinuria with renal artery stenosis: a clinical example of renin-associated proteinuria. *Nephron* 1982; **30**:374–377.
54. Takeda R, Morimoto S, Uchida K, Kigoshi T, Sumitami T, Matsubara F. Effects of captopril on both hypertension and proteinuria. *Arch Intern Med* 1980; **140**:1531–1533.
55. Vea AM, Ruiz CG, Carrera M, Oliver JA, Richart C. Effect of captopril in nephrotic range proteinuria due to renovascular hypertension. *Nephron* 1987; **45**:162–163.
56. Hariharan S, Pandey AP, Shastry JCM, Kirubakaran MG. Nephrotic range proteinuria with renal artery stenosis: its reversal after transluminal angioplasty. *Nephron* 1987; **47**:77.
57. Zimbler MS, Pickering TG, Sos TA, Laragh JH. Proteinuria in renovascular hypertension and the effects of renal angioplasty. *Am J Cardiol* 1987; **59**:406–408.
58. Anderson S, Rennke HG, Brenner BM. Therapeutic advantage of ACE inhibitors in arresting progressive renal disease associated with systemic hypertension in the rat. *J Clin Invest* 1986; **77**:1993–2000.
59. Raij L, Chiou XC, Owens R, Wrigley B. Therapeutic implications of hypertension-induced glomerular injury. *Am J Med* 1985; **79(3C)**:37–41.
60. Zatz R, Dunn BR, Meyer TW, Anderson S, Rennke HG, Brenner BM. Prevention of diabetic glomerulopathy by pharmacological amelioration of glomerular capillary hypertension. *J Clin Invest* 1986; **77**:1925–1930.
61. Meyer TW, Anderson S, Rennke HG, Brenner BM. Reversing glomerular hypertension stabilizes established glomerular injury. *Kidney Int* 1987; **31**:752–759.
62. Bjorck S, Nyberg G, Mulec H, Granerus G, Herlitz H, Aurell M. Beneficial effects of ACE inhibition on renal function in patients with diabetic nephropathy. *Br Med J* 1986; **293**:471–474.
63. Reisch C, Mann J, Ritz E. Konversionenzymhemmer in der antihypertensiven Behandlung nierinsuffizienter Patienten. *Dtsch Med Wschr* 1987; **112**:1249–1252.

SUMMARY

Angiotensin-converting enzyme (ACE) inhibitors are effective antihypertensive agents in patients with renal parenchymal disease. However, caution is needed when administering ACE inhibitors to patients with impaired renal function and dose adjustment may be necessary. Low doses of the drug may be sufficient to maintain adequate blood pressure control, particularly if the patient is on a sodium-restricted diet. Although effective renal plasma flow (ERPF) generally increases in patients with renal parenchymal disease when treated with ACE inhibitors, their effect on glomerular filtration rate (GFR) is variable. Both rises and falls in GFR have been reported, although a fall is more likely in patients on a low-sodium diet. This is in contrast to treatment with ACE inhibitors in patients with normal renal function. Nephrotic range proteinuria is a frequent finding in patients with renal parenchymal disease. The efficacy of ACE inhibitors in reducing proteinuria in these patients is well documented, particularly in patients on a low sodium diet. This antiproteinuric effect appears to be related to a fall in intraglomerular capillary pressure. Animal studies suggest that, unlike conventional antihypertensive agents, ACE inhibitors are able to prevent progressive decline in renal function. Further studies are needed to substantiate these findings in man.

RÉSUMÉ

Les inhibiteurs de l'enzyme de conversion de l'angiotensine sont des antihypertenseurs efficaces chez les patients atteints d'insuffisance rénale parenchymale. Cependant, il faut exercer certaines précautions lorsqu'on administre les inhibiteurs de l'enzyme de conversion de l'angiotensine aux malades atteints d'insuffisance rénale et ajuster la dose selon le cas. Le médicament administré à faible dose peut suffire à maintenir le contrôle de la pression artérielle, surtout si le patient est soumis à une restriction sodée. Alors que l'efficacité du flux plasmatique augmente généralement chez les patients atteints d'insuffisance rénale parenchymale lorsqu'ils sont soumis au traitement d'inhibiteurs de l'enzyme de conversion de l'angiotensine, leurs effets sur la filtration glomulaire rénale est variable. On a noté à la fois des baisses et des hausses de la filtration glomulaire rénale, bien qu'une chute soit plus probable chez les patients sous régime à restriction sodée. Les patients qui ont une fonction rénale normale et qui sont soumis au traitement d'inhibiteurs de l'enzyme de conversion de l'angiotensine ne présentent pas ces caractéristiques. Chez les patients atteints d'insuffisance rénale parenchymale on trouve souvent une protéinurie néphrotique. On a bien mis en valeur l'efficacité des inhibiteurs de l'enzyme de conversion de l'angiotensine chez ces patients. On note une réduction de la protéinurie, en particulier chez les patients soumis à un régime de restriction sodée. L'effet antiprotinéurique semble être lié à une chute de la pression capillaire intraglomérulaire. Comme cela a été montré chez l'animal, les inhibiteurs de l'enzyme de conversion de l'angiotensine, à la différence des antihypertenseurs conventionnels, permettent de prévenir l'évolution vers l'insuffisance rénale chronique. D'autres études sont nécessaires afin d'établir la validité de ces résultats chez l'homme.

ZUSAMMENFASSUNG

Inhibitoren des angiotensinkonvertierenden Enzyms (ACE) sind effektive anti-hypertensive Mittel für Patienten mit renaler parenchymätoser Krankheit. Jedoch sollten ACE-Inhibitoren an Patienten mit behinderter Nierenfunktion nur mit grosser Vorsicht ausgegeben werden, und Anpassung der Dosis könnte nötig sein. In vielen Fällen sind niedrige Dosen der Droge ausreichend für die Aufrechterhaltung einer angemessenen Blutdruckkontrolle; besonders, wenn der Patient eine Natrium-limitierende Diät einhält. Während der effektive Plasmafluss der Niere sich in Patienten mit renaler parenchymätoser Krankheit normalerweise erhöht, sobald sie mit ACE-Inhibitoren behandelt werden, variiert ihr Effekt auf die glomeruläre Filtrationsrate. Sowohl Erhöhungen als auch Verringerungen der glomerulären Filtrationsrate sind berichtet worden, obwohl eine Verringerung in Patienten wahrscheinlicher ist, die sich auf einer niedrigen Natriumdiät befinden. Dies kontrastiert die Behandlung von Patienten mit normaler Nierenfunktion durch ACE-Inhibitoren. Patienten mit renaler parenchymätoser Krankheit zeigen häufig Proteinurie in der nephrotischen Gegend. Die Wirksamkeit der ACE-Inhibitoren für die Reduktion der Proteinurie ist für diese Patienten gut dokumentiert worden, besonders für Patienten auf einer niedrigen Natriumdiät. Dieser anti-proteinurie-Effekt scheint mit einem Abfall des intraglomerulären Kapillardrucks zusammenzuhängen. Tierstudien weisen darauf hin, dass ACE-Inhibitoren im Gegensatz zu konventionellen antihypertonischen Drogen den Fortschritt der nachlassenden Nierenfunktion aufhalten können. Weitere Studien sind nötig, um diese Ergebnisse auf Menschen anwenden zu können.

RIASSUNTO

Gli inibitori dell'enzima isomerizzante dell'angiotensina (EIA) sono agenti antiipertensivi efficaci in pazienti con morbo parenchimale renale. Tuttavia una certa cautela è necessaria nel somministrare inibitori dell'EIA a pazienti con diminuita funzione renale e può essere necessario adattare le dosi. Basse dosi del farmaco possono essere sufficienti a mantenere un controllo adeguato della pressione sanguigna, soprattutto se il paziente segue una dieta che limiti il consumo di sodio. Benché il flusso di plasma renale effettivo (FPRE) generalmente aumenti in pazienti con morbo parenchimale renale quando vengono curati con inibitori dell'EIA, il loro effetto sul TFG è variabile. Sono stati documentati sia aumenti che cadute del TFG, benché una caduta sia più probabile in pazienti con dieta a basso consumo di sodio. Ciò contrasta con la cura mediante inibitori dell'EIA in pazienti con funzione renale normale. La proteinuria nel range nefrosico viene riscontrata frequentemente in pazienti con morbo parenchimale cronico. L'efficacia degli inibitori dell'EIA nel ridurre la proteinuria in tali pazienti è ben documentata, soprattutto in pazienti con dieta a basso consumo di sodio. Questo effetto antiproteinurico appare collegato ad una caduta della pressione capillare intraglomerulare. Studi animali fanno pensare che, contrariamente algi agenti antiipertensivi tradizionali, gli inibitori dell'EIA siano in grado di impedire il degrado progressivo della funzione renale. Sono necessari altri studi per sostanziare tali ipotesi nell'uomo.

SUMÁRIO

Os inibidores da enzima convertidora da angiotensina (ACF) são agentes antihipertensivos eficazes em pacientes com doença renal parenquimatosa. Contudo, precisa-se precaução ao administrarem os inibidores da ACE a pacientes com função renal debilitada e pode ser necessário efetuar ajustes da dose. Doses baixas da droga podem ser suficientes para manter um controle adequado da pressão arterial, particularmente se o paciente se encontrar numa dieta alimentar restringida de sódio. Ainda que o fluxo plasmático renal eficaz (ERPF) geralmente aumenta em pacientes com doença renal parenquimatosa quando se traterem com inibidores da ACE, seu efeito no índice de filtração glomerular (GFR) é variável. Têm-se informado tanto de aumento como de diminuição no GFR, ainda que uma diminuição é mais provável em pacientes com uma dieta alimentar reduzida de sódio. Isto contrasta com o tratamento com inibidores da ACE em pacientes com função renal normal. A proteinúria nefrótica é um achado comum em pacientes com doença renal parenquimatosa. A eficácia dos inibidores da ACE na redução da proteinúria neste tipo de paciente é bem documentada, particularmente em pacientes com uma dieta alimentar reduzida de sódio. Este efeito antiproteinúrico parece estar relacionado com uma diminuição na pressão capilar intraglomerular. Estudos animais sugerem que, ao contrário dos agentes antihipertensivos tradicionais, os inibidores da ACE são capazes de evitar o enfraquecimento progressivo da função renal. Estudos adicionais são necessários para corroborar estes achados no homem.

RESUMEN

Los inhibidores de la enzima convertidora de la angiotensina (ACE) son agentes antihipertensivos eficaces en pacientes con enfermedad renal parenquimatosa. Sin embargo, es necesario tener precaución al administrar los inhibidores de la ACE a pacientes con función renal deteriorada y podría ser necesario efectuar ajustes de la dosis. Volúmenes farmacológicos bajos del podrían ser suficientes para mantener un control adecuado de la presión arterial, particularmente si el paciente se halla en una dieta restringida de sodio. Aunque el flujo eficaz del plasma en el riñón (ERPF) generalmente incrementa en pacientes con enfermedad renal parenquimatosa cuando se tratan con inhibidores de la ACE, su efecto en el índice de filtración glomerular (GFR) es variable. Se ha informado tanto de incremento como de decremento en el GFR, aunque una disminución es más probable en pacientes conuna dieta reducida de sodio. Esto contrasta con el tratamiento con inhibidores de la ACE en pacientes con una función renal normal. La proteinuria nefrótica es un resuetado frecuente en pacientes con enfermedad renal parenquimatosa. La eficacia de los inhibidores de la ACE en la reducción de la proteinuria en este tipo de paciente se ha documentado ampliamente, particularmente en pacientes con una dieta reducida de sodio. Este efecto antiproteinúrico parece estar relacionado con una disminución en la presión capilar intraglomerular. Estudios en animales sugieren que, a diferencia de los agentes antihipertensivos tradicionales, los inhibidores de la ACE son capaces de prevenir la declinación progresiva de la función renal. Ser ́necesario efectuar estudios para corroborar estos resultados en el hombre.

要約

　アンジオテンシン変換酵素（ACE）阻害薬は，腎実質性疾患患者における有効な降圧薬である。しかし，腎機能障害患者に ACE 阻害薬を投与する場合には注意が必要で，用量を調整しなければならない。

　適切な血圧のコントロールの維持には低用量で十分であり，とくに患者が Na 制限食をとっている場合にそうである。有効腎血漿流量（ERPF）は，ACE 阻害薬で治療している腎実質性疾患患者では一般的に上昇し，糸球体濾過値（GFR）に及ぼす影響はさまざまである。GFR の上昇および低下の両方が報告されているが，低 Na 食の患者では低下することが多いようである。この点は，正常腎機能患者での ACE 阻害薬治療の場合と対照的である。

　腎実質性疾患患者では，ネフローゼ症候群をきたすほどのタンパク尿がしばしばみられる。これらの患者でのタンパク尿軽減に関する ACE 阻害薬の効果はよく報告されており，とくに低 Na 食患者では明らかである。この抗タンパク尿効果は，糸球体内毛細管圧の低下に関連しているようである。

　動物実験では，従来の降圧薬とは異なり，ACE 阻害薬は腎機能の進行性の低下を予防できることが示唆されている。このような所見をヒトにおいて実証するためには，さらに研究が必要である。

Cardiac and Renal Failure: An Expanding Role for ACE Inhibitors, edited by C. T. Dollery and L. M. Sherwood, Hanley & Belfus, Inc., Philadelphia.

Potential Renal Protective Effect of ACE Inhibitors in Early and Overt Diabetic Nephropathy as Compared with Other Anti-Hypertensive Agents

Carl Erik Mogensen, Margrethe Mau Pedersen, Jens Sandahl Christiansen, Cramer K. Christensen, Klavs Würgler Hansen, Anita Schmitz, and Leif Thuesen

INTRODUCTION TO DIABETIC NEPHROPATHY

In cross-sectional evaluations of the frequency of nephropathy in a diabetic outpatient clinic, it is likely that the prevalence of diabetic renal disease will not be very high, and, therefore, it could be argued that diabetic nephropathy is not a very important problem in the care of diabetic patients. This, however, would be a serious misunderstanding of the situation, because the reliable parameter is the cumulative incidence of diabetic nephropathy as evaluated in long-term studies with complete follow-up.[1-5] Using this concept, studies from two well-established diabetes clinics, namely the Joslin Clinic in Boston and the Steno Memorial Hospital in Copenhagen (Table I), revealed similar and indeed very high incidences of nephropathy in insulin-dependent diabetes (IDDM) patients. It appears that the 40-year cumulative incidence of nephropathy, as evidenced by proteinuria, is 45–50% when studying IDDM patients whose diabetes was diagnosed around 1940. This very high cumulative incidence is not surprising considering the number of diabetic patients being accepted in renal supportive programs throughout the world.[6] Diabetic nephropathy is now the main cause of end-stage renal failure in many renal clinics, especially in the U.S. but also in parts of Europe, in

287

TABLE I. *Twenty- and forty-year cumulative incidence of nephropathy in IDDM-patients*

Institution	Year of Diagnosis of Diabetes	20-Year Follow-up (%)	40-Year Follow-up (%)
Boston	1939	≈30	≈46
Joslin Clinic	1949	≈18	—
	1959	≈16	—
Copenhagen	1933–1942	≈34	≈47
Steno Hospital	1943–1952	≈24	—
	1953–1962	≈20	—

particular Finland where the prevalence of IDDM is high—probably the highest in the world—and hence the number of patients with end-stage complications is high also.[6]

There is some indication that the cumulative incidence is declining[4] as documented from the 20-year cumulative incidence figures shown in Table I. One out of three insulin-dependent diabetic patients, however, is still likely to develop diabetic nephropathy; at least this would be the situation without any intensified intervention programs.

Clearly end-stage renal failure in diabetes is treatable either by chronic dialysis or renal transplantation, but transplantation is a difficult and dialysis an extremely expensive form of treatment associated with many complications and generally a poorer outcome than in patients with non-diabetic nephropathy at a comparable age.[6] It is important, therefore, to recognize early abnormalities predictive of disease or even involved in the pathogenesis of diabetic renal lesions, with the view to early and effective intervention. Detection of such early abnormalities is now well-established and used in early diagnosis and intervention programs in some centers.[7,8]

The purpose of this paper is to describe briefly early changes in renal function in diabetes, abnormalities that are predictive of late nephropathy, and to evaluate intervention with anti-hypertensive treatment, in particular ACE inhibitors, and compare these with other blood pressure lowering agents or other forms of intervention. It has been clearly established that blood pressure elevation is a very early feature in the development of nephropathy[9-12] and, therefore, very early antihypertensive treatment may be of great clinical importance. In advanced diabetic nephropathy[13,14] antihypertensive treatment is a well-established way of postponing uremia, but it is still not clear exactly when to begin treatment and which agents are most effective and associated with fewest side-effects. Also, the target level for blood pressure is not precisely defined, although some recommendations have already been proposed.[7,15]

PROGRESSION IN NEPHROPATHY AND BLOOD PRESSURE LEVEL ELEVATION IN NON-DIABETIC AND DIABETIC RENAL DISEASES

It seems to be an important clinical observation that reduced kidney function is associated with elevation of blood pressure in most types of nephropathies, including diabetic nephropathy (Figure 1), especially glomerular and small artery diseases, rather than interstitial diseases of the kidney.[16-18] In incipient diabetic nephropathy, progression in microalbuminuria is more rapid in patients with relatively high blood pressure[11] (Figure 2).

It is generally believed that treatment of elevated blood pressure will have a beneficial long-term effect on the rate of deterioration of renal function in all or most kinds of renal diseases.[16-20] However, long-term studies have only been carried out in diabetic nephropathy in insulin-dependent patients.[13,14] In non-diabetic renal diseases there are only a few studies and no detailed long-term follow-up using precise kidney function tests, although evidence suggests that antihypertensive treatment is beneficial with respect to reducing rate of decline in GFR.[16,18,20] No long-term data are available in non-insulin-dependent diabetes.

In essential hypertension it has been shown that the albumin excretion rate is related to blood pressure level,[21] and there are also studies that show that the urinary albumin excretion rate can normalize or partially normalize

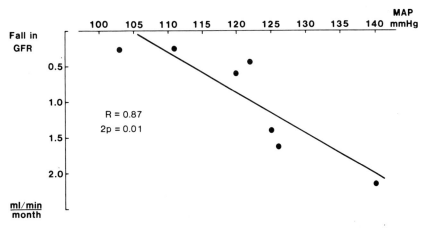

FIG. 1.   Rate of decline in GFR and mean arterial blood pressure (MAP) without antihypertensive treatment in diabetes patients.[72] (·individual patients).

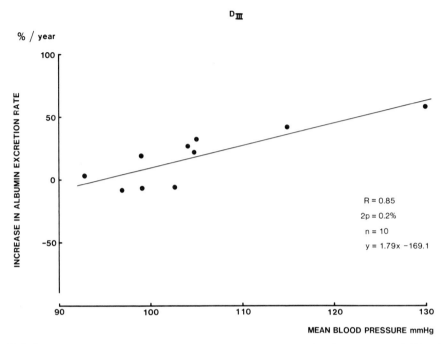

FIG. 2. Rate of increase in urinary albumin excretion rate plotted against mean arterial blood pressure in patients with incipient diabetic nephropathy.[11]

shortly after the start of antihypertensive treatment.[22] Patients with a rather high urinary albumin excretion rate generally respond less well to antihypertensive therapy.[23] Long-term follow-up studies, however, are not yet available.

CLASSIFICATION OF RENAL INVOLVEMENT AND RENAL DISEASE IN IDDM, WITH SPECIAL REFERENCE TO BLOOD PRESSURE LEVEL

Classification of renal involvement in diabetes is clearly important, mainly because of the wide ranges of renal changes seen in diabetic patients.[24] Some patients develop early renal abnormalities (persistent microalbuminuria) after 5 to 10 years of diabetes, whereas others maintain intact renal function and normal blood pressure even after 40 years of metabolic abnormalities.[25] Measurement of urinary albumin excretion rate (UAE) is a key parameter and Table II outlines the different stages of diabetic renal involvement. Usually, blood pressure starts to increase in the phase of incipient diabetic nephropathy. Most authors have found near-normal values in very early stages of microalbuminuria and before the development of microalbuminuria, but when microalbuminuria has been present for a few years blood pressure increases.[26] Typically, blood pressure is 5–10% higher than in normoalbuminuric diabetics, and the rate of increase in blood pressure is around 3–4% per year under conventional insulin treatment, but, of course, without antihypertensive treatment.[27] There is evidence to suggest that blood pressure elevation is secondary to renal changes or to sodium retention,[12] although on the other hand, blood pressure elevation seems to accelerate renal damage thus creating a vicious circle. This is an important observation with respect to therapy, because early antihypertensive treatment can normalize blood pressure in diabetic patients, and thus probably also retard or even prevent early changes in the kidney of diabetic patients (Figure 3).

PATHOGENESIS OF BLOOD PRESSURE ELEVATION IN DIABETES

Sequence of Changes

It has been suggested that a genetic predisposition to hypertension plays an important role in the genesis not only of blood pressure elevation but also nephropathy in IDDM patients (Table III).[28,29] Two recently published studies were in agreement, and the authors were also able to document an increase in sodium lithium counter-transport in the erythrocytes of diabetic patients developing renal disease.[29,30] Therefore pre-disposition to blood pressure elevation could be an important genetic link to development of overt renal disease. It was also reported that poor metabolic control increased several-fold the risk for subsequent development of nephropathy.[29]

New studies from Copenhagen, however, do not confirm these results (T. Deckert, personal communication). The Copenhagen study was very well-planned; the number of patients necessary in order to document differences was determined before the start of study. This included differences in blood pressure elevation in parents of diabetic patients with and without nephropathy, but also the level of sodium lithium counter transport activity in erythrocytes. The reason for the discrepancies is not clear, but no trend at all was observed in the Copenhagen study. It is also clear from another study from Copenhagen that blood pressure was not elevated in patients 10 years prior to nephropathy as could be expected if the "genetic hypertension hypothesis" were correct.[31] It could be suggested that the anxiety of having a diabetic child with nephropathy would tend to cause blood pressure elevation in the parents, especially when blood pressure is measured in a different clinic from the one they usually attended. It seems reasonable to conclude that a genetic predisposition is not important, at least not in all geographical areas.

What is evident, however, is that early detection of blood pressure elevation

TABLE II. *Microalbuminuria and diabetic nephropathy (DN): stages in diabetic renal involvement and nephropathy in IDDM patients*

Stage	Designation	Main Characteristics	Main Structural Changes	GFR (ml/min)	Albumin Excretion (UAE)	Blood Pressure	Suggested Main Pathophysiological Change
Stage I	Hyperfunction and hypertrophy stage*	Large kidneys and glomerular hyperfiltration*	Glomerular hypertrophy; normal basement membrane (BM) and mesangium	≈150	May be increased	N	Glomerular volume expansion and increased intraglomerular pressure
Stage 2 — In short-term diabetes	"Silent" stage with normal UAE but structural lesion present	Normal UAE	Increasing basal membrane thickness and mesangial expansion	With or without hyperfiltration**	N (often increased in stress situations)	N	Changes as indicated above but quite variable (dependent on metabolic control); in addition increased accumulation of BM and BM-like material
In long-term diabetes			No or few studies	With or without hyperfiltration**	N (often in stress situations)	N or slightly elevated	
Stage 3 — Early	Incipient DN (or "at-risk patient'')	Persistently elevated UAE (20–200 μg/min)	Severity probably in between stage 2 and 4	≈160	20–70 μg/min	Often elevated by 5–10% compared with healthy subjects and increasing by 3.5% per year. Blood pressure elevated during exercise	Glomerular closure probably starts in this stage. In some patients high intraglomerular pressure
Late				≈130	70–200 μg/min		

Stage	Clinical	Morphology	GFR (ml/min)	UAE	Blood pressure	Glomerular changes
Stage 4		Further increase in basement membrane thickening and mesangial expansion			Blood pressure increases by ≈ 7% per year.	
Early	Clinical proteinuria or UAE >200 µg/min	Increasing rate of glomerular closure	≈ 130–70	>200 µg/min	Often frank hypertension	High rate of glomerular closure and advancing mesangial expansion
Intermediate —— Overt DN		Hypertrophy of remaining glomeruli	≈ 70–30		Hypertension almost ubiquitous	
Advanced			≈ 30–10		Hypertension almost ubiquitous	Hyperfiltration in remaining glomeruli (deleterious)
Stage 5 / Uremia	End-stage renal failure	Generalized glomerular closure	0–10	Decreasing (due to nephron closure)	High, but often controlled by dialysis treatment	Advanced lesions and glomerular closure

*Changes present probably in all stages when control imperfect.
**Possible marker of future nephropathy (if GFR> 150 ml/min).
GFR = glomerular filtration rate; N = normal; UAE = urinary albumin excretion; DN = diabetic nephropathy.

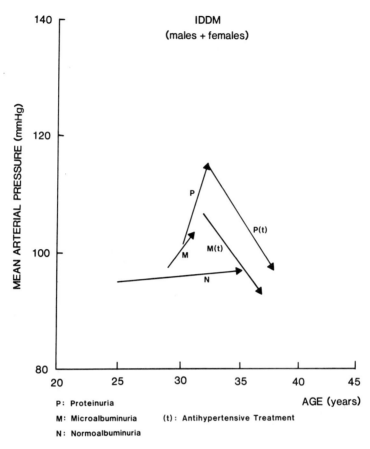

FIG. 3. Increase in blood pressure in male and female IDDM patients with normoalbuminuria, microalbuminuria and clinical proteinuria and effect of antihypertensive treatment. Data compiled from the literature.[9,14,27,36]

is important, although the exact level at which intervention is needed is less clear. It may well be that increase in microalbuminuria occurs along with increase in blood pressure, and the diagnosis of microalbuminuria will thus form a firmer indication for antihypertensive treatment in diabetic patients, especially if a treatment modality without side-effects can be implemented. Another important issue is the technique of blood pressure measurement. Obviously blood pressure measured in an overcrowded diabetic clinic may give spuriously high levels. It is, therefore, of great importance in the future to obtain more reliable blood pressure measurements, e.g., by 24-hour blood-pressure monitoring at home, probably on several occasions. This is very similar to the situation regarding the evaluation of metabolic control. One or two blood-glucose measurements are obviously not sufficient; rather one

TABLE III.   *Abnormalities in incipient diabetic nephropathy and blood pressure elevation*

A. Altered renal hemodynamics (high GFR, high filtration fraction FF). Altered renal structure.
B. Sodium retention.
C. Increased cardiac output.

Genetic Defect

Predisposition to arterial hypertension?

should rely on multiple measurements or exact levels of glycosylated hemoglobin as measured by a reliable technique, and probably on many occasions, using a mean value.[26] Thus, it is likely that in the future 24-hour blood pressure recordings as well as glycosylated hemoglobin values along with microalbuminuria will form the basis for early antihypertensive treatment (and optimized metabolic control) in diabetic patients, followed longitudinally in the diabetic clinic.

It is likely that renal changes play an important role in blood pressure elevation in diabetic patients, but the exact mechanism is not clarified (Table III). Blood pressure certainly rises in diabetic patients long before a substantial decrease in renal function is established, although structural lesions are already likely to be present. There is strong evidence that sodium retention plays a role not only in NIDDM patients[32] but also in IDDM patients.[12] Indeed there is a clear correlation between blood pressure level and sodium retention in patients with incipient diabetic nephropathy.[12]

Increased cardiac output has been documented by ultrasound technique in patients with early microalbuminuria[33] (Figure 4). A similar pattern is seen also when comparing urinary albumin excretion (UAE) with the level of GFR[9] (Figure 5). This increase in UAE is also associated with blood pressure increase, but the exact role of these early cardiac changes in the pathogenesis of blood pressure elevation is not clear. Later, with further increase in albumin excretion and declining renal function, cardiac output decreases as a result of more advanced myocardial damage. Based on the abnormalities mentioned, a combination of an ACE inhibitor, diuretics, and a cardioselective beta-blocker may be an appropriate therapeutic approach (Table IV), as will be discussed later.

ROLE OF BLOOD PRESSURE ELEVATION AND SEQUENCE OF CHANGES, ESPECIALLY THE TRANSITION PHASE FROM NORMO- TO MICROALBUMINURIA

The transition from normoalbuminuria to microalbuminuria is a very important phase in the course of IDDM. Longitudinal studies have now revealed that patients developing microalbuminuria before the microalbuminuric level is reached already show albumin excretion in the upper normal range.[26]

HEART FUNCTION AND KIDNEY FUNCTION IN IDDM

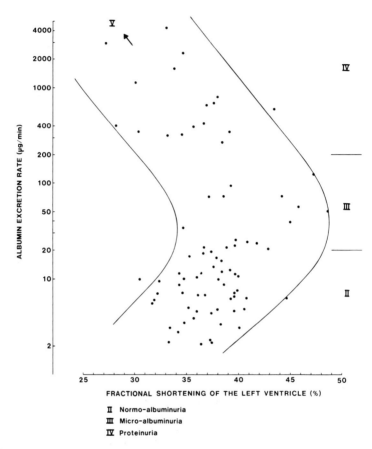

FIG. 4. Fractional shortening of the left ventricle plotted against urinary albumin excretion rate in patients with IDDM. II: normoalbuminuria; III: microalbuminuria; IV: clinical proteinuria.

Therefore, such patients with "high normal" UAE should be followed more carefully. It has also been shown that patients developing microalbuminuria have a higher level of glycated hemoglobin. Indeed the study by Mathiesen *et al.*[26] showed that glycated hemoglobin in these patients is always above 7.5–8%, as evaluated by multiple measurements. If glycated hemoglobin is below 8% the risk of developing microalbuminuria is negligible. On the other hand there are patients whose normal albumin excretion rate remains normal in spite of a rather high value of glycated hemoglobin. The cause of this "protection" is not clear, but low-normal blood pressure may play a role.[25]

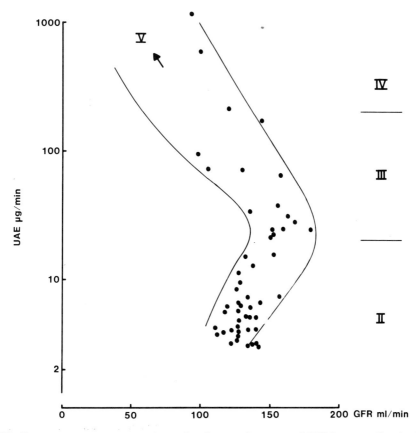

FIG. 5. Relationship between urinary albumin excretion rate and GFR in normoalbuminuric, microalbuminuric and proteinuric patients. II: normoalbuminuria; III: microalbuminuria; IV: overt diabetic nephropathy.

Blood pressure, on the other hand, appears to be quite normal before the development of microalbuminuria but rises a few years after microalbuminuria is clearly established. The data provided by Mathiesen et al.[26] were based on a few measurements of blood pressure in the clinic and not on 24-hour blood pressure recordings. Importantly this study suggests that the early phase of microalbuminuria is more closely related to poor metabolic control than to blood pressure elevation. Soon after development of microalbuminuria, however, an elevation in blood pressure, albeit small, is clearly established.[26,27] The blood pressure rise is only of the order of 2–5% per year, but the *increase* in blood pressure is probably more important than the actual level of pressure. Longitudinal follow-up of blood pressure measurement at regular intervals therefore seems very important.

TABLE IV. *Abnormalities in incipient diabetic nephropathy and modality of antihypertensive treatment*

Abnormality	Potential Treatment
A. Altered renal hemodynamics (high GFR, high FF)	ACE inhibition*
B. Sodium retention	Diuretics*
C. Increased cardiac output	Cardioselective betablockers*

*A combination of these agents seems in many cases rational.

ANTIHYPERTENSIVE TREATMENT IN DIABETES, WITH SPECIAL REFERENCE TO THE CONCEPT OF ACE INHIBITION

The effect of antihypertensive treatment in diabetic nephropathy will be reviewed in the remaining part of this chapter. Much new knowledge has been gained regarding the mechanism of progression of renal disease in general[34] and indeed there are arguments to suggest that ACE inhibition may be important in the treatment in diabetic nephropathy[35] as well as in other renal diseases. Previous intervention studies were performed with beta-blockers and diuretics, because these were the prevailing antihypertensive agents when the studies were initiated.[13,14,36,37]

As discussed previously, marked hyperfiltration in insulin-dependent diabetes is associated with the development of diabetic nephropathy.[38] The pathogenesis of hyperfiltration is not fully understood, but an increase in the hydraulic transcapillary intraglomerular pressure may be an important factor along with increased renal size.[39,40] In experimental diabetes, hyperfiltration has been shown to result from glomerular arteriolar vasodilatation and glomerular hypertension.[41] Recently Zatz and coworkers have reported that ACE inhibition by means of enalapril administered to streptozotocin diabetic rats normalizes the glomerular transcapillary hydrostatic pressure difference as well as the albumin excretion rate.[42] In this study, however, a rather large reduction in mean arterial systemic blood pressure was seen, and this effect could thus account for much of the decline in the transcapillary hydrostatic pressure difference.

Also, inhibition of the ACE system in rats having high glomerular hydrostatic pressure because of partial renal ablation has been shown to lower renal vascular resistance and bring the intraglomerular pressure difference back towards normal levels.[43,44]

Thus, based upon observations in experimental diabetes and other conditions with high intraglomerular pressure, together with theoretical considerations concerning the initiation and progression of the glomerular lesions, the concept of ACE inhibition in diabetes seems to be an attractive avenue for further experimental and clinical studies.

Important studies have appeared regarding the effect of ACE inhibition in normal subjects,[45-48] and also in essential hypertension and various renal diseases associated with hypertension and proteinuria.[49-52] Interesting results have also been published regarding the efficacy of ACE inhibition in hypertensive diabetic patients.[53-57] With the perspective of reducing high glomerular pressure, studies have also been carried out in young diabetic patients with hyperfiltration but a normal or near normal albumin excretion rate.[58-60] More attention has been focused on diabetic patients with microalbuminuria or incipient diabetic nephropathy.[61-63] Important studies have also appeared on the possible effect of ACE inhibition in overt diabetic nephropathy.[64-69] Some of these studies will be reviewed below in conjunction with data from our laboratory.

ACUTE ACE INHIBITION IN NORMAL SUBJECTS

In normotensive normal subjects acute ACE inhibition has been consistently shown to induce a rise in renal plasma flow and a decrease in renal vascular resistance. Hollenberg and coworkers have reported decreased renal resistance after oral administration of captopril.[45,46] Enalapril has been shown to have a similar and significant action on renal hemodynamics — after both oral and intravenous administration in normal subjects.[47] A significant increase in fractional sodium excretion and in urate and phosphate excretion seems to be the uniform finding in several studies.[45-48]

We administered 10 mg of enalaprilat in 10 ml isotonic sodium chloride (MSD, West Point PA., USA) to eight normal subjects and measured kidney function before and during this intravenous injection.[58] GFR was unchanged, but there was an increase in renal plasma flow from 592 to 642 ml/min and consequently a significant decline in filtration fraction from 0.210 to 0.188 (2 $p < 0.02$). Also the total renal resistance declined from 0.156 mm Hg ml/min to 0.135 mm Hg/ml/min (2 $p < 0.05$). The significant enhancing effect on natriuresis was confirmed showing an increase in fractional excretion of sodium from 1.00 to 1.50% (2 $p < 0.01$). Diuresis was unchanged and there were no significant changes in the beta-2-microglobulin excretion rate, indicating that the acute renal effect of ACE inhibition is primarily glomerular.[58]

Figure 6 compares the effect on blood pressure and renal function of enalapril and felodipine[70] in normal subjects. Probably more generalized vasodilatation is seen with the calcium-antagonist as evidenced by the marked increase in heart rate and a considerable fall in diastolic pressure. The effect on the kidney is very similar (Table V).

POSSIBLE INTERVENTION IN NORMOALBUMINURIC DIABETIC SUBJECTS: ACUTE AND LONG-TERM STUDIES

The acute effect of ACE inhibition in uncomplicated normotensive, normoalbuminuric insulin-dependent diabetics has been investigated recently.[58]

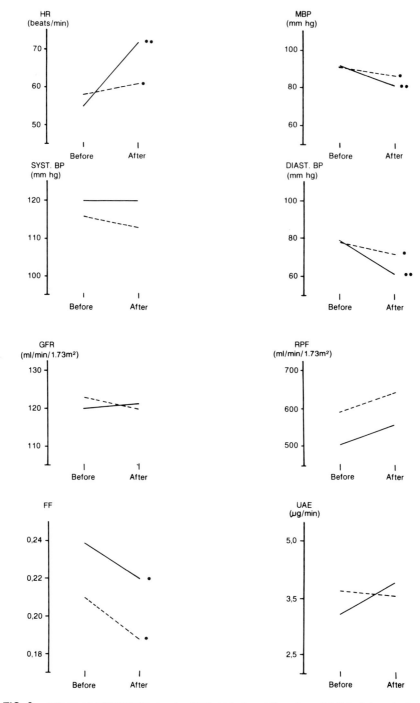

FIG. 6. Effects of ACE inhibitor (enalapril 10 mg i.v.) and Ca antagonist (felodipine, single oral dose of 0.15 mg/kg) in normal subjects. -----Enalapril, ——— felodipine. Significant differences from basal values are indicated as xx = p < 0.01 and * = p < 0.05.[58,70]

TABLE V.   *Acute effects of ACE inhibition and calcium antagonist administration in normal individuals*

Drug	Heart Rate	Mean BP	Syst. BP	Diast. BP	RPF	GFR	FF	TRR	UAE
Enalapril	↑5%	↓5%	—	↓8%	↑8%	—	↓10%	↓13%	—
Felodipine	↑31%	↓12%	—	↓23%	—	—	↓8%	↓21%	—

— No change.
↑↓ Significant change (2p < 5%);
%Indicate degree of change in percent.

Glomerular filtration rate, renal plasma flow, and urinary albumin excretion were measured before and after the intravenous injection of 10 mg of enalaprilat in ten diabetics (mean age 27 years) with duration of diabetes between 1 and 15 years. None of the patients had clinical evidence of diabetic microangiopathy. An acute reduction in systolic (116 to 114 mm Hg) as well as diastolic (77–69 mm Hg) blood pressure (2 p < 0.01) was seen following the administration of enalapril (Table VI). This reduction in blood pressure was accompanied by a small but significant rise in heart rate from 56 to 58 beats/min. A small but significant increase in GFR from 127 to 132 ml/min (2 p < 0.02) (Figure 7a) and a considerable rise in renal plasma flow from 499 to 572 ml/min (2 p < 0.01) (Figure 7b) were seen. Consequently, a highly significant fall in filtration fraction from 0.259 to 0.237 was found after intravenous enalaprilat administration (Figure 7c). The total renal resistance was also markedly reduced from 0.187 mm Hg/ml/min to 0.154 mm Hg/ml/min (Table VI).

It can thus be concluded that the acute renal hemodynamic response to ACE inhibition is identical in normal subjects and in relatively short-term uncomplicated normotensive insulin-dependent diabetics.

There are very few data on the effect of more longstanding ACE inhibition in normoalbuminuric diabetic subjects. Voja and coworkers reported in abstract form that 2 weeks of captopril treatment (50 mg/daily) did not change renal plasma flow or GFR in six diabetics as compared with six patients receiving placebo.[60]

We conducted a 3-month prospective trial on the effect of enalapril administration (30 mg/day) to 10 normoalbuminuric diabetic patients. The study was designed as a double-blind, randomized cross-over study using enalapril and placebo, each for 3 months[58] (Table VI). After 3 months of enalapril treatment, filtration fraction decreased from 0.253 to 0.235 (2 p < 0.05) and urinary albumin excretion rate declined significantly from 5.6 to 4.3 μg/min. Interestingly, the fractional albumin clearance was also significantly reduced from 1.22 to 0.92 · 10^{-6} (2 p < 0.02).[58] During long-term ACE inhibition in these diabetics, no statistically significant rise in renal plasma flow or fall in total renal resistance was seen. Furthermore there was no lowering effect on blood pressure. Thus, one could speculate on the occurrence of adaptive

TABLE VI. Acute and chronic effects of β-blockade and ACE inhibition in normoalbuminuric IDDM patients

Acute Effects

Drug	Heart Rate	Mean BP	Syst. BP	Diast. BP	RPF	GFR	FF	TRR	UAE	Exerc. UAE	Exerc. BP
Metoprolol	—	—	↓4%	—	(↓)6%	—	—	—	—	—	↓13%
Enalapril	↑4%	↓7%	↓3%	↓10%	↑15%	↑4%	↓8%	↓18%	—	?	?

Chronic Effect (3 months)

Drug	Heart Rate	Mean BP	Syst. BP	Diast. BP	RPF	GFR	FF	TRR	UAE	Exerc. UAE	Exerc. BP	Fall Rate of GFR
Metoprolol	not studied											
Enalapril	—	—	—	—	—	—	↓7%	—	↓21%	?	?	—

— no change
↑↓ significant change (2p < 5%)
(↑)(↓) borderline chance (2p = 5–10%)
% indicate degree of change in per cent

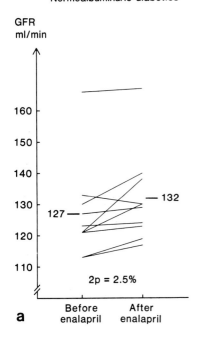

Normoalbuminuric diabetics

GFR
ml/min

160
150
140
130   — 132
127 —
120
110

2p = 2.5%

Before   After
enalapril   enalapril

a

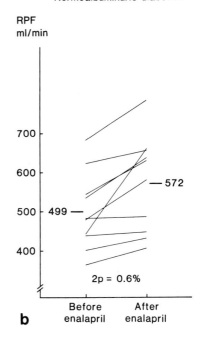

Normoalbuminuric diabetics

RPF
ml/min

700
600   — 572
499 —
500
400

2p = 0.6%

Before   After
enalapril   enalapril

b

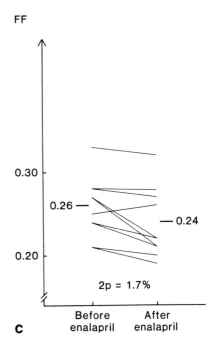

Normoalbuminuric diabetics

FF

0.30
0.26 —   — 0.24
0.20

2p = 1.7%

Before   After
enalapril   enalapril

c

FIG. 7 a, b, c. Acute effect of enalapril in normoalbuminuric diabetics (GFR, RPF, FF).

303

changes secondary to long-term inhibition of the renin angiotensin system in these patients on a free sodium intake. The important thing demonstrated in this study, in our opinion, is the reduction in filtration fraction and fractional albumin excretion rate. These changes cannot be explained by changes in glycemic control, since blood glucose and HbA_{1c} were unchanged. The possibility that significant alterations in the diet might change renal hemodynamics also seems to be ruled out by the randomized cross-over design.

We believe that the decline in fractional albumin excretion and filtration fraction seen in this long-term study suggests that ACE inhibition lowers glomerular capillary hydrostatic pressure. This is probably due to a reduced resistance of the efferent arteriole. Similar changes could perhaps be induced by a fall in the ultrafiltration coefficient, but experimental studies give reason to believe that ACE inhibition will not reduce the ultrafiltration coefficient.[71]

It is also noteworthy that the general antihypertensive effect would not explain the changes in renal function, as no significant impact on blood pressure was seen during 3 months of ACE inhibition. This seems to be an important observation, since the initial findings in experimental diabetic rats demonstrating a lowering of the intraglomerular capillary pressure following ACE inhibition was seen in animals where a highly significant reduction took place.[42]

From the present results it can be concluded that short-term use of ACE inhibitors in normotensive normoalbuminuric insulin-dependent diabetics provides an interesting opportunity to test the hypothesis that long-term reduction in intracapillary glomerular pressure might be beneficial to patients through a possible protection against the development of clinical renal disease. At the present time, however, there is no clinical indication to treat these patients.

INTERVENTION IN INCIPIENT OR EARLY
DIABETIC NEPHROPATHY

Table VII reviews both the acute, short-term (6-week), and long-term (6-month) effect of different antihypertensive programs, namely cardioselective beta-blockers and ACE inhibitors and calcium antagonists. In a recent study from our laboratory, we compared the acute effect on renal function and blood pressure of metoprolol 10 mg i.v., enalapril 10 mg i.v., and enalapril + metoprolol, 5 mg of each i.v. There appears to be important differences in the acute response of these two different classes of antihypertensive agents.

Both drugs, singly and in combination, reduce blood pressure almost equally, although enalapril may be more effective in the acute reduction of diastolic blood pressure in the above doses. When given in combination, the same effect on blood pressure is seen, a reduction of about 5%, which is more than after placebo. Not surprisingly, heart rate is suppressed after cardioselective beta blockade. The response with respect to the kidney is clearly different

(Figure 8). Metoprolol reduces renal plasma flow and increases renal resistance, but filtration fraction is also increased. On the other hand enalapril, as might be expected, increases renal plasma flow and reduces filtration fraction and renal resistance. Interestingly, there is no acute effect on urinary albumin excretion rate by any of the drugs.

By using a combination of an ACE inhibitor and a cardioselective beta-blocker, the opposing effects on renal function seem to outweigh each other. It would be of interest to know what the effect is on transglomerular pressure. It may still be reduced using the combined injection, but this parameter is not measurable in humans.

When an ACE inhibitor is added acutely to conventional treatment, approximately the same picture as combined injection is seen as with the combined injection of enalapril and a beta-blocker; however, urinary albumin excretion rate is slightly reduced and so is total renal resistance.

The effect at 6 months is also shown in Table VII. In the table the data by M. Marre *et al.* on enalapril treatment are presented and compared with our own results. A similar technique is used with respect to renal function measurement, namely constant infusion technique with labelled iothalamate and hippuran. In the study by Marre,[61] placebo administration is also included. Interestingly, approximately the same reduction in blood pressure is seen with the two agents, metoprolol and enalapril. Giving enalapril to metoprolol-treated patients causes only a small reduction in systolic pressure and no effect on diastolic blood pressure. On long-term metoprolol treatment, no effect on GFR and renal plasma flow is noted, but an increase is seen using enalapril (Figure 9). With both drugs a fall in urinary albumin excretion rate is seen. Importantly, during placebo administration a considerable increase was observed.[61] This increase is higher than usually observed in the spontaneous course of diabetic patients with incipient diabetic nephropathy.[11,27]

After a 6-month period of treatment with metoprolol, exercise-induced increase in blood pressure is reduced, but no effect on albumin excretion rate was noted. In a more long-term study using metoprolol over 6 years,[36] a continuous reduction in urinary albumin excretion rate was seen and exercise-induced microalbuminuria was ameliorated after a few years of treatment.[37] In this study patients were used as their own controls, with a mean 2.5 year observation period without treatment before administration of beta-blockers.[36]

When enalapril is added to metoprolol and diuretics, we showed in an open study that GFR was reduced by 8%. This reduction in GFR, seen after 3 months with no further reduction after 6 months, is probably an indication of reduction of glomerular hyperfiltration, an effect that is likely to be beneficial in the long term. Albumin excretion rate was reduced by 56% on this combination therapy. No notable side-effects were seen. An open design was employed because of the number of drugs used, the known spontaneous course, and the objective measurements.

Table VII also included data from a short-term study over 6 weeks com-

TABLE VII. *Acute and chronic effects of β-blockade, ACE inhibition, calcium antagonism and combination therapy in IDDM patients with incipent diabetic nephropathy or early diabetic nephropathy*

Drug	Acute Effects										
	Heart Rate	Mean BP	Syst. BP	Diast. BP	RPF	GFR	FF	TRR	UAE	Exerc. UAE	Exerc. BP
Metoprolol	↓9%	—	↓3%	—	↓6%	—	↓5%	↑6%	—	—	↓15%
Enalapril	—	(↓)3%	—	↓6%	(↑)6%	—	(↓)6%	↓10%	—	?	?
Metoprolol + Enalapril	—	↓5%	↓5%	↓5%	—	—	—	—	—	?	?
No active substance	—	(↓)2%	↓3%	—	—	—	—	—	—	?	?
Enalapril added to Metoprolol + diuretic	—	↓3%	—	↓4%	—	—	—	↓6%	↓18%	?	?

	Chronic Effect (6 months)											
(Drug regimen needs to be tested)	Heart Rate	Mean BP	Syst. BP	Diast. BP	RPF	GFR	FF	TRR	UAE	Exerc. UAE	Exerc. BP	Decline in GFR
Metoprolol	↓11%	↓7%	—	↓9%	—	—	—	?	↓34%	—	↓13%	?
Enalapril	?	↓10%	↓9%	12%	↑10%	↑8%	—	↓22%	↓70%	?	?	? (Ref 61)
Placebo	?	—	—	—	—	—	—	—	↑126%	?	?	(Ref 61)
Enalapril added to Metoprolol + diuretic	—	—	↓5%	—	—	↓8%	—	?	↓56%	?	?	?
						Short-term Effect (6 weeks)						
						S-crea-tinine						
Captopril	—	↓6%	↓7%	↓5%	?	—	?	?	↓41%	?	?	? (Ref 63)
Nifedipine	—	↓5%	↓5%	↓5%	?	—	?	?	↑42%	?	?	? (Ref 63)
Placebo	—	—	—	—	?	—	?	?	—	?	?	? (Ref 63)

— no change
↑↓ significant change (2p < 5%)
(↑)(↓) borderline chance (2p = 5–10%)
% indicate degree of change in per cent

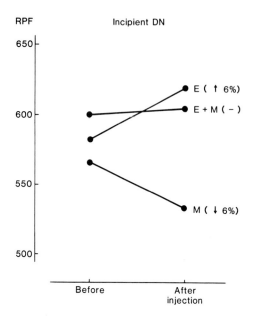

FIG. 8. The acute effect on renal plasma flow (RPF) of metoprolol (M), enalapril (E), and enalapril plus metoprolol (E+M) as a combined injection, in patients with incipient diabetic nephropathy.

paring captopril with the calcium antagonist nifedipine and placebo administration.[63] No change was seen after placebo, but both captopril and nifedipine reduced blood pressure by about 5–7%. GFR was unchanged as evaluated by measurement of serum creatinine. Interestingly, captopril reduced microalbuminuria by 41%, whereas nifedipine increased microalbuminuria by 42%. No change was noted in UAE after placebo.

It can be concluded that during incipient diabetic nephropathy antihypertensive treatment with beta-blockers and ACE inhibitors, either alone or in combination, is able to reduce microalbuminuria considerably (Figure 10). GFR is maintained at the same level or is only slightly changed during such therapy. There is only one long-term study (5–6 years) on a small series of patients indicating that during long-term administration of metoprolol and diuretics renal function is maintained[36] and is accompanied by a continuous reduction of urinary albumin excretion rate of the order of 20% per year. It is important to bear in mind that without intervention an increase could be expected in these patients. In all the studies mentioned glycemic control was evaluated either by multiple measurements of blood glucose or glycosylated hemoglobin, and no change was seen. Dietary intake of proteins was not recorded carefully, but patients were asked to continue their usual dietary habits and it is unlikely that any major change in a dietary protein intake took place.

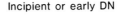

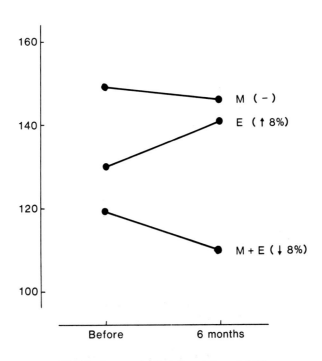

FIG. 9. The effect of antihypertensive treatment (AHT) on GFR in patients with incipient or early diabetic nephropathy. Metoprolol (M) enalapril (E) and metoprolol plus enalapril (M+E) a 6-month study.[36,61]

INTERVENTION IN OVERT DIABETIC NEPHROPATHY

The first study suggesting a beneficial effect on renal function of antihypertensive treatment in diabetic nephropathy was published in 1976, when little attention was being paid to problems related to hypertension in diabetes and its possible relationship to rate of decline in renal function.[72,73] In two studies it was documented that antihypertensive treatment with beta-blockers and diuretics not only reduced albumin excretion[72] but also seemed to reduce the rate of decline of GFR.[73] Long-term studies, where patients were followed for several years, have since been published, confirming the beneficial effect.[13,14] No data are available in NIDDM patients.[74]

Figure 10 summarizes all available results on the reduction in urinary

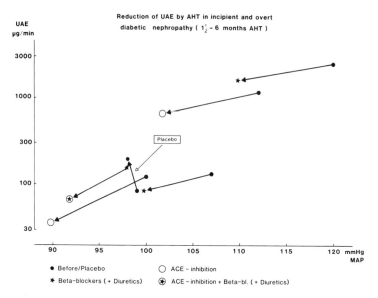

FIG. 10. Reduction in urinary albumin excretion (UAE) rate by antihypertensive treatment (AHT) in incipient and overt diabetic nephropathy: treatment period 1.5 to 6 months. With placebo an increase in urinary albumin excretion rate is seen at 6 months follow-up.[13,36,61,66]

albumin excretion rate in incipient and overt diabetic nephropathy after 1.5 to 6 months of antihypertensive therapy. A similar reduction is seen irrespective of which antihypertensive drug is used, beta-blocker or ACE inhibitor, or these two agents combined with diuretics. A similar drop is also seen when combining ACE inhibitors, beta-blockers and diuretics.

Figure 11 summarizes studies on the effect of blood pressure reduction on the rate of decline in GFR. Related data are also summarized in Table VIII. Although the number of patients studied in these reports is not large, they present statistical evidence that a reduction of blood pressure causes a reduction in rate of decline of GFR. In the first published study, beta-blockers and diuretics were used, sometimes in combination with vasodilators. In this initial study[12] blood pressure was quite high before treatment, and rate of decline of GFR, although reduced considerably, was still quite marked during treatment. By introducing an ACE inhibitor, usually combined with beta-blockers and diuretics, a reduction in both blood pressure and rate of decline of GFR is also seen, as documented in the study by Björk and coworkers.[64,68] Two studies by Parving and coworkers show similar results. The administration of beta-blockers and diuretics reduces blood pressure considerably, as well as rate of decline of GFR.[14] A similar, although not so pronounced, effect is seen with ACE inhibition alone, or combined with diuretics.[75] In this latter study, patients on ACE inhibitors were carefully matched to historical con-

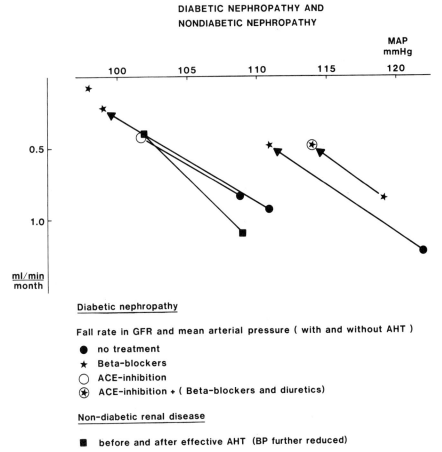

DIABETIC NEPHROPATHY AND
NONDIABETIC NEPHROPATHY

FIG. 11.   Rate of decline in GFR and mean arterial blood pressure with and without antihypertensive treatment (AHT).[13,14,20,36,64,75]

trols. In the only long-term study in incipient diabetic nephropathy,[36] urinary albumin excretion rate was reduced, and rate of decline in GFR was not significantly different from zero (the upper left * in Figure 11). Diabetes-related side-effects are summarized in Table IX.

BLOOD PRESSURE INTERVENTION AS COMPARED WITH OTHER TYPES OF TREATMENT

Table X summarizes and compares the effect of optimal insulin treatment, antihypertensive treatment, with and without ACE inhibition, and low protein diet.

TABLE VIII.   *Rate of decrease in GFR during antihypertensive treatment*

Study	Treatment	BP During Treatment mmHg	Years of Treatment/ Observation	Decrease in GFR ml/min/month
Mogensen[13] (ODN)	β-blockers +diuretics (+vasodilatators)	144/95	6	0.49
Parving et al.[14] (ODN)	"	124/85	6	0.22
Parving et al.[75] (ODN)	ACE inhibitors +diuretics	136/85	2.5	0.40
Christensen & Mogensen[36] (IDN)	β-blockers +diuretics	125/85	5	0.07
Parving et al.[75] (ODN)	Untreated historical controls	137/95, and increasing by 6%/2.5 yr	2.5	0.83

IDN = incipient diabetic nephropathy
ODN = overt diabetic nephropathy

In patients with hyperfiltration alone in association with increased filtration fraction, optimal insulin treatment with insulin pumps reduces hyperfiltration, but only to a minor degree—about 5% after 2 years of intervention—compared with a control group.[76] With ACE inhibition no effect on hyperfiltration was seen, but filtration fraction and UAE (in the normal range) were reduced in accordance with the concept of ACE inhibition.[58] There are no long-term studies on the effect of beta-blockers, but it has been shown that hyperfiltration can be reduced by a moderate protein restriction in the diabetic diet.[77] An interesting observation appeared from the Oslo study. After 4

TABLE IX.   *Diabetes related side-effects by antihypertensive treatment in diabetes*

	Diuretics	Beta-blockers	ACE-inhibition
Glucose intolerance	Yes, NIDDM	No problem	No side-effects
Hypoglycemic unawareness	No	Yes, in IDDM	No side-effects
Unfavorable lipid profits	Yes	Possibly?	No side-effects

TABLE X. Effects of intervention modalities

Test Parameter	Metabolic Intervention Insulin Pump Treatment	Antihypertensive Intervention ACE Inhibition (+diuretics in some case)	β-Blockers +Diuretics	ACE Inhibitors +β-blockers +Diuretics (small doses)	Dietary Intervention Low-protein Diet
Hyperfiltration (and elevated filtration fraction)	GFR rduced by about 5% in long-term studies (Aarhus)	Filtration fraction may be reduced by ACE inhibition (Aarhus)	No studies	No studies	Hyperfiltration reduced (Aarhus)
Borderline elevated UAE	Total normalization in a 4-yr follow-up study (Oslo)	No studies	No studies	No studies	No studies
Persistent microalbuminuria (30–300 mg/24 h)	Stabilization (Gentofte)	Microalbuminuria reduced (Paris)	Long-term regression of microalbuminuria (Aarhus)	Regression in a 6 months study (Aarhus)	Reduced in a small series on a short-term basis (3 weeks) (London)
Proteinuria without high BP, possibly with reduced GFR	No effect seen in a small series (does not rule out an effect) (London)	Studies ongoing	No studies	No studies	Reduction of decline in GFR and reduced proteinuria according to preliminary studies (London)
Proteinuria, high BP, reduced GFR	No effect seen in a small series (does not rule out an effect) (London)	Rate of decline in GFR lower than in historical controls (Hvidöre)	Long-term treatment with cardioselective β-blockers, diuretics and vasodilators reduces decline in GFR considerably (Aarhus/Hvidöre)	In patients conventionally treated, additional ACE-inhibitor may reduce progression (Göteborg)*	Reduction in decline in GFR and reduced proteinuria according to preliminary studies (London)

*The combination not used in all patients.

years of optimal insulin treatment using pumps, a normalization of border-line elevated urinary albumin excretion rate was seen.[78] No studies are available on other forms of intervention in these patients.

In patients with persistent microalbuminuria, a stabilization or reduction of microalbuminuria is observed on optimal insulin treatment.[27] With ACE inhibition and reduction in blood pressure, microalbuminuria is reduced in a 6–12 month study.[61,62] On long-term treatment with beta-blockers and diuretics, microalbuminuria is reduced considerably, and in these patients GFR is maintained at a high and even supranormal level as mentioned above.[36] Regarding low protein diet, a short-term study (3 weeks) from London has documented a reduction in microalbuminuria on a low-protein diet, but so far there are no long-term studies,[79] perhaps because of compliance problems. In patients without raised blood pressure or patients being treated effectively for hypertension, optimal insulin treatment has not been documented to have a beneficial effect on rate of decline in GFR.[80] At present only a small series has been published, and therefore, no definitive answer can be given as yet regarding the role of optimal insulin treatment in patients with overt diabetic nephropathy. It should be mentioned that a correlation has been found between rate of decline in GFR and glycemic control.[81] New studies from the Guy's Hospital in London suggest that the rate of fall of GFR can be reduced by reduction of protein intake.[82,83] Similar studies are in progress elsewhere.

In patients with overt nephropathy (with proteinuria, blood pressure increase, and fall in GFR), the most convincing studies are those using antihypertensive agents as summarized above. Irrespective of modality of treatment, rate of decline in GFR can be reduced considerably, thereby probably postponing end-stage renal failure (Figure 11). Indeed, new follow-up studies at the Steno Memorial Hospital have shown that survival of diabetic patients with proteinuria has markedly improved after the implementation of effective antihypertensive treatment (T. Deckert, personal communication). In the 1960s when no antihypertensive treatment was given, the 10-year survival for patients with proteinuria was very poor, only about 40% of patients survived for this period. Now, after implementation of effective antihypertensive treatment, 10-year survival in these patients is greater than 90–95%. It is unlikely that glycemic control has changed very much, since patients with overt nephropathy are quite often difficult to control from the metabolic point of view. It is presumed, therefore, that antihypertensive treatment is the main cause of this very striking improvement in survival.

Thus, effective antihypertensive treatment programs should be implemented in diabetic patients with proteinuria. It may even be that treatment should be started in the phase of early microalbuminuria, because it is quite likely that patients with early microalbuminuria subsequently go on to develop raised blood pressure as well as an increase in microalbuminuria, and after a few years GFR might start to decline.

RECOMMENDATIONS

Based on pathophysiological knowledge of early renal involvement in diabetes, it is now possible to monitor patients carefully in the diabetes clinic with emphasis on metabolic control as measured by glycosylated hemoglobin, blood pressure measurements, and early renal involvement, as evaluated by measurement of urinary albumin excretion rate.

Antihypertensive treatment is an important element, because many patients with diabetic renal involvement and disease show blood pressure rises. Consequently it is important to select antihypertensive agents with few side-effects. Although important new information will be gained by ongoing trials, it is now possible to propose guidelines for the management of IDDM patients with respect to early treatment of complications.

PROPOSAL FOR PRACTICAL GUIDELINES IN THE MANAGEMENT OF YOUNG IDDM PATIENTS

A treatment policy has to be adapted on the basis of present knowledge, while awaiting the results of the large Diabetes Control and Complications Trial (DCCT) of primary and secondary intervention of diabetic renal and retinal complications[84,85] and the British Microalbuminuria Collaborative Study,[86] both running for 5 years or more. Large multicenter studies on the effect of ACE inhibition in incipient diabetic nephropathy are also in progress.

Based upon recent studies, as summarized in this chapter, the following guidelines with regard to glycemic, antihypertensive, dietary intervention and finally renal supportive treatment may be recommended:

Glycated hemoglobin, apart from multiple blood glucose measurements, is a key parameter for glycemic control and the reference level for HbA_{1c} is clearly important. It has been found that the reference is 5.4 ± 1.0% ($\overline{X}$± 2SD) using both the BIO-RAD HbA_{1c} mini-columns and a method using high-pressure liquid chromatography.[87,88] Thus, the level 7.5% is roughly equal to 4 standard deviations above the mean of the reference value, when reliable methods are used.

Likewise, urinary albumin excretion is the key parameter with respect to early renal involvement, and patients will, therefore, be classified here as proposed in Table II. Patients should be regularly checked for microalbuminuria, e.g., every year or even at every visit to the clinic.[15]

The Normoalbuminuric Patient (<20 μg/min or <30 mg/24h period)

$$HbA_{1c} < 7.5 – 8\%$$

Let the patients continue present treatment. Continuing diabetes education is important and at least yearly measurement of glycated hemoglobin (with reliable methods) and frequent blood-glucose measurements should be performed in monitoring patients. Care should be taken that glycemic control does not deteriorate.

The level of 7.5–8% was chosen because hyperfiltration is rarely seen below this level.[89,90] Also, patients with HbA_{1c} below this level are generally stable without progression in the Steno studies.[26,27] Patients with glucose intolerance rarely show microangiopathy and HbA_{1c} is usually below 7.5% in these patients.[91,92]

$$HbA_{1c} > 7.5-8.0\%$$

Try to obtain better control either by conventional insulin treatment or by multiple daily injections, for instance by the new insulin pen systems, which are easy to handle (in contrast to insulin pumps). In our experience both severe hypoglycemia and ketoacidosis are rarely seen on such a pen program. General diabetes education is always extremely important and should always be conducted along with introduction of all new types of treatment. Otherwise patients may "relax" on the pen program, without achieving better control. Insulin-pump treatment might be considered, but should only be introduced in highly motivated and well-disciplined adult diabetics. Patients are at risk for ketosis, due to pump or catheter failure.

Hypertension or borderline hypertension (BP ≥140/90 mm Hg) is rarely seen in normoalbuminuric patients and should be managed as indicated below.

Patients with Persistent or Increasing Microalbuminuria (20 → 200 μg/min or 30 → 300 mg/24 h by Repeated Measurements)

Glycemic control should be achieved as in the normoalbuminuric patients, but even more aggressively in view of the results of the Steno Study II.[27] This study showed that microalbuminuria could be arrested by good metabolic control ($HbA_{1c} \leq 7.5-8\%$) accompanied by low blood pressure. As indicated above, insulin-pump treatment might be introduced, but only in very selected diabetics. Blood pressure elevation is often found in these patients, and blood pressure should be reduced to less than 140/90. Elevation of diastolic pressure is particularly characteristic in these patients, and slight systolic blood pressure elevation is probably not very important. This means that patients defined as WHO-borderline hypertensive should be treated. A pressure of 130–135/80–85 in young persons is probably appropriate, but it should also be born in mind that blood pressure should not be too low as this may result in renal ischemia and other side effects. Blood pressure and urinary albumin excretion rates should be monitored to document the effect of treatment, short-term and long-term. Initially, a nonpharmacological approach may be attempted. If pharmacological intervention is required, side-effects should be minimized by using low doses of cardioselective betablockers and/or diuretics, usually with potassium supplementation and/or ACE inhibitors as single, dual, or triple therapy. Frequent evaluation of other complications is required, especially in retinopathy. Which antihypertensive agent should be used initially is still under discussion, but the treatment of choice would be the drug or the combination of drugs effective in lowering blood pressure with fewest side-effects. The long-term effect on renal function of different antihypertensive agents seems rather similar (Figures 10 and 11).

The Proteinuric Patients

Elevated blood pressure is a very consistent finding in patients with diabetic nephropathy, and the glycemic and antihypertensive treatment program, as indicated above, should be adopted, although good glycemic control may be very difficult to obtain. Higher dosages of antihypertensive drugs and/or triple therapy are often needed to reduce blood pressure to $\leq 135/85$ mm Hg. Loop diuretics should be used in patients with advanced nephropathy, and ACE inhibitors may be useful. Hypoglycemic unawareness (especially with betablockers) and orthostatic hypotensive discomfort or other side-effects may be a problem, especially in patients with advanced neurological or vascular involvement, and treatment in such patients may be difficult. Again an effective antihypertensive program with the fewest side-effects should be chosen. In most patients antihypertensive treatment will slow progression of the nephropathy, and thus end-stage renal failure will be considerably postponed. Regarding the dietary approach, long-term results are not yet available, but a high protein diet (previously and still often recommended to diabetics) should certainly not be advocated, but a rather low-normal protein diet as recommended by the American Diabetes Association. Such a diet should probably be recommended throughout the course of diabetes (around 0.8 g protein per kilo body weight per 24 h for adults).

As soon as reduced renal function is demonstrated, the patient should be evaluated by a nephrologist, who, in close collaboration with the diabetologist, must plan future strategy concerning symptomatic and antihypertensive treatment, monitoring progression of renal insufficiency and planning renal replacement therapy.

Patients Just Before Start of Renal Replacement Therapy

Control of hypertension and glycemia should proceed. HbA_{1c}, as determined by standard techniques, is of no value at this stage. Fluid retention in patients can generally be controlled by sodium restriction and furosemide. In the uremic stage there is no place for diets with a protein content of less than 40–50 g/day. Commencement of dialysis is advised before serum creatinine reaches a level of 600 to 750 μmol/l. Renal transplantation is recommended earlier, especially in those individuals who have a related donor. In this case transplantation should be performed when the creatinine is around 450 μmol/l, or even sooner or if the patient is symptomatic. A vascular access should be established approximately 6 to 9 months prior to this point. Renal transplantation is the treatment of choice when a living donor is available especially in younger patients.

GUIDELINES FOR BLOOD PRESSURE AND ANTIDIABETIC TREATMENT IN THE OLDER NIDDM-PATIENT

At present, there are no clinical trials on the long-term effect of antihypertensive treatment, optimal metabolic control, and low protein diet in patients with non-insulin-dependent diabetes mellitus (NIDDM), but from a theoretical point of view the same guidelines can be used as in insulin-dependent diabetes mellitus (IDDM) patients with respect to metabolic control. Of course, higher blood pressure values should be accepted in the case of patients above the age of 45, with allowance for increasing blood pressure levels before the start of pharmacological treatment. One may add 5 mm Hg per decade after the age of 45 with regard to the above criteria, so that a patient aged 65 should be treated if the diastolic blood pressure exceeds 100 mm Hg on repeated measurements. However, it must be stressed that there are no longitudinal follow-up studies showing that antihypertensive treatment affects morbidity and mortality, and, therefore, such a treatment modality will be a matter of further debate until studies are available. Mortality in these patients is clearly related to level of UAE,[93,94] but not to blood pressure or level of glycemic control. Guidelines for nondiabetic hypertensives of the same age may be used and, likewise, guidelines for elderly nondiabetics regarding renal supportive therapy may also be used in diabetics.

REFERENCES

1. Knowler WC, Kunzelman CL. Population comparisons of the frequency of diabetic nephropathy. In Mogensen CE, ed. *The Kidney and Hypertension in Diabetes Mellitus.* Boston, Martin Nijhoff Publishing, 1988; 25–32.
2. Krolewski AS, Warram JH, Rand LI, Kahn CR. Epidemiologic approach to the etiology of type I diabetes mellitus and its complications. *N Engl J Med* 1987; 317:1390–1398.
3. Borch-Johnsen K, Kreiner S, Deckert T. Diabetic nephropathy—susceptible to care? A cohort-study of 641 patients with type I (insulin-dependent) diabetes. *Diabetes Res* 1986; 3:397–400.
4. Kofoed-Enevoldsen A, Borch-Johnsen K, Kreiner S, Nerup J, Deckert T. Declining incidence of persistent proteinuria in type I (insulin-dependent) diabetic patients in Denmark. *Diabetes* 1987; 36:205–209.

5. Borch-Johnsen K. Incidence of nephropathy in insulin-dependent diabetes as related to mortality. In Mogensen CE, ed. *The Kidney and Hypertension in Diabetes Mellitus.* Boston, Martinus Nijhoff Publishing, 1988; 33–40.

6. Challah S, Brunner FP, Wing AJ. Evolution of the treatment of patients with diabetic nephropathy by renal replacement therapy in Europe over a decade: Data from the EDTA registry. In Mogensen CE, ed. *The Kidney and Hypertension in Diabetes Mellitus.* Boston, Martinus Nijhoff Publishing, 1988; 365–378.

7. Mogensen CE. Management of diabetic renal involvement and disease. *Lancet* 1988; I:867–870.

8. Mogensen CE. Microalbuminuria as a predictor of clinical diabetic nephropathy. *Kidney Int* 1987; 31:673–689.

9. Mogensen CE, Christensen CK. Predicting diabetic nephropathy in insulin-dependent patients. *N Engl J Med* 1984; 311:89–93.

10. Wiseman M, Viberti G, MacKintosh D, Jarrett RJ, Keen H. Glycaemia, arterial pressure and micro-albuminuria in type 1 (insulin-dependent) diabetes mellitus. *Diabetologia* 1984; 26:401–405.

11. Christensen CK, Mogensen CE. The course of incipient diabetic nephropathy: Studies of albumin excretion and blood pressure. *Diabetic Medicine* 1985; 2:97–102.

12. Feldt-Rasmussen B, Mathiesen ER, Deckert T, Giese J, Christensen NJ, Bent-Hansen L, Nielsen MD. Central role for sodium in the pathogenesis of blood pressure changes independent of angiotensin, aldosterone and catecholamines in type 1 (insulin-dependent) diabetes mellitus. *Diabetologia* 1987; 30:610–617.

13. Mogensen CE. Long-term antihypertensive treatment inhibiting progression of diabetic nephropathy. *Br Med J* 1982; 285:685–688.

14. Parving H-H, Andersen AR, Smidt UM, Hommel E, Mathiesen ER, Svendsen PAA. Effect of antihypertensive treatment on kidney function in diabetic nephropathy. *Br Med J* 1987; 294:1443–1447.

15. Mogensen CE. Diabetic renal involvement and disease in patients with insulin-dependent diabetes. In Alberti KGMM, Krall LP, eds. *The Diabetes Annual/4.* Elsevier Science Publishers, B.V., 1988; 409–448.

16. Blythe WB. Natural history of hypertension in renal parenchymal disease. In *Hypertension and the Kidney: Proceedings of a Symposium.* The National Kidney Foundation, 1985; A50–A56.

17. Hasslacher C, Ritz E, Tschöpe W, Gallasch G, Mann JFE. Hypertension in diabetes mellitus. *Kidney Int* 1988; 34(suppl. 25):S133–S137.

18. Shimamatsu K, Onoyama K, Harada A, Kumagai H, Hirakata H, Miishima C, Inenaga T, Fujimi S, Fujishima M, Omae T. Effect of blood pressure on the progression rate of renal impairment in chronic glomerulonephritis. *J Clin Hypertens* 1985; 3:239–244.

19. Narins RG, Krishna GG. Development and progression of chronic renal disease: can it be prevented or attenuated? *Am J Cardiol* 1987; 60:531–561.

20. Alvestrand A, Gutierrez A, Bucht H, Bergström J. Reduction in blood pressure retards progression of chronic renal failure in man. *Nephrol Dial Transplant* 1988; 3:624–631.

21. Christensen CK, Krusel LR, Mogensen CE. Increased blood pressure in diabetes: essential hypertension or diabetic nephropathy? *Scand J Clin Lab Invest* 1987; 47:363–370.

22. Christensen CK. Rapidly reversible albumin and β-2-microglobulin hyperexcretion in recent severe essential hypertension. *J Hypertens* 1983; 1:45–51.

23. Pedersen EB, Mogensen CE. Effect of antihypertensive treatment on urinary albumin excretion, glomerular filtration rate, and renal plasma flow in patients with essential hypertension. *Scand J Clin Lab Invest* 1976; 36:231–237.

24. Mogensen CE. Definition of diabetic renal disease in insulin-dependent diabetes mellitus based on renal function. Mogensen CE, ed. *The Kidney and Hypertension in Diabetes Mellitus.* Boston, Martinus Nijhoff Publishing, 1988; 7–16.

25. Borch-Johnsen K, Nissen H, Nerup J. Blood pressure after forty years of insulin-dependent diabetes. *Diabetic Nephropathy* 1985; 4:11–12.

26. Mathiesen ER, Ronn B, Jensen T, Storm B, Deckert T. Microalbuminuria precedes elevation in blood pressure in diabetic nephropathy. *Diabetologia* 1988; 31:519A.

27. Feldt-Rasmussen B, Mathiesen E, Deckert T. Effect of two years of strict metabolic control on the progression of incipient nephropathy in insulin-dependent diabetes. *Lancet* 1986; I:1300–1304.

28. Viberti GC, Keen H, Wiseman MJ. Raised arterial pressure in parents of proteinuric insulin dependent diabetics. *Br Med J* 1987; **295**:515–517.
29. Krolewski AS, Canessa M, Warram JH, Laffel LMB, Christlieb AR, Knowler WC, Rand LI. Predisposition to hypertension and susceptibility to renal disease in insulin-dependent diabetes mellitus. *N Engl J Med* 1988; **318**:140–145.
30. Mangili R, Bending JJ, Scott G, Li LK, Gupta A, Viberti GC. Increased sodium-lithium countertransport activity in red cells of patients with insulin-dependent diabetes and nephropathy. *N Engl J Med* 1988; **318**:146–150.
31. Jensen T, Borch-Johnsen K, Deckert T. Changes in blood pressure and renal function in patients with type I (insulin-dependent) diabetes mellitus prior to clinical diabetic nephropathy. *Diabetes Res* 1987; **4**:159–162.
32. Weidmann P, Beretta-Piccoli C, Trost BN. Pressor factors and responsiveness in hypertension accompanying diabetes mellitus. *Hypertension* 1985; **7**:II-33–II-42.
33. Thuesen L, Christiansen JS, Mogensen CE, Henningsen. Cardiac hyperfunction in insulin dependent diabetic patients developing microvascular complications. *Diabetes* 1988; **37**:851–856.
34. Klahr S, Schreiner G, Ichikawa I. The progression of renal disease. *N Engl J Med* 1988; **318**:1657–1666.
35. Narins RG, Kirshna GG. Diabetic nephropathy. The basis for dietary and converting enzyme inhibitor therapy. *Am J Hypertension* 1988; **1**:215–220.
36. Christensen CK, Mogensen CE. Antihypertensive treatment: long-term reversal of progression of albuminuria in incipient diabetic nephropathy. A longitudinal study of renal function. *J Diabetic Complications* 1987; **1**:45–52.
37. Christensen CK, Mogensen CE. Acute and long-term effect of antihypertensive treatment on exercise-induced albuminuria in incipient diabetic nephropathy. *Scand J Clin Lab Invest* 1986; **46**:553–559.
38. Mogensen CE. Early glomerular hyperfiltration in insulin-dependent diabetics and late nephropathy. *Scand J Clin Lab Invest* 1986; **46**:201–206.
39. Hostetter TH, Rennke HG, Brenner BM. The case for intrarenal hypertension in the initiation and progression of diabetic and other glomerulopathies. *Am J Med* 1982; **72**:375–380.
40. Parving H-H, Viberti GC, Keen H, Christiansen JS, Lassen NA. Hemodynamic factors in the genesis of diabetic microangiopathy. *Metabolism* 1983; **32**:943–949.
41. Hostetter TH, Troy JL, Brenner BM. Glomerular haemodynamics in experimental diabetes mellitus. *Kidney Int* 1981; **19**:410–415.
42. Zatz R, Dunn BR, Meyer TW, Andersson S, Rennke HG, Brenner BM, Troy JL, DeGraphenried RL, Noddin JL, Nunn AW, Sandstrom D. Prevention of diabetic glomerulopathy by pharmacological amelioration of glomerular capillary hypertension. *J Clin Invest* 1986; **77**:1925–1930.
43. Meyer TW, Andersson S, Rennke HG, Brenner BM. Control of glomerular hypertension retards progression of established glomerular injury in rats with renal ablation. *Kidney Int* 1985; **27**:247.
44. Anderson S, Meyer TW, Rennke HG, Brenner BM. Control of glomerular hypertension limits glomerular injury in rats with reduced renal mass. *J Clin Invest* 1985; **76**:612–619.
45. Hollenberg NK, Meggs GL, Williams GH, Katz J, Garnic JD, Harrington DP. Sodium intake and renal responses to captopril in normal man and in essential hypertension. *Kidney Int* 1981; **20**:240–245.
46. Hollenberg NK. Angiotensin-converting enzyme inhibition: renal aspects. *J Cardiovasc Pharmacol* 1985; **7**:S40–S44.
47. Lant AF, McNabb RW, Noormohamed FH. Kinetic and metabolic aspects of enalapril action. *J Hypertension* 1984; **2(suppl 2)**:37–42.
48. McNabb WR, Noormohamed FH, Brooks BA, Till AE, Lant AF. Effects of repeated doses of enalapril on renal function in man. *Br J Clin Pharmacol* 1985; **19**:353–361.
49. Marre M, Sassano P, Corvol P, Passa P, Menard J. Microalbuminuria in uncomplicated essential hypertension and its reduction by antihypertensive treatment. *Diabete & Metabolisme* 1988; **14**:232–234.
50. Bauer JH, Reams GP. Renal effects of angiotensin converting enzyme inhibitors in hypertension. *Am J Med* 1986; **81(suppl. 4C)**:19–27.

51. Bauer JH, Reams GP, Lal SM. Renal protective effect of strict blood pressure control with enalapril therapy. *Arch Intern Med* 1987; **147**:1397–1400.
52. Heeg JE, de Jong PE, van der Hem GK, de Zeeuw D. Reduction of proteinuria by angiotensin converting enzyme inhibition. *Kidney Int* 1987; **32**:78–83.
53. Sullivan PA, Kelleher M, Twomey M, Dineen M. Effect of converting enzyme inhibition on blood pressure, plasma renal activity (PRA) and plasma aldosterone in hypertensive diabetics compared to patient with essential hypertension. *J Hypertens* 1985; **3**:359–363.
54. D'Angelo A, Giannini S, Benetollo P, Castrignano R, Lodetti MG, Malvasi L, Pati T, Crepaldi G. Efficacy of captopril in hypertensive diabetic patients. *Am J Med* 1988; **84(suppl. 3A)**:155–158.
55. Passa P, LeBlanc H, Marre M. Effects of enalapril in insulin-dependent diabetic subjects with mild to moderate uncomplicated hypertension. *Diabetes Care* 1987; **10**:200–204.
56. Dominguez JR, de la Calle H, Hurtado A, Robles RG, Sancho-Rof J. Effect of converting enzyme inhibitors in hypertensive patients with non-insulin-dependent diabetes mellitus. *Postgr Med J* 1986; **62(suppl. 1)**:66–68.
57. Matthews DM, Wathen CG, Bell D, Collier A, Muir AL, Clarke BF. The effect of captopril on blood pressure and glucose tolerance in hypertensive non-insulin dependent diabetics. *Postgrad Med J* 1986; **62(suppl. 1)**:73–75.
58. Pedersen MM, Schmitz A, Pedersen EB, Danielsen H, Christiansen JS. Acute and long-term renal effects of angiotensin converting enzyme-inhibition in normotensive, normoalbuminuric insulin-dependent diabetic patients. *Diabetic Med* 1988; **5**:562–569.
59. Levy-Marchal C, Drummond K, Laborde K, Dechaux M, Czernichow P. Enalapril in normotensive type 1 (insulin-dependent) diabetes: a double blind cross-over study in children with elevated glomerular filtration rate. *Diabetologia* 1988; **31**:514A.
60. Vora J, Owens DR, Luzio S, Atiea J, Ryder REJ, Williams S, Haes TM: Glomerular function during angiotensin converting enzyme (ACE) inhibition in early insulin dependent diabetes (IDDs). *Diabetic Medicine* 1986; **4**:584A.
61. Marre M, Leblanc H, Suarez L, Guyenne T-T, Ménard J, Passa P. Converting enzyme inhibition and kidney function in normotensive diabetic patients with persistent microalbuminuria. *Br Med J* 1987; **294**:1148–1452.
62. Passa Ph, Marre M, Menard J. One year effect of enalapril in diabetic patients with microalbuminuria and no hypertension. *Diabete & Metabolisme* 1988; **14**:230–231.
63. Mimran A, Insua A, Ribstein J, Monnier L, Bringer J, Mirouze J. Contrasting renal effects of captopril and nifedipine in normotensive patients with incipient diabetic nephropathy. *J Hypertens* 1988 (in press).
64. Björck S, Nyberg G, Mulec H, Granerus G, Herlitz H, Aurell M. Beneficial effects of angiotensin converting enzyme inhibition on renal function in patients with diabetic nephropathy. *Br Med J* 1986; **293**:471–474.
65. Taguma Y, Kitamoto Y, Futaki G, Ueda H, Monma H, Ishizaki M, Takahashi H, Sekino H, Sasaki Y. Effect of captopril on heavy proteinuria in azotemic diabetics. *N Engl J Med* 1985; **313**:1617–1620.
66. Hommel E, Parving HH, Mathiesen E, Edsberg B, Nielsen MD, Giese J. Effect of captopril on kidney function in insulin-dependent diabetic patients with nephropathy. *Br Med J* 1986; **293**:479–480.
67. Hay U, Ludvik B, Gisinger Ch, Schernthaner G. Fehlender Effekt der ACE-Inhibition auf dei Makroproteinurie bei diabetischer Nephropathie—eine Langzeitstudie über 6 Monate. *Schweiz Med Wschr* 1988; **118**:165–169.
68. Nyberg G, Nordén G, Björck S, Larsson O. Progression of diabetic nephropathy—a multifactorial process. *Scand J Urol Nephrol* 1988; **(suppl. 108)**:35–40.
69. Ahmad S. Beneficial effects of angiotensin converting enzyme inhibition on renal function in patients with diabetic nephropathy. *Br Med J* 1986; **293**:1028.
70. Schmitz A. Acute renal effects of oral felodipine in normal man. *Eur J Clin Pharmacol* 1987; **32**:17–22.
71. Dworkin LD, Ichikawa I, Brenner BM. Hormonal modulation of glomerular function. *Am J Physiol* 1983; **244**:F95–F104.
72. Mogensen CE. Progression of nephropathy in long-term diabetics with proteinuria and effect of initial anti-hypertensive treatment. *Scand J Clin Lab Invest* 1976; **36**:383–388.
73. Mogensen CE. Renal function changes in diabetes. *Diabetes* 1976; **25**:872–879.

74. Mogensen CE, Schmitz A, Christensen CK. Comparative renal pathophysiology relevant to IDDM and NIDDM patients. *Diabetes/Metabolism Reviews* 1988; **4**:453–483.
75. Parving H-H, Hommel E, Smidt UM. Angiotensin converting enzyme inhibition protects kidney function and reduces albuminuria in diabetic nephropathy. *Diabetologia* 1988; **31**:530A.
76. Christensen CK, Christiansen JS, Schmitz A, Christensen T, Hermansen K, Mogensen CE. Effect of continuous subcutaneous insulin infusion on kidney function and size in IDDM patients—a two year controlled study. *J Diab Complications* 1987; **1**:91–95.
77. Pedersen O, Jørgensen FS, Pedersen MM, Møller B, Lykke G, Mogensen CE. The effect of moderate protein restriction on kidney function in normoalbuminuric Type 1 (insulin-dependent) diabetic patients. *Diabetologia* 1988; **31**:530A.
78. Dahl-Jørgensen K, Hanssen KF, Kierulf P, Bjøro T, Sandvik L, Aagenæs Ø. Reduction of urinary albumin excretion after 4 years of continuous subcutaneous insulin infusion in insulin-dependent diabetes mellitus. *Acta Endocrinol (Copenh)* 1988; **117**:19–25.
79. Cohen D, Dodds R, Viberti GC. Effect of protein restriction in insulin dependent diabetics at risk of nephropathy. *Br Med J* 1987; **294**:795–798.
80. Viberti GC, Bilous RW, Mackintosh D, Bending JJ, Keen H. Long term correction of hyperglycaemia and progression of renal failure in insulin dependent diabetes. *Br Med J* 1983; **286**:598–602.
81. Nyberg G, Blohmé G, Nordén G. Impact of metabolic control on progression of clinical diabetic nephropathy. *Diabetologia* 1987; **30**:82–86.
82. Bending JJ, Dodds R, Keen H, Viberti GC. Lowering protein intake and the progression of diabetic renal failure. *Diabetologia* 1986; **29**:516A.
83. Viberti GC, Bending JJ, Dodds R. Protein restriction, blood-pressure and the progression of diabetic nephropathy. *Blood Purif* 1988; **6**:315–323.
84. The DCCT Research Group. Diabetes control and complications trial (DCCT): Results of feasibility study. *Diabetes Care* 1987; **10**:1–19.
85. The DCCT Research Group: Are continuing studies of metabolic control and microvascular complications in insulin-dependent diabetes justified? *N Engl J Med* 1988; **318**:246–250.
86. Microalbuminuria Collaborative Study Group, UK. Microalbuminuria and glycaemic control. In *Diabetic Complications '87. Multicentre and/or Prospective Study Session on Diabetic Complications.* Rome, Italy, Consiglio Nazionale delle Ricerche, 1987.
87. Ellis G, Diamandis EP, Giesbrecht EE, Daneman D, Allen LC. An automated "high-pressure" liquid-chromatographic assay for hemoglobin A1c. *Clin Chem* 1984; **30**:1746–1752.
88. Goldstein DE, Little RR, Wiedmeyer H-M, England JD, McKenzie EM. Methodologies and clinical applications. *Clin Chem* 1986; **32**:B64–B70.
89. Mogensen CE, Christensen CK, Christiansen JS, Boye N, Pedersen MM, Schmitz A. Early hyperfiltration and late renal damage in insulin-dependent diabetes. *Pediat Adolesc Endocr* 1988; **17**:197–205.
90. Christiansen JS. Early renal hyperfunction and hypertrophy in insulin-dependent patients: changes found at diagnosis and early in the course of diabetes. In Mogensen CE, ed. *The Kidney and Hypertension in Diabetes Mellitus.* Boston, Martinus Nijhoff Publishing, 1988; 157–164.
91. Jarrett RJ, Keen H. Hyperglycaemia and diabetes mellitus. *Lancet* 1976; **II**:1009–1012.
92. Svendsen PAA, Jørgensen J, Nerup J. HbA$_{1c}$ and the diagnosis of diabetes mellitus. *Acta Med Scand* 1981; **210**:313–317.
93. Schmitz A, Væth M. Microalbuminuria a major risk factor in non-insulin-dependent diabetes. A 10-year follow-up study of 503 patients. *Diabetic Medicine* 1988; **5**:126–134.
94. Damsgaard EM, Frøland A, Mogensen CE. Microalbuminuria is a strong predictor of 6-year mortality of elderly type 2 (non-insulin-dependent) diabetic patients and non-diabetic subjects. A prospective study. *Diabetologia* 1988; **31**:483A.

SUMMARY

This review deals with early abnormalities in renal function in diabetes and the possibility of intervention with ACE inhibition. In patients with a normal albumin excretion rate, the only abnormality is increased GFR (hyperfiltration) and increased filtration fraction, suggesting high intraglomerular pressure. New studies by ACE inhibition, carried out over 3 months show, that filtration fraction could be reduced, and also in this study urinary albumin excretion rate was reduced, although the excretion rate was quite normal before treatment. These findings suggest that ACE inhibition may be useful in these patients, but certainly further studies have to be conducted. In incipient diabetic nephropathy, characterized by persisting microalbuminuria, longitudinal studies have shown that many years of treatment by conventional antihypertensive agents such as cardioselective beta-blockers and diuretics are able to reduce microalbuminuria considerably, while maintaining quite normal or supranormal GFR. Also ACE inhibition in such patients is able to reduce microalbuminuria, and probably is also able to maintain glomerular filtration rate, although further studies have to be conducted. The reduction in microalbuminuria, however, is certainly a positive sign. In overt diabetic nephropathy, reduction of proteinuria is associated with preservation of glomerular function and conventional antihypertensive treatment is able to reduce proteinuria considerably; longitudinal studies have also shown that the rate of decline in GFR can be reduced considerably by antihypertensive treatment. Pretreatment values are compared with values after antihypertensive therapy, so in these studies patients were used as their own control. Similar studies have been published recently, using ACE inhibition, with similar results. In some studies ACE inhibitors were combined with beta-blockers and diuretics, again resulting in reduction in fall rate of GFR, thus postponing uremia. Therefore, it can be concluded that antihypertensive treatment including ACE inhibition is able to reduce not only microalbuminuria and proteinuria, but also to reduce considerably the rate of decline in GFR.

RÉSUMÉ

Cette étude traite des premiéres anomalies de la fonction rénale chez les diabétiques et de la possibilité d'intervenir avec les inhibiteurs de l'enzyme de conversion de l'angiotensine. Chez les patients qui ont un taux d'excrétion normal d'albumine la seule anomalie est l'augmentation de la filtration glomérulaire ainsi que l'augmentation de la fraction de filtration, ce qui indique une pression intraglomérulaire élevée. De nouvelles études, sur une période de 3 mois, utilisant l'inhibition de l'enzyme de conversion de l'angiotensine montrent que la fraction de filtration peut être diminuée; dans cette même étude le taux d'excrétion urinaire d'albumine a aussi diminué, bien que le taux d'excrétion ait été tout à fait normal avant le traitement. Ces résultats soulignent les effets bénéfiques de l'inhibition de l'enzyme de conversion de l'angiotensine chez ces malades, mais il est certain que des études plus approfondies doivent être menées. Dans la néphropathie diabétique débutante, qui se caractérise par une microalbuminurie persistante, des études longitudinales ont montré qu'au bout de nombreuses années de traitement par des antihypertenseurs conventionnels, tels que les bêtabloquants cardiotoniques et les diurétiques, on arrive à réduire considérablement la microalbuminurie, tout en maintenant un taux de filtration glomérulaire tout à fait normal et même audessus de la normale. L'inhibition de l'enzyme de conversion de l'angiotensine peut aussi réduire la microalbuminurie, et probablement maintenir également le taux de filtration glomérulaire de ces patients. Cependant, des études plus approfondies restent à faire. La réduction de microalbuminurie est, cependant, un signe prometteur. Dans les néphropathies diabétiques avancées, la réduction de la protéinurie est liée au maintien de la fonction glomérulaire. Dans les néphropathies diabétiques avancées le traitement antihypertensif conventionnel peut réduire considérablement la protéinurie, et des études longitudinales ont également montré que le traitement antihypertenseur peut réduire considérablement le taux de chute de la filtration glomérulaire. On compare les résultats de traitements avant et après utilisation d'antihypertenseurs. Dans ces études les patients étaient donc leur propre contrôle. Ces résultats sont comparables à ceux d'autres études récentes utlisant l'inhibition de l'enzyme de conversion de l'angiotensine. Dans quelques études les inhibiteurs de l'enzyme de conversion de l'angiotensine étaient combinés avec des bêtabloquants et des diurétiques, entraînant à nouveau une réduction du taux de chute de la filtration glomérulaire, différant ainsi l'urémie. On peut donc en conclure que les traitements antihypertenseurs y compris l'inhibition de l'enzyme de conversion de l'angiotensine, peuvent réduire non seulement la microalbuminurie et al protéinurie, mais ils peuvent aussi réduire significativement le taux de chute de la filtration glomérulaire.

ZUSAMMENFASSUNG

Diese Veröffentlichung behandelt frühe Abnormalitäten der Nierenfunktion bei Diabetes und die mögliche Intervention mit Inhibitoren des angiotensinkonvertierenden Enzyms (ACE).

In Patienten mit normaler Albuminausscheidungsrate besteht die einzige Abnormalität in erhöhter Hyperfiltration (GFR) und einer grösseren Filtrationsfraktion, was auf einen hohen intraglomerulären Druck hinweist. Neue Studien der ACE-Inhibition über einen Zeitraum von drei Monaten zeigen, dass die Filtrationsfraktion reduziert werden könnte; in dieser Studie wurde auch die Rate der Albuminabscheidung reduziert, obwohl die Abscheidungsrate vor der Behandlung ganz normal war. Diese Ergebnisse liefern einen Hinweis darauf, dass die ACE-Inhibition für diese Patienten nützlich sein kann, aber weitere Studien sind mit Sicherheit notwendig. Bei der beginnenden diabetischen Nephropathie, charakterisiert durch andauernde Mikroalbuminurie, haben Longitudinalstudien gezeigt, dass eine Behandlung mit konventionellen antihypertonischen Mitteln wie kardioselektiven Beta-

Rezeptorenblockern und Diuretika über einen Zeitraum von vielen Jahren in der Lage ist, die Mikroalbuminurie beträchtlich zu verringern und gleichzeitig ganz normale oder supranormale glomeruläre Filtrationsraten aufrechtzuerhalten. In solchen Patienten kann die ACE-Inhibition auch die Mikroalbuminurie reduzieren und wahrscheinlich auch die glomeruläre Filtrationsrate aufrechterhalten, obwohl weitere Studien durchgeführt werden müssen. Jedoch ist die Reduktion der Mikroalbuminurie sicherlich ein positives Zeichen. Bei offener diabetischer Nephropathie erscheint die Reduktion der Proteinurie zusammen mit der Erhaltung der Glomerularfunktion. Liegt offene diabetische Nephropathie vor, kann konventionelle antihypertonische Behandlung die Proteinurie beträchtlich verringern; und Longitudinalstudien haben ausserdem gezeigt, dass die Reduktionsrate der glomerulären Filtration durch antihypertonische Behandlung beträchtlich reduziert werden kann. Die Werte vor Beginn der Behandlung sind verglichen worden mit den Werten nach der antihypertonischen Therapie, so dass in dieser Studie die Patienten ihre eigene Kontrollgruppe darstellten. Kürzlich sind ähnliche Untersuchungen veröffentlicht worden, die ACE-Inhibition mit ähnlichen Resultaten benutzten. In einigen Studien wurden ACE-Inhibitoren mit Beta-Rezeptoren-blockern und Diuretika kombiniert, wieder mit dem Resultat einer Reduktion der glomerulären Filtrationsrate und damit eine Urämie hinausschiebend. Man kann daher schliessen, dass antihypertonische Behandlung mit ACE-Inhibition in der Lage ist, nicht nur Mikroalbuminurie und Proteinurie zu reduzieren, sondern auch die Reduktion der glomerulären Filtrationsrate beträchtlich zu reduzieren.

RIASSUNTO

Questo articolo tratta delle anormalità iniziali della funzione renale nel diabete e la possibilità di intervento mediante gli inibitori dell'enzima isomerizzante dell'angiotensina (EIA). In pazienti con tasso di escrezione d'albumina normale, l'unica anormalità è un aumento del TFG (iperfiltrazione) ed un aumento della frazione di filtrazione, cosa che fa pensare ad un'alta pressione intraglomerulare. Nuovi studi sull'inibizione dell'EIA, eseguiti nel corso di 3 mesi, dimostrano che la frazione di filtrazione può essere ridotta; in questo studio anche il tasso di escrezione urinaria dell'albumina è stato ridotto benché il tasso d'escrezione urinaria dell'albumina è stato ridotto benché il tasso d'escrezione fosse piuttosto normale prima della cura. Queste scoperte fanno pensare che l'inibizione dell'EIA possa essere utile in tali pazienti ma è certo che ulteriori studi devono essere compiuti. Nella nefropatia diabetica incipiente, caratterizzata da microalbuminuria persistente, degli studi longitudinali hanno mostrato che molti anni di di cura mediante agenti antiipertensivi quali beta-bloccanti e diuretici sono in grado di ridurre considerevolmente la microalbiminuria pur mantenendo un TFG normale o sopranormale. Anche l'inibizione dell'EIA in tali pazienti è in grado di ridurre la microalbuminuria e probabilmente anche a mantenere il tasso di filtrazione glomerulare, benché sia necessario compiere ulteriori studi. La riduzione della microalbuminuria è comunque un segno positivo. Nella nefropatia diabetica manifesta, la riduzione della proteinuria è associata alla preservazione della funzione glomerulare. Nella nefropatia diabetica manifesta la cura antiipertensiva tradizionale è in grado di di ridurre considercvolmente la proteinuria e studi longitudinali hanno anche mostrato che il tasso di diminuzione del TFG può essere notevolmente ridotto da terapia antiipertensiva. I valori di prima della cura vengono paragonati a quelli dopo terapia antiipertensiva, per cui in queti studi i pazienti venivano usati come controllo di sé stessi. Studi analoghi sono stati pubblicati di recente in cui è stata usata l'inibizione dell'EIA con simili risultati. In alcuni stati gli inibitori dell'EIA erano combinati a beta-bloccanti e diuretici, ottenendo anche qui una riduzione del tasso di diminuzione di TFG e posponendo quindi l'uremia. Si può quindi concludere che la terapia antiipertensiva, inibizione dell'EIA compresa, e in grado non solo di ridurre la microabluminuria e la proteinuria ma anche di ridurre considerevolmente il tasso di degrado del TFG.

SUMÁRIO

Este trabalho trata de anormalidades precoces da função renal no diabetes e a possibilidade de intervenção com inibidores da enzima convertidora da angiotensina (ACE). Em pacientes com um índice normal de excreção de albumina, a única anormalidade é um GFR aumentado (hiperfiltração) e uma fração aumentada de filtração, o que sugere uma elevada pressão intraglomerular. Novos estudos de inibição da ACE, efetuados durante 3 meses, mostram que a fração de filtração poderia ser reduzida; também observou-se uma redução no índice de excreção urinária de albumina, ainda que o índice de excreção foi muito normal antes do tratamento. Estos achados sugerem que a inibição da ACE pode ser útil nestos pacientes, mas será necessário realizar estudos adicionais. Na nefropatia diabética incipiente, caracterizada por microalbuminúria persistente, os estudos longitudinais têm demonstrado que muitos anos de tratamento com agentes antihipertensivos tradicionais, tais como betabloqueadores cardioseletivos e diuréticos, são capazes de reduzir consideravelmente a microalbuminúria, ao mesmo tempo que mantêm um GFR normal ou supranormal. Além disso, a inibição da ACE em tais pacientes é capaz de reduzir a microalbuminúria e provavelmente também manter o índice de filtração glomerular, ainda que será necessário efetuar estudos adicionais. Contudo, a redução na microalbuminúria certamente é um sinal positivo. Na nefropatia diabética manifesta, a redução da proteinúria encontra-se associada com a preservação da função glomerular. Na nefropatia diabética manifesta, o tratamento com antihipertensivos tradicionais é capaz de reduzir a proteinúria consideravelmente, e estudos longitudinais também têm demonstrado que o índice de decremento no GFR pode reduzir-se consideravelmente pelo tratamento com antihipertensivos. Os valores pré-tratomento comparam-se com os valores após do tratamento antihipertensivo, de maneira que nestos estudos os pacientes se utilizaram como seus próprios controles. Recentemente têm-se publicado estudos semelhantes utilizando inibidores da ACE, com resultados semelhantes. Em alguns estudos, os inibidores da ACE combinaram-se com betabloquedores e diuréticos, resultando novamente numa redução no índice de decremento do GFR, assim adiando a uremia. Deste modo, pode concluir-se que o tratamento antihipertensivo, inclusive a inibição da ACE, é capaz de reduzir não somente a microalbuminúria e proteinúria, senão também de reduzir consideravelmente o índice de decremento do GFR.

RESUMEN

Este trabajo examina anormalidades tempranas de la función renal en la diabetes y la posibilidad de intervención con inhibidores de la enzima convertidora de la angiotensina (ACE). En pacientes con un índice normal de excreción de albúmina, la única anormalidad es un incremento en el GFR (hiperfiltración) y un incremento en la fracción de filtración, lo que es sugestivo de una elevada presión intraglomerular. Nuevos estudios de inhibición de la ACE, efectuados durante 3 meses, muestran que la fracción de filtración podría ser reducida; también se observó una reducción en el índice de excreción urinaria de albúmina, aunque el índice de excreción fue normal antes del tratamiento. Estos resultados sugieren que la inhibición de la ACE podría ser útil en estos pacientes, pero será necesario efectuar estudios adicionales. En la nefropatía diabética incipiente, caracterizada por microalbuminuria persistente, los estudios longitudinales han demostrado que muchos años de tratamiento con agentes antihipertensivos tradicionales, tales como betabloqueadores cardioselectivos y diuréticos, son capaces de reducir considerablemente la microalbuminuria, al mismo tiempo que mantienen un GFR normal o supranormal. Además, la inhibición de la ACE en tales pacientes es capaz de reducir la microalbuminuria y probablemente también mantener el índice de filtración glomerular, aunque será necesario efectuar estudios posteriores. Sin embargo, la reducción en la microalbuminuria ciertamente es un signo positivo. En la nefropatía diabética manifiesta, la reducción de la proteinuria se halla asociada con la preservación de la función glomerular. Por otro lado, en la nefropatía diabética manifiesta el tratamiento con antihipertensivos tradicionales es capaz de reducir la proteinuria considerablemente, y estudios longitudinales también han demostrado que el índice de decremento en el GFR puede reducirse considerablemente por el tratamiento con antihipertensivos. Los valores pretratamiento se comparan con los valores después del tratamiento antihipertensivo, de modo que en estos estudios los pacientes se emplearon como sus propios controles. Recientemente se han publicado estudios similares empleando inhibidores de la ACE, con resultados similares.

En algunos estudios los inhibidores de la ACE se combinaron con betabloqueadores y diuréticos, resultando nuevamente en una reducción en el índice
de decremento del GFR, posponiendo así la uremia. De modo que se puede
concluir que el tratamiento antihipertensivo, incluyendo la inhibición de la
ACE, es capaz de reducir no solamente la microalbuminuria y proteinuria,
sino también reducir considerablemente el índice de decremento del GFR.

要約

　この総説では，糖尿病における腎機能の早期異常とこれに対するアンジオテン
シン変換酵素（ACE）阻害薬の介在の可能性について論ずる。

　正常なアルブミン排泄率をもつ患者では，唯一の異常所見は糸球体濾過値
（GFR）の上昇（過剰濾過）と濾過率(filtration fraction; FF)の上昇で，これは糸
球体内圧が高いことを示唆している。ACE阻害薬を用いた新しい研究では，3カ
月以上の治療後にFFを減少しえた。ここでは同時に，治療前に正常であったアル
ブミン尿中排泄率も治療後低下した。この知見は，ACE阻害薬が上記のような患
者に有用であることを示すものであるが，さらに検討が必要であると考えられる。

　持続するミクロアルブミン尿を特徴とする初期の糖尿病性腎症においては，長
期臨床試験で，選択的 β 遮断薬や利尿薬などの従来の降圧薬で長年にわたって治
療すると，ミクロアルブミン尿をかなり軽減させることができ，しかもGFRをほ
とんど正常または正常以上の状態に維持することが示されている。ACE阻害薬も
また，このような患者で，ミクロアルブミン尿を軽減し，おそらくGFRを正常に
保つと考えられるが，さらに検討が必要であろう。確かにミクロアルブミン尿の
軽減は1つの改善の指標ではある。

　明らかな糖尿病性腎症では，糸球体機能の維持に伴ってタンパク尿が減少する。
明白な糖尿病性腎症での従来の降圧薬治療はタンパク尿を相当に軽減させること
ができ，長期試験では，GFRの低下の速度を降圧療法によってかなり遅らせうる
ことが示されている。なおここでは，治療前と治療後の値を比較しており，治療
対象患者自身が対照とされていた。最近，ACE阻害薬を用いた同様の研究が報告
され，同じような結果が得られている。また，ある研究においては，ACE阻害薬
と β 遮断薬および利尿薬との併用が試みられ，ここでもGFRの低下の抑制と尿
毒症発現の遅延が認められている。したがって，ACE阻害薬を含む降圧療法はミ
クロアルブミン尿やタンパク尿を軽減しうるばかりでなく，GFRの低下をかなり
抑制できると考えられる。

Cardiac and Renal Failure: An Expanding Role for ACE Inhibitors, edited by C. T. Dollery and L. M. Sherwood, Hanley & Belfus, Inc., Philadelphia.

Discussion

SHERWOOD: Dr. Mogensen, in your triple therapy studies, with beta-blockers known to mask the symptoms of hypoglycemia and diuretics potentially aggravating hyperglycemia, did you run into any difficulties using this combined approach in diabetic patients?

MOGENSEN: It is important to use low doses of beta-blockers. Problems with hypoglycemic unawareness may occur in some patients. You should explain carefully to your patients that the nature of their hypoglycemic attacks may change. It is important to use diuretic therapy in patients with hypertension and nephropathy. Insulin-dependent diabetics characteristically have sodium retention; there isn't necessarily a worsening of glycemic control. There may be less adequate blood sugar control in non-insulin-dependent diabetics but you can then intensify their diabetic treatment. I am inclined to believe that the dangers of using beta-blockers and diuretics in diabetic patients have been overestimated. However, there may be fewer side-effects with ACE inhibitors.

GANTEN: There have been reports that ACE inhibitors improve metabolic control in diabetic patients. There is an effect on glucose utilization, possibly related to kinins. Have you seen any improvement in the metabolic status of your patients, Dr. Mogensen? What about insulin requirements?

MOGENSEN: We were unable to detect changes in the levels of glycated hemoglobin in our patients. Although there may be slight changes in glycemic control, I do not think this is clinically relevant because the effects are minor.

IMURA: You have said that ACE inhibitors lower GFR in the initial stages of treatment, and may aggravate a decline in renal function. How did you evaluate the effect on renal function in your patients?

MOGENSEN: It is important to titrate the blood pressure levels carefully. With all kinds of antihypertensive treatment there is initially a small drop in GFR. This effect is particularly noticeable with beta-blockers. The effect is probably beneficial as hyperfiltration in the individual glomerus is reduced. The initial drop in GFR does not worry me, but if the drop continues then this may be due to the blood pressure being lowered too much. Usually, the rate of decline in GFR is reduced considerably.

IMURA: In this situation would you reduce your drug dosage?

MOGENSEN: Yes. When ACE inhibitors were first introduced high doses were used. I would not recommend this now.

IMURA: In advanced nephropathy postural hypotension is a problem. How do you use ACE inhibitors in these patients?

MOGENSEN: Careful monitoring of therapy is essential in patients with advanced diabetic nephropathy. If postural hypotension occurs the dose must be reduced, or short-acting agents used, e.g., during night.

THURAU: I would like to ask Dr. Keane about the effect of ACE inhibition on protein excretion. You have related this phenomenon to reduced glomerular capillary pressure. Are there studies which indicate that this effect is due to a change in the electrical barrier of the basement membrane? There is a preferential effect on negatively charged proteins.

KEANE: I do not know of any specific studies, although angiotensin II is a cationic peptide and could possibly alter the filtration barrier. Our recent experimental data in the Zucker rat treated with enalapril suggest that there is modification of protein excretion independent of changes in glomerular hemodynamics. That raises the possibility that there are other effects on the membrane itself. The gel constituency of the filtration barrier may be changed, thus affecting pore size, or pore density in the glomerular filtration barrier. This has not been explored to my knowledge.

GANTEN: Proteinuria was a problem with high doses of ACE inhibitor therapy. Now we hear that protein excretion is decreased. How can this be explained? Even with low doses I understand that there is a 1 – 1.5% induction of proteinuria.

DE JONG: I think you are referring to earlier studies with captopril reporting the induction of membranous nephropathy. These patients were given very high doses of the drug. There is no evidence now that this is a clinical problem with enalapril, or any of the other ACE inhibitors, at lower doses.

MOGENSEN: In our acute studies using enalapril in patients with early diabetic neuropathy, we found in a single patient that when there was a marked drop in blood pressure there was also a dramatic, but reversible, drop in renal plasma flow and GFR, and a marked increase in albumin excretion. The effect would seem to be caused by renal ischemia and is a reflection of overdosage.

JOHNSTON: Although the ACE inhibitors have not been shown selectively to affect the filtration barriers, the reverse was shown by Sir George Pickering in the 1940s. He showed that renin produced proteinuria, and this has been confirmed with intrarenal angiotensin, independent of its hemodynamic effects. It changes the basement membrane barrier, and this has been known for many years.

SONNENBLICK: I would like to ask a broader pathological question. How do changes affecting the kidney relate to the interstitial fibrosis one sees in the heart? Is there a more general vascular pathology?

DE JONG: There are no demonstrable pathological changes in the kidney with the longer term use of ACE inhibitors. In animal studies you can prevent glomerular sclerosis. This is dependent on long-term treatment with the ACE inhibitor.

ROCHA: I would like to ask Dr. Mogensen whether we have unequivocal data that ACE inhibitors can prevent the progression of Stage 3 diabetes with microproteinuria to Stage 4 with overt proteinuria?

MOGENSEN: There are new data from Michel Marre and Philippe Passa which show that patients with Stage 3 diabetic nephropathy microalbuminuria who have been treated with ACE inhibitors for one year maintain stable renal function.[1] Enalapril was compared with placebo. It could be suggested that diabetic patients might need to be monitored very closely for the early development of microproteinuria, and such patients should be treated routinely by these agents. It is too early, however, to make this a general policy, but it may certainly be the approach for the future. Also exercise-induced microalbuminuria can be reduced by ACE inhibition.[2]

MIMRAN: I want to comment on the data published by Dr. Mogensen and Michel Marre in the Paris group. This study compared placebo with enalapril without any other treatment being used. We have also carried out a trial in patients with incipient nephropathy. We compared placebo, captopril, and nifedipine. We were surprised to find that in the placebo group, who were all normotensive, there were insignificant changes in urinary albumin excretion, but in the captopril group there was a 40% reduction in urinary albuminuria. Nifedepine increased excretion. ACE inhibitors seem to cause a persistent reduction, and the 40% reduction was maintained at one year.

MOGENSEN: There is a long-term reduction in microalbuminuria when you follow patients for a number of years during antihypertensive treatment.

DOLLERY: Blood pressure is also important. There is continuing evidence, when you take into account retinal changes, that it is the combination of diabetic vascular changes, together with hypertension, that causes much more rapid progression. You can prevent this, at least in part, by control of blood pressure, and this is a main effect of the ACE inhibitor.

MOGENSEN: Experimental studies in humans demonstrate that permeability changes can be reversed by the use of ACE inhibitors in diabetic retinopathy.

REFERENCE

1. Marre M, Passa P. *Br Med J.* 1988; **297**:1092–1095.
2. Romanelli G, Giustina G. *Br Med Jr* 1989; **298**:284–289.
3. Hominel E, Parving HH. *Diabetologia* 1988; **31**:502A.

Cardiac and Renal Failure: An Expanding Role for ACE Inhibitors, edited by C. T. Dollery and L. M. Sherwood, Hanley & Belfus, Inc., Philadelphia.

Angiotensin-Converting Enzyme Inhibitors in Renovascular Hypertension and Hypertension of Renal Transplant Recipients

Albert Mimran, Jean Ribstein, and Georges Mourad

INTRODUCTION

Although the prevalence of renovascular hypertension may be as high as 30% in patients with accelerated or malignant hypertension,[1] it is estimated to be less than 4% in the large population of hypertensive patients that are referred to care centers. In addition, renal artery stenosis may be found in normotensive subjects in whom arteriography is performed for other reasons such as renal donation or peripheral occlusive arterial disease.[2] At the present time, the screening of patients with renal artery stenosis and the criteria for predicting a favorable outcome following correction of the stenosis are not well defined. Following the advent of orally-active angiotensin I-converting enzyme (ACE) inhibitors, a large number of papers appeared on the use of these agents in patients with severe resistant hypertension and subsequently in those with moderate essential hypertension. In the last five years, several groups reported on ACE inhibitor induced deterioration in renal function in patients with bilateral stenosis or stenosis of a single functioning kidney and the possible extinction of function of the stenotic side in patients with unilateral renal artery stenosis. These observations cast some doubts on the usefulness of ACE inhibitors in such patients.

CONVERTING ENZYME INHIBITION IN THE DETECTION OF PATIENTS WITH RENAL ARTERY STENOSIS

High circulating renin levels are found in approximately 60% of patients with renovascular hypertension; however about 20% of essential hypertensives

333

present with elevated renin levels.[3,4] If a high renin level is defined as a value higher than that observed in 95% of essential hypertensives, only 27% of patients with renal artery stenosis meet this criterion.[5] Although, it has been extensively argued that the effect of specific angiotensin II antagonists as well as angiotensin-converting enzyme inhibitors (ACEIs) may be influenced by the existence of a partial agonistic activity of saralasin and accumulation of kinins or prostaglandins during ACE inhibition, it is widely accepted that the change in arterial pressure associated with acute administration of either agent is closely correlated with the basal renin level. During the last decade, several studies were reported on the value of pharmacological blockade of the renin-angiotensin system in the diagnosis of renovascular hypertension. In 1979, Case et al[5] assessed the acute effect of saralasin and ACEI in 44 patients with renal artery stenosis (RVH) and 100 patients with essential hypertension (74 normal renin and 26 high renin subjects) maintained on a normal sodium intake and after being off medication for at least 2 weeks. The diagnosis of functionally significant renal artery stenosis was based on the existence of lateralization of renin secretion towards the stenotic kidney, along with arteriographic confirmation of the stenosis. It was found that 95.4% of RVH patients had a positive depressor response to angiotensin blockade (maximum percent decrease in diastolic pressure equal to or greater than 9.3 with saralasin, 9.4 after teprotide and 8.5 after captopril) whilst 65% and 26% of patients with high and normal renin essential hypertension (EH) respectively also had a positive depressor response. In contrast, when the increase in plasma renin activity (PRA) resulting from inhibition of the negative feedback loop between angiotensin II and renin secretion was considered, an excessive response was found in 98% of RVH and 12% and 0% of high and normal renin EH patients respectively. They concluded that reactive hyperreninemia resulting from inhibition of the renin-angiotensin system was a more specific test for identifying patients with functionally significant renal artery stenosis. In a recent report,[6] the same group observed that a 100% specificity of and a 100% sensitivity to the captopril test was achieved when excessive post-captopril PRA level as well as an increase in PRA of more than 150% in response to captopril were taken as criteria for a positive test in patients with RVH and normal renal function. These investigators also insisted on the fact that prior sodium depletion abolished the specificity of the renin and depressor responses to angiotensin blockade for identification of RVH. Similar conclusions were reached by other groups.[4]

In a personal study,[7] the acute effect of captopril on blood pressure and PRA was assessed in 81 EH and 56 RVH patients on unrestricted sodium intake and off medications for at least 2 weeks. A fall in mean arterial pressure, more marked than that observed in normal persons (−10 mm Hg), was found in 77% of RVH and 38% of EH patients; however, when a positive response was defined as a response higher than that obtained in EH patients, only 40% of RVH fulfilled this criteria. In addition, when considering the PRA response to captopril, 74% of RVH had a more marked response than

EH patients (+5.4 ng/ml/h). In an attempt to improve the sensitivity of the captopril test, patients with EH were divided according to age. We observed that the magnitude of the fall in mean arterial pressure as well as the rise in PRA induced by captopril tended to be blunted with increasing age in EH patients. When a positive response to captopril in terms of depressor effect or reactive hyperreninemia was defined as a response more marked than that observed in EH patients in the same age group, 52 and 80% of RVH patients respectively were considered as positive. These results demonstrated that the sensitivity of the test for identifying RVH patients was improved (from 40 to 52% for the depressor response and from 74 to 80% for the PRA response) when responses to captopril were analyzed according to age (Figure 1).

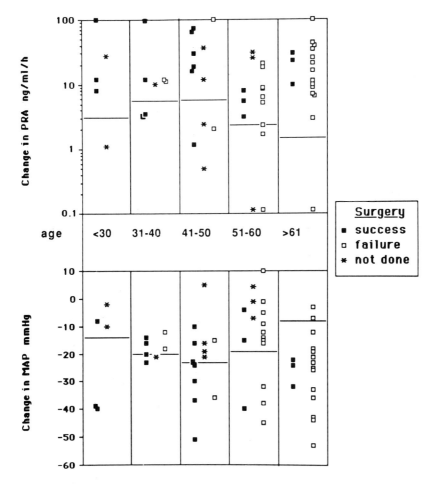

FIG. 1. Acute effect of captopril on mean arterial pressure (MAP) and plasma renin activity (PRA) and the detection of renovascular hypertension. Horizontal bars denote maximum change observed in patients with essential hypertension. Note that the effect of captopril on MAP and PRA is blunted with increasing age in essential hypertension.

In 1984, Wenting et al[8] reported on the acute effect of captopril on individual kidney function as assessed by the renal uptake of 99 mTc-DTPA (a reliable index of glomerular filtration rate) in 14 patients with unilateral renal artery stenosis. They observed that in 50% of patients, DTPA uptake of the affected side fell to almost zero; however, in the other half, no change in DTPA uptake occurred after administration of captopril. These two groups were indistinguishable with respect to the fall in arterial pressure induced by captopril, the degree of lateralization of renin secretion and the proportion of patients with atherosclerotic disease (6/7 in each group). In two recently reported studies, a positive scintigraphic acute captopril test (defined as a decrease in DTPA uptake of the stenotic side by more than 20%) was observed in 10/12[9] and 14/21[10] patients with unilateral renal artery stenosis; no change in DTPA uptake was observed in EH patients. In both studies, no false positive test was found; however, the incidence of false negative results was 17[9] and 43%[10]. In contrast with this rather high incidence of false negative scintigraphic tests, Miyamori et al[11] and Jackson et al[12] showed that chronic ACEI therapy for 1 and 6 weeks respectively was associated with a constant fall in the glomerular filtration rate of the stenotic side in patients with unilateral renal artery stenosis.

Overall, no relationship between the change in glomerular filtration rate (GFR) of the stenotic side and changes in systemic pressure induced by ACEI was demonstrated. Since the degree of anatomical stenosis was not reported, it is possible to speculate that profound changes in the filtration rate of the stenotic kidney, only occur in patients with tight narrowing of the renal artery.

In conclusion, the observation of a lateralized fall in DTPA uptake following acute or chronic CEI in a hypertensive patient is highly suggestive of the existence of renal artery stenosis; however, a negative test does not exclude it.

CONVERTING ENZYME INHIBITION IN THE PREDICTION OF CURABILITY OF RENOVASCULAR HYPERTENSION

In contrast to the rather poor diagnostic usefulness of acute blockade of the renin-angiotensin system in the diagnosis of unilateral renal artery stenosis, a good relationship between the level of arterial pressure achieved during chronic ACE inhibition and after correction of the stenosis by surgery or percutaneous transluminal angioplasty (PTA) was found by Atkinson et al[13] and Staessen et al.[14]

In a recent study, Geyskes et al[10] observed that a consistent fall in the glomerular filtration rate of the stenotic kidney occurred in response to acute administration of captopril in 12/15 patients with unilateral RVH who were cured by PTA. A negative test was found in 6/6 patients who did not respond favorably to PTA. This suggests that an initially normal captopril renogram is highly predictive of a poor effect of PTA on arterial pressure in patients with unilateral renal artery stenosis.

ANGIOTENSIN-CONVERTING ENZYME INHIBITORS AS LONG TERM TREATMENT IN PATIENTS WITH UNILATERAL RENAL ARTERY STENOSIS

There are a few reports on the effect of long-term ACEIs in patients with unilateral renal artery stenosis or occlusion. In the study of Atkinson et al[13] on 15 patients, treatment with captopril as monotherapy was associated with no change in serum creatinine; similar results were obtained by Reams et al.[15] In contrast with these results, a slight decrease in the overall GFR was observed after 48 weeks of treatment in 3/5 patients with unilateral stenosis; split renal function studies showed that captopril induced a slight fall in the GFR of the stenotic kidney with no change in the function of the non-stenotic side.[11] In a larger trial comparing the effect of 6 weeks treatment with enalapril plus hydrochlorothiazide (49 patients) and standard triple therapy (STT, hydrochlorothiazide, timolol and hydralazine, 39 patients) a rise in serum creatinine of more than 0.3 mg/100 ml was observed in 20% of patients in the enalapril group and 3% of patients in the STT group. The hallmark in enalapril-treated patients (7/10 with unilateral lesions) who developed a deterioration in renal function, was evidence of 80–100% renal artery stenosis.[16]

Taken together, these observations suggest that an ACE inhibitor induced reduction in the function of the stenotic kidney may not be fully compensated for by a rise in the GFR in the contralateral kidney despite a consistant increase in renal plasma flow of both kidneys.[11] The concomitant use of diuretics may facilitate a change in overall renal function. Finally, the fall in GFR in the stenotic kidney is rapidly reversible upon discontinuation of ACEI treatment.[8] Nevertheless, occlusion of the stenotic kidney was reported in a few patients with RVH during chronic ACE inhibitor therapy. Such a complication was observed in 1/15 patients with unilateral stenosis treated with enalapril for 3 months.[17] Three other cases were reported in patients with 75–90% atherosclerotic stenosis, and a 13–21-week period of treatment with captopril plus hydrochlorothiazide was associated with a marked fall in systemic pressure.[18] It is rather difficult to prove that ACEI treatment contributed to the occlusion of the severely stenotic renal arteries in these patients. It has been reported that administration of the beta-blocker, atenolol, associated with an acute and profound fall in systemic pressure was complicated by anuria resulting from thrombosis of a single functioning stenotic kidney.[19] In addition, the possibility that occlusion of a stenotic renal artery occurs as a consequence of the natural course of the disease has to be considered. In a report on long-term follow up of 169 patients with renal artery stenosis treated by antihypertensive medications only, Schreiber et al[20] observed that 16% of 85 patients with atherosclerotic stenosis progressed to occlusion within a follow-up period of 52 months; however, 39% of cases with 75–99% initial stenosis developed total occlusion within a mean follow-up period of 13 months. No difference in the blood pressure level achieved during treatment was found between those patients in whom disease progressed and those in whom it did not. By contrast, in none of the 84 patients with fibrous dysplasia did their disease progress to renal artery occlusion within a 45-month period of follow-up. These authors concluded that the risk of progression to total occlusion was particularly high in atherosclerotic renal arteries with more than 75% stenosis on the initial angiogram and the greater the degree of stenosis, the more quickly total occlusion occurred.

In favor of a role of ACEI in the development of profound functional deterioration of the clipped kidney are experimental studies conducted in rats with 2-kidney-1-clip hypertension. Michel et al[21] and Jackson et al[22] showed that irreversible cessation of renal function and atrophy of the clipped kidney only developed during treatment with ACE inhibitors in contrast to minoxidil therapy; however, ACE inhibitors but not the association of clonidine, hydralazine and furosemide prevented the development of hypertensive microangiopathy of the unclipped kidney.[21] Such observations suggest that inhibition of the circulating renin-angiotensin system may have a deleterious effect on the stenotic kidney whilst protecting the intact contralateral kidney against the development of nephroangiosclerosis in unilateral renal artery stenosis in experimental animals. Transposition of these results to human renovascular hypertension remains to be demonstrated.

CONVERTING ENZYME INHIBITORS IN BILATERAL RENOVASCULAR HYPERTENSION

In 1983, Hricik et al[23] reported on the occurrence of reversible and non-oliguric acute renal failure in seven patients with bilateral renal artery stenosis and three patients with stenosis of a single functioning kidney. In all cases, captopril was given in patients already receiving a diuretic and in whom renal function was abnormal prior to ACEI treatment. Arterial pressure consistently fell in response to ACEI in six of these ten patients thus suggesting that a decrease in systemic pressure may not be a prerequisite for the development of acute renal failure. It appeared, however, that the most critical factor was the presence in all patients of very tight narrowing of the renal arteries (more than 90%). Such an observation was followed by several concurring reports.[11,12,15,16,24] The incidence of renal deterioration associated with the use of ACEI in patients with bilateral renal artery stenosis is variable as shown in Table I; however, in only four studies[12,16,24,25] was a systematic assessment of the effect of ACEI on renal function performed.

Bilateral renal artery stenosis is four times less frequent than the unilateral form and is usually found in patients with atherosclerotic disease; in addition, approximately 15% of patients with renovascular hypertension present with a single functioning kidney.[4] It has been shown that 48% of patients with bilateral stenosis present with a deterioration of renal function, in contrast with only 16% of patients with essential hypertension.[26] This suggests that in

TABLE I. *Incidence of deterioration in renal function induced by converting-enzyme inhibitor (CEI) treatment in bilateral renal artery stenosis*

	CEI-Induced Renal Failure	Prior Renal Failure	Diuretic Treatment
Hricik et al. (1983)	7/7	7/7	All
Reams et al. (1986)	0/4	Not reported	All
Jackson et al. (1986)	3/11	3/3	Not mentioned
Franklin et al. (1986)	3/10	3/3	All
Miyamori et al. (1986)	3/3	3/3	None
Dominiczak et al. (1988)	13/14	7/14	50% of patients
Ribstein et al. (1988)	5/12	10/12	None

patients who present with hypertension resistant to conventional triple therapy and with impaired renal function, the use of ACE inhibitors should be carefully monitored especially if diuretic treatment is continued and regardless of the effect of ACEI on arterial pressure. If renal function rapidly deteriorates, and this deterioration can be reversed after discontinuation of ACEI, then the existence of bilateral renal artery stenosis or stenosis of a single functioning kidney should be suspected. In fact, ACEI-induced renal failure may be reversible even after prolonged use of up to two years as reported by Salahudeen and Pingle.[27] The possibility exists, however, that ACEI-induced renal failure could develop in patients without renovascular disease who are sodium-depleted prior to ACEI and in whom arterial pressure decreases in response to ACEI.[28,29]

At the present time, no study on the prevalence of bilateral stenosis or stenosis of a single functioning kidney in patients who develop renal deterioration during ACEI treatment has been reported. Such a study could be helpful in order to avoid systematic angiography in those patients at risk of developing contrast medium-induced renal failure because of age and prior sodium depletion.

CONVERTING ENZYME INHIBITORS IN RENAL TRANSPLANTATION

The overall incidence of hypertension 6–12 months after grafting varies between 40 and 60%; however, it is lower in recipients of living donors and in subjects who have undergone bilateral nephrectomy prior to transplantation.[30,31] A direct relationship between prednisone dosage and blood pressure was found by some groups; however, others denied a role for steroids in patients followed for a longer period.[31] In recent years, the use of cyclosporin was associated with a significant increase in the overall incidence of hypertension.[32] Although the most frequent cause of post-transplant hypertension is chronic rejection, excessive renin secretion by the native kidneys and stenosis of the transplant renal artery are important in the development of hypertension. The incidence of transplant renal artery stenosis is variable, ranging from 2 to 20%; a significant number of patients, however, may still be normotensive despite significant (more than 50%) narrowing of the renal artery.[33] Transplant renal artery stenosis usually occurs within 6 months after operation and is associated with a slight decrease in renal function when narrowing of more than 80% exists; an improvement in renal function is often observed following correction of the stenosis by surgery or PTA.

1 Converting Enzyme Inhibition in Patients Without Renal Artery Stenosis

In this situation, the presence of host kidneys as well as chronic rejection are considered the most frequent causes of hypertension. In recent reports, it was demonstrated that excision[34] or embolization[35] of native kidneys is associated with a fall in arterial pressure and renal vasodilatation whilst GFR remains unchanged. A similar effect was observed following acute administration of captopril[34] in transplant recipients maintained on conventional immunosuppressive agents (azathioprine and prednisone). These findings prompted us to assess the long-term action of ACE inhibition by enalapril in a group of six hypertensive transplant recipients in whom renal artery stenosis had been ruled out by digitalized intravenous angiography in order to prevent the often-reported occurrence of ACEI-induced acute renal failure.[36] As shown in Table II, acute ACE inhibition by captopril was associated with a significant fall in arterial pressure, a rise in renal plasma flow by approximately 50% and no change in GFR; as a consequence, calculated filtration fraction decreased markedly. After a mean period of 22 ± 3 months of enalapril treatment, arterial pressure remained well controlled whilst the renal vasodilatory effect of ACEI was maintained and GFR was unaffected. These results demonstrate

TABLE II. *Effect of acute and chronic (16–35 months) converting-enzyme inhibitor treatment in 6 hypertensive renal transplant recipients on conventional immunosuppressive therapy (azathioprine and prednisone)*

	Control	Acute Captopril	Chronic Enalapril
Mean arterial pressure, mmHg	119 ± 3	$104 \pm 2^*$	$101 \pm 5^*$
Creatinine clearance, ml/min/1.73 m²	77 ± 3	81 ± 10	82 ± 7
Effective renal plasma flow, ml/min/1.73 m²	227 ± 14	$344 \pm 35^*$	$334 \pm 36^*$
Filtration fraction	0.35 ± 0.01	$0.21 \pm 0.03^*$	$0.25 \pm 0.02^*$
Plasma renin activity, ng/ml/h	14.8 ± 3.3	$25.8 \pm 6.1^*$	18.8 ± 1.4

Values are expressed as mean $\pm$ sem.
*$p < 0.05$ when compared to control.

that the systemic and renal effects of enalapril were sustained over a period of up to 35 months; the observed fall in filtration fraction suggests that endogenous generation of angiotensin II predominantly constricts the efferent glomerular arteriole of the transplanted kidney. Such a fall in post-glomerular tone may probably result in a decrease in intraglomerular capillary pressure, an effect that could ultimately be potentially beneficial for the survival of the transplanted kidney. There are similarities between the effect of ACEI and the renal functional changes associated with removal of host kidneys reported by Curtis *et al.*[34] It is then logical to assume that in the absence of any deleterious effect of chronic ACEI treatment, this drug may be considered as a good alternative to nephrectomy in hypertensive transplant recipients without renal artery stenosis. It should, however, be mentioned that, in addition to renal artery stenosis, ACEI treatment may be complicated by reversible deterioration of renal function in transplant patients with chronic rejection,[37] a situation associated with multiple narrowing of intrarenal small vessels.

In the future, it would be interesting to assess the effect of ACEI treatment in hypertensive patients maintained on cyclosporin, an immunosuppressive regimen associated with lower levels of renin when compared to patients on conventional treatment.[38]

2 Converting Enzyme Inhibition in Transplant Renal Artery Stenosis

There are numerous reports on the occurrence of acute renal deterioration during ACEI treatment in transplant renal artery stenosis.[23,25,39,40,41] As summarized in Table III, a decrease in GFR of more than 20% was observed in almost all patients in three studies during acute[41] or chronic[39,40] ACEI. In our experience, acute administration of captopril was associated with a fall in GFR of more than 20% in 7/8 patients and anuria developed in one patient in whom no fall in arterial pressure occurred (Figure 2). In contrast with most reports, Schwietzer et al[42] observed no change in GFR after acute ACEI in eight patients. Analysis of cases of ACEI-induced acute renal deterioration shows that this complication may occur in the absence of a fall in systemic pressure and is facilitated by the concomitant use of diuretics.[43]

TABLE III. *Converting-enzyme inhibition (CEI) in transplant renal artery stenosis: incidence of renal function deterioration*

	Number of Patients	CEI Treatment	Diuretic Treatment	Deterioration of GFR
Curtis et al. (1983)	9	Chronic	1/9	9/9 (3 anuric)
Van der Woude et al. (1985)	4	Chronic	4/4	4/4 (nonoliguric)
Schweitzer et al. (1985)	8	Acute	4/4	0/8
Mourad et al. (1988)	8	Acute	0/8	7/8 (1 anuric)

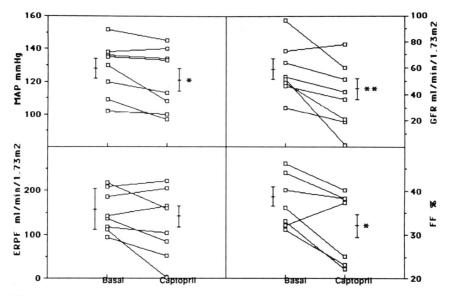

FIG. 2. Acute effect of converting-enzyme inhibitor (captopril) on mean arterial pressure (MAP), creatinine clearance (glomerular filtration rate — GFR), hippuran clearance (effective renal plasma flow — ERPF), and filtration fraction (FF) in transplant renal artery stenosis.

It is reasonable to assume that the development of renal failure after acute ACEI or within a few days of treatment, is highly suggestive of the existence of significant narrowing of the transplant renal artery. Such a complication should lead to renal angiography and ultimately correction of the stenosis by percutaneous angioplasty or surgery; a procedure often associated with a consistent improvement in GFR,[41] and the subsequent possibility of using ACE inhibitors without a risk of deterioration in renal function.[10,41] In a few transplant patients who developed acute renal impairment during ACEI treatment, no evidence of significant renal artery stenosis was found when arteriographic study was performed; such a situation may be encountered in chronic rejection.[37]

MECHANISM OF IMPAIRMENT IN RENAL FUNCTION ASSOCIATED WITH ACEI TREATMENT

Acute or chronic treatment with ACE inhibitors is usually associated with no change in GFR, renal vasodilatation and consequently a fall in the filtration fraction in patients with essential hypertension.[44] In subjects with moderate renal impairment of non-stenotic origin, a rise in GFR may be observed during chronic ACE inhibition.[45] In the presence of renal artery stenosis, of

MAP: mean arterial pressure; GFR: glomerular filtration rate;
ERPF: effective renal plasma flow; FF Filtration fraction
■ SK solitary kidney; □ BS bilateral renal artery stenosis
changes are expressed in percent and shown as mean ± sem

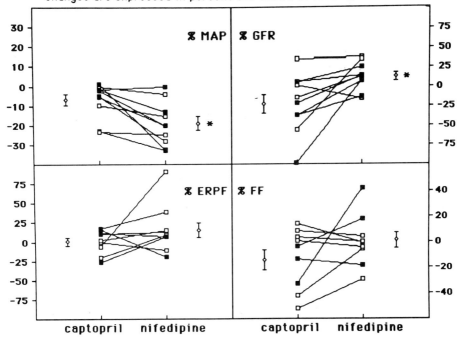

FIG. 3. Comparison of the acute effect of captopril and nifedipine on renal function in patients with bilateral artery stenosis and stenosis of a solitary kidney.

sufficient degree, the GFR of the stenotic kidney is often impaired, sometimes leading to cessation of function during treatment with ACE inhibitors in some patients with unilateral renal artery stenosis or in the kidney with the most marked arterial narrowing in bilateral disease. As emphasized by several groups, the ACE inhibitor-induced fall in GFR is usually associated with no change or an increase in renal plasma flow and it is not correlated with changes in systemic pressure.[25] In addition, the change in GFR induced by ACE inhibition is inversely correlated with the pretreatment filtration fraction (ie GFR decreased in patients with a high basal filtration fraction) in patients with bilateral stenosis and stenosis of single functioning kidney including renal transplant recipients.[25] These observations are compatible with an important role of intrarenal angiotensin II generation in the regulation of GFR through a marked tonic effect on the efferent glomerular arteriole in a situation associated with a decrease in intrarenal perfusion pressure below a critical level (ie significant renal artery stenosis).

It has been shown, in experimental sodium-depleted two-kidney, two-clip hypertensive rats that a similar reduction of arterial pressure by inhibitors of the renin-angiotensin system or direct vasodilators (hydralazine or minoxidil) is associated with renal function impairment only during treatment with ACE inhibitors.[46] In patients with bilateral renal artery stenosis[25] or stenosis of a transplanted kidney,[41] it was observed that despite a more marked fall in arterial pressure associated with the acute administration of the calcium entry blocker nifedipine, no consistent change in GFR occurred, whilst acute ACE inhibitors induced a marked fall in GFR in most patients (Figure 3). Such a contrasting effect of ACE inhibitors and calcium blockers on renal function in patients with renovascular hypertension probably results from a difference in their intrarenal site of action. Both agents are renal vasodilators; ACE inhibitors, however, predominantly dilate the efferent arteriole thus lowering glomerular capillary pressure and ultimately GFR whilst calcium antagonists preferentially dilate the afferent arteriole, thus resulting in an unchanged intraglomerular capillary pressure.[47] Thus, in the presence of a fall in systemic pressure, the site of action of the antihypertensive agent is probably critical with regard to its ability to induce a deterioration of GFR.

REFERENCES

1. Davis BA, Crook JE, Vestal RE, Oates JA: Prevalence of renovascular hypertension in patients with grade III or IV hypertensive retinopathy. *N Engl J Med* 1979; **301**:1273–1276.
2. Dustan HP, Humphries AW, De Wolfe VG, Page IH: Normal arterial pressure in patients with renal arterial stenosis. *J Am Med Assoc* 1964; **187**:138–143.
3. Marks LS, Maxwell MH: Renal vein renin value and limitations in the prediction of operative results. *Urol Clin N Am* 1975; **2**:311–325.
4. Grim CE, Weinberger MH: Renal artery stenosis and hypertension. Semin Nephrol 1983; **3**:52–64.
5. Case DB, Atlas SA, Laragh JH: Reactive hyperreninaemia to angiotensin blockade identifies renovascular hypertension. *Clin Sci* 1979; **57**:313s–316s.
6. Muller FB, Sealey JE, Case DB, Atlas SA, TG Pickering, Pecker MS, Preibisz JJ, Laragh JH: The captopril test for identifying renovascular disease in hypertensive patients. *Am J Med* 1986; **80**:633–644.
7. Mimran A, Klouche K, Beigbeder JY, Ribstein J: Acute effect of captopril in the detection of renovascular hypertension. In Noninvasive Investigations in Hypertension Evaluation and Prospective Views. Proceedings of Symposium. Courchevel France, 25–27 January 1985, pp 155–160.
8. Wenting GJ, Tan-Tjiong HL, Derkx FHM, De Bruyn JHB, Man in't Veld AJ, Schalekamp MADH: Split renal function after captopril in unilateral renal artery stenosis. *Br Med J* 1984; **288**:886–890.
9. Fommei E, Ghione S, Palla L, Mosca F, Ferrari M, Palombo C, Giaconi S, Gazzetti P, Donato L: Renal scintigraphic captopril test in the diagnosis of renovascular hypertension. *Hypertension* 1987; **10**:212–220.
10. Geyskes GG, Oei HY, Puylaert BAR, Mees EJD: Renovascular hypertension identified by captopril-induced changes in the renogram. *Hypertension* 1987; **9**:451–458.
11. Miyamori I, Yasuhara S, Takeda Y, Koshida H, Ikeda M, Nagal K, Okamoto H, Morise T,

Takeda R, Aburano T: Effects of converting enzyme inhibition on split renal function in renovascular hypertension. *Hypertension* 1986; **8**:415–421.

12. Jackson B, McGrath BP, Matthews P, Wong C, Johnston CI: Differential renal function during angiotensin converting enzyme inhibition in renovascular hypertension. *Hypertension* 1986; **8**:650–654.

13. Atkinson AB, Brown JJ, Cumming AMM, Fraser R, Lever AF, Leckie BJ, Morton JJ, Robertson JIS: Captopril in renovascular hypertension: long-term use in predicting surgical outcome. *Br Med J* 1982; **284**:689–693.

14. Staessen J, Bulpitt C, Fagard R, Lijnen P, Amery A: Long-term converting enzyme inhibition as a guide to surgical curability of hypertension associated with renovascular disease. *Am J Cardiol* 1983; **51**:1317–1322.

15. Reams GP, Bauer JH, Gaddy P: Use of the converting enzyme inhibitor enalapril in renovascular hypertension. Effect on blood pressure, renal function, and the renin-angiotensin-aldosterone system. *Hypertension* 1986; **8**:290–297.

16. Franklin SS, Smith RD: A comparison of enalapril plus hydrochlorothiazide with standard triple therapy in renovascular hypertension. *Nephron* 1986; **44 (suppl 1)**:73–82.

17. Hodsman GP, Brown JJ, Cumming AMM, Davies DL, East BM, Lever AF, Morton JJ, Murray GD, Robertson I, Robertson JIS: Enalapril in the treatment of hypertension with renal artery stenosis. *Br Med J* 1983; **287**:1413–1417.

18. Hoefnagels WHL, Thien T: Renal artery occlusion in patients with renovascular hypertension treated with captopril. *Br Med J* 1986; **292**:24–25.

19. Shaw AB, Gopalka SK: Renal artery thrombosis caused by antihypertensive treatment. *Br Med J* 1982; **285**:1617.

20. Schreiber MJ, Pohl MA, Novick AC: The natural history of atherosclerotic and fibrous renal artery disease. Urol Clin North Am 1984; **11**:383–392.

21. Michel JB, Dussaule JC, Choudat L, Auzan C, Nochy D, Corvol P, Menard J: Effects of antihypertensive treatment in one-clip, two-kidney hypertension in rats. *Kidney Int* 1986; **29**:1011–1020.

22. Jackson B, Franze L, Sumithran E, Johnston CI: Pharmacologic nephrectomy with chronic angiotensin converting enzyme inhibitor treatment in the 2-kidney 1-clip hypertensive rat. Kyoto, International Society of Hypertension (Abstract 919), 1988.

23. Hricik DE, Browning PJ, Kopelman R, Goorno WE, Madias NE, Dzau VJ: Captopril-induced functional renal insufficiency in patients with bilateral renal-artery stenoses or renal-artery stenosis in a solitary kidney. *N Engl J Med* 1983; **308**:373–376.

24. Dominiczak A, Isles C, Gillen G, Brown JJ: Angiotensin converting enzyme inhibition and renal insufficiency in patients with bilateral renovascular disease. *J Human Hypertens* 1988; **2**:53–56.

25. Ribstein J, Mourad G, Mimran A: Contrasting acute effects of captopril and nifedipine on renal function in renovascular hypertension. *Am J Hypertens* 1988; **1**:239–244.

26. Ying CY, Tifft CP, Gavras H, Chobanian AV: Renal revascularization in the azotemic hypertensive patient resistant to therapy. *N Engl J Med* 1984; **311**:1070–1075.

27. Salahudeen AK, Pingle A: Reversibility of captopril-induced renal insufficiency after prolonged use in an unusual case of renovascular hypertension. *J Human Hypertens* 1988; **2**:57–59.

28. Murphy BF, Whitworth JA, Kincaid-Smith P: Renal insufficiency with combinations of angiotensin converting enzyme inhibitors and diuretics. *Br Med J* 1984; **288**:844–845.

29. Thind GS: Renal insufficiency during angiotensin-converting enzyme inhibitor therapy in hypertensive patients with no renal artery stenosis. *J Clin Hypertens* 1985; **4**:337–343.

30. Cohen S: Hypertension in renal transplant recipients: role of bilateral nephrectomy. *Br Med J* 1973; **3**:78–81.

31. Bachy C, Alexandre GPJ, Van Ypersele de Strihou C: Hypertension after renal transplantation. *Br Med J* 1976; **2**:1287–1289.

32. Chapman JR, Marcen R, Arias M, Raine AEG, Dunnill MS, Morris PJ: Hypertension in renal transplantation: a comparison of cyclosporine and conventional immunosuppression. *Transplantation* 1987; **43**:860–864.

33. Nerstrom B, Ladefoged J, Lund F: Vascular complications in 155 consecutive kidney transplantations. *Scand J Urol Nephrol* 1972; **6(suppl 15)**:65–74.

34. Curtis JJ, Luke RG, Diethelm AG, Whelchel JD, Jones P: Benefits of removal of native kidneys in hypertension after renal transplantation. *Lancet* 1985; **2**:739–742.

35. Thompson JF, Fletcher EWL, Wood RFM, Chalmers DHK, Taylor MH, Benjamin IS: Control of hypertension after renal transplantation by emolisation of host kidneys. *Lancet* 1987; **2**:424–427.
36. Ribstein J, Mourad G, Mion C, Mimran A: Chronic angiotensin converting enzyme inhibition as an alternative to native kidneys removal in post-transplant hypertension. *J Hypertens* 1986; **4(suppl 5)**:255–257.
37. Nath KA, Crumbley AJ, Murray BM, Sibley RK: Captopril and renal insufficiency. *N Engl J Med* 1983; **309**:666.
38. Bantle JP, Nath KA, Sutherland DER, Najarian JS, Ferris TF: Effects of cyclosporine on the renin-angiotensine-aldosterone system and potassium excretion in renal transplant recipients. *Arch Intern Med* 1985; **145**:505–508.
39. Curtis JJ, Luke RG, Whelchel JD, Jones P, Dustan HP: Inhibition of angiotensin-converting enzyme in renal-transplant recipients with hypertension. *N Engl J Med* 1983; **308**:377–381.
40. Van der Woude FJ, Van Son WJ, Tegzess AM, Donker AJM, Sloff MJH, Van der Slikke LB, Hoorntje SJ: Effect of captopril on blood pressure and renal function in patients with transplant renal artery stenosis. *Nephron* 1985; **39**:184–188.
41. Mourad G, Ribstein J, Argiles A, Mimran A, Mion C: Contrasting effects of acute angiotensin converting enzyme inhibitors and calcium antagonists in transplant renal artery stenosis. *Nephrol Dial Transplant* 1988 (in press).
42. Schwietzer G, Laass C, Kampf D, Bahr V, Schultze G, Molzahn M, Distler A: Does captopril reduce renal function in renovascular disease by postglomerular vasodilatation? *J Hypertens* 1985; **3(suppl 2)**:S139–S141.
43. Hricik DE: Captopril-induced renal insufficiency and the role of sodium balance. *Ann Intern Med* 1985; **103**:222–223.
44. Mimran A, Brunner HR, Turini GA, Waeber B, Brunner D: Effect of captopril on renal vascular tone in patients with essential hypertension. *Clin Sci* 1979; **57**:421s–423s.
45. Bauer JH: Role of angiotensin converting enzyme inhibitors in essential and renal hypertension. *Am J Med* 1984; **77**:43–51.
46. Helmchen U, Grone HJ, Kirchertz EJ, Bader H, Bohle RM, Kneissler U, Khosla M: Contrasting renal effects of different antihypertensive agents in hypertensive rats with bilaterally constricted renal arteries. *Kidney Int* 1982; **22(suppl 12)**:198–205.
47. Loutzenhiser RD, Epstein M: Calcium antagonists and renal hemodynamics. *Am J Physiol* 1985; **249**:F619–F629.

SUMMARY

At the present time, it is reasonable to assert that angiotensin converting enzyme (ACE) inhibitors are useful in the detection of patients with renovascular hypertension despite the rather large proportion of positive vasopressor responses in patients with essential hypertension. The occurrence of a positive response to acute administration of an ACE inhibitor in a patient with hypertension of recent onset, or accelerated hypertension and a significant difference in kidney size, is highly suggestive of unilateral renal artery stenosis. Such a combination should discourage the use of these agents as long-term treatment although no definite evidence has been provided that administration of ACE inhibitors is responsible for the rare cases of total renal occlusion. On the other hand, the acute development of a deterioration of renal function following administration of ACE inhibitors, especially in patients with already impaired renal function, should encourage a search for bilateral stenosis or stenosis of a single functioning kidney. In the latter condition, ACE inhibitor-induced renal failure almost always occurs when functionally significant renal artery narrowing is present. In the last few years, the occurrence of ACE inhibitor-associated renal impairment has been helpful, particularly in renal transplant recipients and patients with a single functioning kidney, because correction of the stenosis often results in a significant improvement in renal function. In such patients with a reduced number of functioning nephrons, correction of the stenosis may allow long-term treatment with ACE inhibitors in an attempt to protect function of the remaining nephrons through a reduction in intraglomerular capillary pressure. Further studies are needed to document this assumption.

RÉSUMÉ

Il est raisonnable, à présent, d'affirmer que les inhibiteurs de l'enzyme de conversion de l'angiotensine sont utiles pour la détection de patients atteints d'hypertension rénovasculaire en dépit du nombre important de réponses favorables aux vasopresseurs parmi les hypertendus essentiels. Une réponse positive à une administration aigue d'un inhibiteur de l'enzyme de conversion de l'angiotensine dans le cas d'une hypertension à un stade précoce ou d'une hypertension accélérée et une importante différence de la taille du rein font évoquer une sténose unilatérale des artères rénales. Une telle combinaison devrait décourager l'utilisation de ces agents pour les traitements à long terme bien que jusqu'à présent rien ne prouve que l'administration d'inhibiteurs de l'enzyme de conversion de l'angiotensine soit responsable des rares cas d'occlusion rénale complète qui se soient porduits. D'un autre côté, le développement aigu d'une dégradation de la fonction rénale à la suite de l'administration d'inhibiteurs de l'enzyme de conversion de l'angiotensine, en particulier chez les malades déjà atteints d'insuffisance rénale, devrait encourager la recherche d'une sténose bilatérale ou d'une sténose sur rein unique. Dans le deuxième cas, l'insuffisance rénale induite par l'inhibiteur de l'enzyme de conversion de l'angiotensine se produit presque toujours lorsqu'il y a un rétrécissement important de l'artère rénale. Ces dernières années, l'apparition de l'insuffisance rénale associée à l'inhibiteur de l'enzyme de conversion de l'angiotensine s'est avéré utile, en particulier dans le cas des transplantés rénaux et des patients à rein fonctionnel unique, parce que la correction de la sténose entraîne souvent une importante amélioration de la fonction rénale. Parmi les patients à masse néphronique réduite, la correction de la sténose peut permettre un traitement à long terme avec les inhibiteurs de l'enzyme de conversion de l'angiotensine. Ils auront pour effet de protéger la fonction des néphrons restants par une réduction capillaire intraglomérulaire. Il s'avère nécessaire de faire des études complémentaires afin d'établir la validité de ces hypothèses.

ZUSAMMENFASSUNG

Zum gegenwärtigen Zeitpunkt ist es vernünftig, davon auszugehen, dass Inhibitoren des angiotensinkonvertierenden Enzyms (ACE) nützlich sind für die Diagnose von Patienten mit reno-vaskulärer Hypertonie, trotz des ziemlich grossen Anteils an positiven Vasopressor-Reaktionen bei Patienten mit essentieller Hypertonie. Das Vorliegen einer positiven Reaktion auf akute Zufuhr eines ACE-Inhibitors in einem Patienten mit kürzlichem Einsetzen der Hypertonie oder beschleunigte Hypertonie und eine deutliche Differenz in der Nierengrösse macht es sehr wahrscheinlich, dass eine unilaterale renale Arterienstenose vorliegt. Solch eine Kombination sollte die Verwendung von diesen Mitteln als Langzeitbehandlung nicht empfehlen, obwohl andererseits kein definitiver Beweis dafür vorliegt, dass Behandlung mit ACE-Inhibitoren für die seltenen Fälle totaler Nierenokklusion verantwortlich ist. Andererseits sollte die akute Entwicklung einer Verschlechterung der Nierenfunktion als Reaktion auf die Zufuhr von ACE-Inhibitoren, besonders in Patienten mit schon vorher krankhafter Nierenfunktion, eine Suche nach bilateraler Stenose oder Stenose einer einzigen funktionierenden Niere einleiten. Liegt der letztere Fall vor, dann tritt Nierenversagen, durch ACE-Inhibitoren hervorgerufen, fast immer in Erscheinung, wenn auch eine funktional signifikante Nieren-Arterienverengung anwesend ist. In den letzten paar Jahren ist die Erscheinung der ACE-Inhibitor-induzierten Nierenverletzung hilfreich gewesen, besonders bei Empfängern eines Nierentransplantats und bei Patienten mit nur einer funtionierenden Niere, denn die Korrektur der Stenose hat oft eine bedeutende Verbesserung der Nierenfunktion zur Folge. In solchen Patienten, die eine begrenzte Anzahl funktionierender Nephronen zur Verfügung haben, kann die Korrektur der Stenose eine Langzeitbehandlung mit ACE-Inhibitoren möglich machen, indem man versucht, die Funktion der verbleibenden Nephronen durch eine Reduktion des intraglomerulären Kapillardrucks zu schützen. Um diese Annahme zu stützen, sind weitere Studien nötig.

RIASSUNTO

Al presente, è ragionevole asserire che gli inibitori di enzima angiotensin-convertente (EAC) sono utili nella scoperta di pazienti con ipertensione renovascolare malgrado la proporzione assai grande di positive risposte vasopressori nei pazienti con ipertensione essenziale. L'evento di una risposta positiva all'acuta somministrazione di un inibitore EAC in un paziente con ipertensione di attacco recente, oppure con ipertensione accelerata e una differenza significativa della grandezza del rene, è molto suggestivo di stenosi unilaterale dell'arteria renale. Tale combinazione dovrebbe scoraggiare l'uso di questi agenti come trattamento di lunga durata, benché non si sia provvista nessun evidenza definita che la somministrazione degli inibitori EAC è responsabile per i rari casi di totale occlusione renale. Per contro, l'acuto sviluppo di una deteriorazione di funzione renale dopo la somministrazione degli inibitori EAC, particolarmente nei pazienti con funzione renale giá indebolita, dovrebbe incoraggiare una ricerca di stenosi bilaterale oppure di stenosi di un solo rene funzionale. Nella seconda condizione, il fallimento renale indotto dagli inibitori EAC accade quasi sempre quando è presente un restringimento funzionalmente significativa dell'arteria renale. Negli ultimi anni, l'evento di debolezza renale associata con l'inibitore EAC è stato utile, particolarmente nei ricevitori di trapianti renali eppure nei pazienti con un solo rene funzionale, perchè la correzione della stenosi risulta spesso in un miglioramento significativo di funzione renale. In tali pazienti con un numero ridotto di nefroni funzionali, la correzione della stenosi permetta un trattamento di lunga durata con gli inibitori EAC in un tentativo di proteggere la funzione dei nefroni rimanenti tramite una riduzione nella pressione capillare intraglomerulare. Ulteriori studi sono necessari per documentare quest'-assunzione.

SUMÁRIO

Atualmente, é razoável afirmar que os inibidores da enzima convertidora da angiotensina (ACE) são úteis na detecção de paceintes com hipertensão renovascular, apesar da proporção bastante elevada de respostas vasopressoras positivas em pacientes com hipertensão essencial. A ocorrência de uma resposta positiva à administração aguda de um inibidor da ACE a um paciente com hipertensão de início recente, ou uma hipertensão acelerada com uma diferença significativa no tamanho do rim, é muito sugestiva de uma estenose unilateral da arteria renal. Tal combinação deve desaconselhar o uso destes agentes como tratamento a largo prazo, ainda que não tem-se proporcionado evidência definitiva de que a administração de inibidores da ACE seja responsável dos casos raros de oclusão renal total. Por outro lado, o desenvolvimento agudo de debilitação da função renal após da administração de inibidores da ACE, especialmente em pacientes com função renal já debilitada, deve estimular a busca de estenose bilateral ou estenose do único rim em funcionamento. Nesta última condição, a insuficiência renal induzida por inibidores da ACE quase sempre ocorre quando houver um estreitamento funcionalmente significativo da arteria renal. Nos últimos anos, a presença de debilitação renal associada com inibidores da ACE têm sido útil, particularmente em receptores de transplantes renais e pacientes com um único rim em funcionamento, porque a correção da estenose muitas vezes resulta numa melhoria significativa da função renal. Em tais pacientes com um reduzido número de nefros em funcionamento, a correção da estenose poderia permitir o tratamento a largo prazo com inibidores da ACE num intento de proteger a função dos restantes nefros através da redução da pressão capilar intraglomerular. Precisam-se estudos adicionais para documentar esta hipótese.

RESUMEN

En estos momentos es razonable asegurar que los inhibidores de la enzima convertidora de la angiotensina (ACE) son útiles en la detección de pacientes con hipertensión renovascular, a pesar de la proporción bastante elevada de respuestas vasopresoras positivas en pacientes con hipertensión esencial. La obtención de una respuesta positiva a la administración aguda de un inhibidor de la ACE a un paciente con hipertensión de reciente aparición, o una hipertensión acelerada con una diferencia significativa en el tamaño del riñón, es muy sugestiva de una estenosis unilateral de la arteria renal. Tal combinación debería desalentar el empleo de estos agentes como tratamiento a largo plazo, aunque no se han proporcionado evidencias definitivas de que la administración de inhibidores de la ACE sea responsable de los pocos casos de oclusión renal total. Por otro lado, el desarrollo agudo de deterioro de la función renal después de la administración de inhibidores de la ACE, especialmente en pacientes con función renal ya deteriorada, debe alentar la búsqueda de estenosis bilateral o estenosis del único riñón en funcionamiento. En esta última condición, la insuficiencia renal inducida por inhibidores de la ACE casi siempre ocurre cuando se halla presente un estrechamiento funcionalmente significativo de la arteria renal. En los últimos años, la presencia de deterioro renal asociado con inhibidores de la ACE ha sido útil, particularmente en receptores de transplantes renales y pacientes con un único riñón en funcionamiento, debido a que la corrección de la estenosis a menudo resulta en una mejoría significativa de la función renal. En tales pacientes con un reducido número de nefrones en funcionamiento, la corrección de la estenosis podría permitir el tratamiento a largo plazo con inhibidores de la ACE en un intento de proteger la función de los restantes nefornes a través de la reducción de la presión capilar intraglomerular. Se necesitan estudios adicionales para documentar esta presunción.

要約

本態性高血圧患者でも血圧反応陽性率がかなり高いが, 現在, 腎血管性高血圧患者の発見にはアンジオテンシン変換酵素（ACE）阻害薬が有用であると考えられ れている。最近発症したか進行性の高血圧患者あるいは左右の腎の大きさが明らかに異なる高血圧患者において, ACE阻害薬の急性投与に対して陽性反応を示せば, 片側性腎動脈狭窄が強く示唆される。

　ACE 阻害薬が腎動脈の完全閉塞というまれな症例に関与しているという明らかな証拠はないが，このような高血圧と腎動脈狭窄の合併症では，長期治療にこれらの薬剤を使用することには問題がある。一方，すでに腎機能障害を有する患者で，ACE 阻害薬の投与後に腎機能低下が急速にすすむ場合には，両側性の腎動脈狭窄あるいは単腎性の腎動脈狭窄を考慮する必要がある。後者の場合，ACE 阻害薬誘発性の腎不全は，機能的に有意な腎動脈狭窄がある場合には必ず起こる。

　ここ数年，とくに腎移植患者や片側の腎しか機能しない患者などにおいて，ACE 阻害薬に伴う腎障害の発生が参考になるようになった。というのは，狭窄の修復が腎機能の著明な改善をしばしばもたらすからである。機能するネフロン数が減少している患者では，狭窄の修復によって，糸球体内毛細管圧を下げることにより，残存ネフロンの機能の保護をはかるという ACE 阻害薬の長期治療の可能性がでてきた。この仮説を証明するためには，さらに研究が必要である。

Cardiac and Renal Failure: An Expanding Role for ACE Inhibitors, edited by C. T. Dollery and L. M. Sherwood, Hanley & Belfus, Inc., Philadelphia.

Roundtable 3: *Role of ACE Inhibitors in Renal Disease*

Chairman: John G. G. Ledingham
Panelists: Paul De Jong, William Keane, J. Derek K. North, D. Keith Peters, Ronald D. Smith

The commonest causes of death in chronic renal failure are myocardial infarction, cardiac failure and stroke. The main risk factor for death in the dialysis and transplant population is probably high blood pressure. Dr. Ledingham summed this up by saying: "Blood pressure control is essential, whether or not it has a beneficial effect on the kidney."

Does Control of Hypertension Have a Beneficial Effect on Renal Function?

Dr. Smith suggested that the data on this aspect of antihypertensive therapy are mixed. In malignant hypertension it is undoubtedly beneficial, but other studies suggest that there is no such effect in the benign phase of the disease. He went on to describe these studies—Pettinger demonstrated no advantage of clonidine over diuretic plus vasodilator therapy; neither therapy prevented a decline in GFR. A study by Lundjund *et al.* showed that, despite control of blood pressure, GFR declined over a 7-year period in hypertensive males being treated with metoprolol. GFR also continued to decline in a series of diabetic patients being treated with captopril (Valvo), and blood pressure control in patients with renal disease other than with diabetes has failed to produce obvious benefit.

The difficulties involved in assessing the effect of antihypertensive treatment on renal function were underscored by Dr. North. He emphasized that there is a lack of good prospective studies involving large numbers of patients. He said, "There are no sound studies in which patients were grouped by the initial blood pressure and then followed to see if there were different rates of deterioration of renal function." Professor Dollery disagreed with this, and said, "I think there are substantial data, although not from randomized studies." He cited the records of patients attending a group of hypertension clinics, which together cover 10,000 patients. Analysis of death certificates showed renal failure to be an exceedingly rare cause of death in the 1000 chronically treated hypertensives who have died. Before antihypertensive treatment was available, renal failure was a fairly common cause of death in the moderately hypertensive population. There was agreement that renal failure was now an uncommon consequence of benign-phase hypertension, but this did not bear directly on the different question of whether or not blood pressure reduced the rate of loss of renal function in patients in whom hypertension was a consequence of primary and ongoing renal disease.

Assessment of such patients will be complicated by variations in the rate of deterioration of renal function, depending on the activity of the underlying disease. Although there is evidence supporting a beneficial effect of antihypertensive treatment in the earlier stages of diabetic nephropathy, this may not be obvious in advanced cases. Dr. Smith emphasized that there is a need to understand whether there is a common pathway for the progression of renal disease after the initial insult. Studies are underway to attempt to determine the mechanisms involved in renal failure of various etiologies, and these are linked with studies analyzing the specific effect of control of arterial pressure.

RELATIONSHIP OF RENAL FUNCTION WITH BLOOD PRESSURE

There is a need to control blood pressure to prevent stroke and heart disease. Dr. Ledingham posed the problem of the patient with progressive renal failure of glomerulonephritic origin, a GFR of 30 ml/min, and severe hypertension. "We know," he said, "in this context that in some situations the blood pressure can be lowered too far with respect to the cerebral [Ledingham and Rajagopalan, 1979] and perhaps also the coronary circulation [Hall et al., 1979; Cruikshank et al., 1987]. Might it be that lowering pressure beyond a certain point is also harmful to renal function?" In response to this, Dr. Mogensen suggested that data from young patients with diabetic nephropathy suggest that a target blood pressure should be 135/85 mm Hg. At this level, the progression of renal failure is very slow, provided that the diabetes is controlled. Dr. Keane's response to this question was that there is a range over which high blood pressure does cause damage to endothelial cells and vascular structures. The critical blood pressure above which this occurs in the kidney is not known.

Is One Treatment More Effective than Another?

Dr. Smith cited on-going studies in post-transplant and diabetic patients that compare the results of standard therapy with those achieved using enalapril. In the controlled study of type II diabetics (Lebowitz et al.), the standard

354 LEDINGHAM ET AL.

therapy group had a decrease in GFR of 14% over 12 months, in accordance with the literature. In contrast, the group treated with the ACE inhibitor had a GFR decline of only 5%. This is a significant difference, even though numbers are small. In response to this, Dr. Johnston doubted whether significant results can be obtained with small numbers of patients. "There are problems with the variability in proteinuria in these patients, and differences between treatments are likely to be small," he said. He went on "I believe that all the drugs slow the progression, so that [to detect] differences between them will require many patients and a long time."

DIETARY CONTROL AND RENAL FUNCTION

"Studies of protein restriction have not been successful because of problems with patient compliance and due to the confounding issue of blood pressure and its control," said Dr. Keane. Further discussion produced the consensus that, since control of blood pressure does seem to have a beneficial effect on renal function, antihypertensive treatment is a factor that must be taken into account in future studies of dietary effects. Other confounding factors include the diet itself—whether lipid, protein or both are controlled, and how the caloric intake is made up.

THE HYPERFILTRATION HYPOTHESIS

Some physicians believe that animal models of hyperfiltration are applicable to man. However, Dr. Keane doubted this and cited animal studies in various strains of rat, dogs, rabbits, and monkeys that suggest that it is not a universal mechanism. Micropuncture techniques have shown the presence of single nephron hyperfiltration in these animal models. Dr. Keane emphasized that "there are no studies in man which can approach this." However, giant glomeruli have been described in patients who have had 75% of their kidneys irradiated. "There may be some correlation," he said, "but data are sketchy." Glomerular sclerosis can be seen in type I diabetic patients, and a study by Myers has shown adaptive increases in glomerular size in biopsies from patients with various kidney diseases.

In response to this statement, Dr. Mogensen described long-term studies in patients who have undergone unilateral nephrectomy. These patients showed "profound hyperfiltration," with a GFR per nephron in the remaining kidney of twice the expected level. Dr. Ledingham confirmed that there are other data from trauma victims to support this finding. There does not appear to be an increase in proteinuria or in arterial blood pressure in these patients. Dr. Mimran stated that the data from transplant donors are quite variable—30–40% develop proteinuria >150 mg/day, and about 30% develop hypertension by 10 years. He suggested that there might be a "minimal microalbuminuric phase," and that age might also be involved.

THE PATHOLOGY OF MICROALBUMINURIA

Dr. Sonnenblick brought up the subject of pathology, saying that the diabetic rat develops very few vascular changes, and those that do occur are reversible with insulin therapy. The same is true of experimental renal hypertension. However, combining the two diseases leads to serious vascular abnormalities that affect many organs. How does the pathology relate to the presence of albumin in the urine?

Dr. Mogensen underlined the importance of microalbuminuria, which is often the first abnormality to be detected in diabetes and is a predictor of later changes. A "vicious circle" develops, in which albuminuria is followed by an increase in blood pressure. The greater this increase, the more rapid the increase in microalbuminuria. "Patients with microalbuminuria have quite advanced renal changes, both diffuse and nodular, and this had been shown in a study from Japan," he said.

How Might ACE Inhibitors Affect Glomerular Disease?

Dr. Ledingham outlined a number of potential ways in which an ACE inhibitor might reduce the rate of loss of renal function other than by reducing hyperfiltration by reduction of intraglomerular pressure and flows. These include:

- the influence of angiotensin II (ANG II) on the passage of macromolecules
- its role as a growth factor, or tissue mitogen
- its effects on tissue prostanoids
- an effect mediated via heparans and glomerular charge
- the local effects of lipoproteins in the glomerulus.

There is also some evidence to suggest that anaemia might preserve renal function (Brenner et al. Proc NY Acad Sci 1988).

Dr. Keane began the discussion on the mechanisms of ACE inhibition by considering the first of Dr. Ledingham's points—that ANG II may modulate the increased flux of macromolecules across the mesangium. Inhibition of ANG II by ACE inhibitors would therefore have an effect on this process. The effects have yet to be fully elucidated in terms of structural damage to the glomerulus, but in all experimental models mesangial expansion with proliferation of mesangial cells and increased numbers of monocytes and macrophages in the mesangium occur prior to the development of irreversible structural damage. Lipids also appear to affect this process, and the mesangial proliferation and accumulation of cells can be reduced by lipid lowering agents. Dr. Keane emphasized that most of these studies have been performed in animal models of the nephrotic syndrome and it is not known how they relate to man.

Dr. Thurau and Dr. Mogensen discussed this in relation to the interpretation of microalbuminuria. In healthy individuals, the transglomerular passage of albumin is very much higher than the amount seen in the urine. The presence of normal beta-2 microglobulin excretion in patients with microalbuminuria suggests that the defect is glomerular and not tubular. This was confirmed by Dr. Smith, who stated that "the resorptive capacities of the tubules are indeed intact in microproteinuria." He went on to cite a study which indicates that there might be important changes in the basement membrane. This study suggests that enalapril may alter the pattern of proteinuria towards greater selectivity.

SUMMARY

There was general agreement that control of blood pressure is likely to retard development of renal disease, but there was doubt as to the mechanisms underlying this. A need was also felt for more studies into the effectiveness of different antihypertensive agents in slowing the rate of renal deterioration.

Cardiac and Renal Failure: An Expanding Role for ACE Inhibitors, edited by C. T. Dollery and L. M. Sherwood, Hanley & Belfus, Inc., Philadelphia.

Pan-European Trials: Their Design, Execution and Relevance

Paul G. Hugenholtz, Jacobus Lubsen, Jan G.P. Tijssen, and John Lennane

THE TREATY OF ROME AND THE SINGLE EUROPEAN ACT

When it was signed in 1957, the Treaty of Rome expressed the deep desire of the major European nations to put an end to the fratricidal strife that had caused the deaths of millions of men and women, and wreaked irreparable destruction in recent wars. The hope was that complete and irreversible integration of the means of production would create conditions such as might prevent a repetition of such conflicts.

Furthermore, Jean Monnet, its architect, drew from his experience at the heart of combined allied operations in both World Wars the knowledge that interlocking the human and production resources of more than 300 million people could be the way forward for Western Europe. Initial high hopes and early successes, however, gave way, in the early seventies, to the virtual halting of the process of building the European Community as had been intended under the provisions of the Treaty of Rome; the oil crisis, partly responsible for the delay, brought with it world recession from which Western economies only began to emerge in 1984–85.

This disconcerting stagnation in progress towards a united Europe provoked in most of the countries involved a certain weary skepticism. Nevertheless, there was a spectacular change with the signature of the Single European Act; the headline of the *International Herald Tribune* of 18 May 1988 announced: "1992, the World's rendezvous with Europe." The year 1992 is the target date on which the European Commission in Brussels, under the leadership of Jacques Delors as current President of the European Commission, and Lord Cockfield, as Commissioner for the Internal Market, have clearly indicated various directives they wish to implement. The West German Chancellor Helmut Kohl, Britain's Prime Minister Margaret Thatcher, and France's recently re-elected President François Mitterand have strongly backed these moves.

Following this major step forward, the medical profession needs to make its own in-depth examination of the medium- and long-term consequences of European integration.

INCREASED CARDIOVASCULAR KNOWLEDGE, CO-OPERATION WITH THE PHARMACEUTICAL INDUSTRY, AND IMPROVED COST-EFFECTIVENESS

Cardiology and its related sciences, such as cardiac surgery, physiology, pharmacology, medical technology, biochemistry have in the Western World in the past decade distanced themselves from many other disciplines in the medical sciences. This is because, with the prevalence of cardiovascular disorders, rapid advances in scientific knowledge were embraced by the cardiovascular specialities much earlier and more fully than by any other medical discipline. The rapid development of many powerful drugs and techniques in the last two decades (by the European pharmaceutical industry in particular), the availability of a large group of well-trained specialists in the various countries of Europe, and a strong tradition of clinical research have propelled this movement forward.

We have now, either in hand or in sight, the means to modify and avoid hypertension, atherosclerosis, and the various acquired forms of heart disease with such efficacy that it would not surprise me if the total health expenditure for cardiovascular-related disorders after 2010 were half what it is now. Others will say that costs can only increase as new inventions keep piling up. But both opinions concur that it requires forward-looking cooperation to channel these forces and use them wisely to improve the cost-effectiveness of our management of the largest epidemic of our time.

With the recent advances in cardiology, it is important to develop a good understanding of the costs versus benefits early on. Otherwise newer and — medically but not economically — better techniques will replace older ones too rapidly, and by the year 2000 may have become too expensive even to contemplate, let alone implement. Nevertheless, the job of cardiologists is the same as that of all other specialists in medicine: to provide the best care to the patient, to prevent or shorten illness, and to promote a long and healthy life. So where is the balance? Who decides the trade off? And how can we continue to search for better products and techniques? What is the place of the multi-center, randomized clinical trial in Europe?

Let us look at a few examples of common cardiovascular disorders, on which the pharmaceutical industry of today and tomorrow is concentrating its efforts.

Angina Pectoris

As far as angina pectoris is concerned, it will become rapidly evident from the contributions in the recent annual congress of the European Society of Cardiology (which more than 8,500 cardiac scientists attended), that the diagnosis of angina pectoris and related syndromes has now advanced so far that with a relatively modest investment in terms of careful history taking, proper use of the electrocardiogram and the standardized exercise test, and, in rare instances where needed, nuclear techniques, this diagnosis can be made with a high degree of accuracy in most cases. Its prevalence (together with the silent forms) may be as high as 10% of the male population between 35 and 70 years of age. It has become equally clear that current policy all over Europe is to attempt therapy first by pharmacological means. Only if such therapy fails, so that there is increasingly severe exertional angina or rapidly progressing, pharmacologically refractory, unstable angina should a coronary angiogram be obtained. In that case, earlier rather than later "definitive" intervention such as percutaneous transluminal coronary angioplasty (PTCA) or coronary artery bypass grafting (CABG) becomes essential to save lives. Current and past investments in most of the Western European countries have made such facilities generally available for those who require them. A host of effective therapies thus present themselves.

It is remarkable how much agreement there is among European cardiologists about the available pharmacological armamentarium of nitrates, calcium antagonists and beta-blockers. Those compounds, now used worldwide, have all been found, developed, and perfected in Europe by the giants of the European pharmaceutical industry. It would be a great pity if the search for newer and better cardiovascular drugs were to be thwarted by plans now pending in several countries to require such stringent pricing structures that funds for further research dry up. Ideas, such as decreeing one price for all beta-blockers or all calcium-channel antagonists, are not only highly illogical, as these compounds vary greatly in their chemical composition, effects and side-effects, but would also penalize the inventiveness of the pharmacological research institutes, which are mostly driven by input from the cardiological community. The ESC, through its contacts in Brussels, will lobby strongly against such ill-conceived and destructive ideas, as these would be opposed to the proper interpretation of the Single European Act.

In fact, most patients with angina pectoris can be treated pharmacologically. Eventually, however (that is to say within the 12 months following onset of symptoms), a more definite procedure is required in nearly half of them. Although at first sight, pharmacological therapy, together with conservative measures such as changes in life-style, stopping cigarette smoking, dietary changes, and adjustment in work load would appear to be the more "economic" manner to proceed, ultimately a more cost-effective approach in many patients may consist of an intensive pharmacological trial followed by PTCA in single and two-vessel disease, with bypass grafts (preferably with mammary artery implantation for multivessel disease) in the subset that does not respond well to drugs. This is based on the now increasing evidence that such procedures, although still palliative, usually extend a useful and economically-beneficial life. Particularly with PTCA, the period of being out of work for the "operation" is negligible. A small initial increase in cost turns out to be cost-saving in the long run. Even with the increasing evidence that some 30% of patients with initially successful PTCA or CABG will ultimately require a repeat procedure, the benefits in terms of cost still outweigh the disadvantages, as is evident from Table I.

Acute Myocardial Infarction

A major revolution is now also underway in the management of acute myocardial infarction (MI). Long gone are the days when we could treat our patients' symptoms with morphine and await the outcome of acute or subacute obstruction of a major nutrient artery, whether it be death, a failing heart, or spontaneous recovery. Now it is scientifically feasible to treat patients who can reach a medical support system within the first few hours after the onset of symptoms typical of MI with a strategy aimed at early reperfusion in an effort to salvage as much myocardial tissue as possible. Data have now been presented from both sides of the Atlantic, with the European evidence most strongly indicating that early intravenous therapy with a thrombolytic agent — recombinant tissue plasminogen activator (rt-PA) being the leading contender at present — can achieve lysis of obstructing thrombi with consequent major saving of myocardial tissue (in fact the studies by the European Cooperative Study Group on rt-PA having provided an excellent example). This in turn limits infarct size and maintains both regional and global function. In the European randomized studies, there has been a consequent

TABLE I. *Comparison of cost effectiveness in 1986 of various therapies expressed as cost (in \$U.S.) per year of life gained (derived from data by Bigger, AHA; Kelly, J Am Coll Cardiol; ICIN data)*

1. Coronary artery bypass procedure	44,200
2. Cardiac transplantation	26,850
3. Treatment of mild hypertension	23,200
4. Treatment of moderate to severe hypertension	11,400
5. PTCA for stable/unstable angina	7,700
6. Thrombolysis and PTCA for inferior infarction	6,600
7. Thrombolysis and PTCA for anterior infarction	2,100

From this table it is evident that early reperfusion in myocardial infarction is the most economical of all seven major cardiac treatments when expressed as cost per year of life gained.

reduction in the death rate of as much as 50% both in the short- and long-term in those patients who were treated early. No other therapy has demonstrated such a large reduction in mortality of acute MI.

Furthermore, data from the Netherlands ICIN[2] trial have shown that there was a marked reduction in the rates of costly late complications that attend MI, both in the short and long term. Thus, ventricular fibrillation, congestive heart failure, and cardiogenic shock were considerably less in the treated groups (Table II). These highly beneficial results translate to longer life and less disability, which can be achieved at relatively modest costs, as was demonstrated by The Netherlands trial (provided the subgroups showing the greatest benefit — those with the greatest area at risk and treated earliest — are selected for this therapy and those least likely to benefit are excluded) (Table III).

It is attractive to postulate that since at least 40% of the population in Europe suffering an MI under 75 years of age could reach the hospital in time to receive such beneficial therapy, the ultimate outcome would indeed be cheaper than if one had persisted with the conventional "modern" therapy of admission to a CCU, the administration of beta-blockers, antiarrhythmic agents, eventually leading to costly therapy for (avoidable) later complications. Thus, as was the case for angina pectoris with early treatment by PTCA or CABG (rather than sustaining economic losses for being out of work too long), economic arguments are now creeping into the equation for MI, although the final answers are not yet in. Indeed, it was argued in Mainz during the ESC Congress discussions in 1986 that when physicians, the health care agencies, and the pharmaceutical industry decide to make recommendations to the new 1992 European policy makers,[1] they would be wise to formulate a policy that, although cost-saving in the long run, allows for initial extra expenditures to provide these facilities.

One other example of an adverse outcome of cost benefit consideration is the recently published Helsinki trial.[3] In this meticulously executed primary

TABLE II. *Data condensed from the ICIN trial[3] display the acute consequences of ischemia within 2 weeks after acute myocardial infarction with and without thrombolytic therapy*

	Thrombolytic Therapy	P Value	Conventional Therapy
Patients	269	—	264
2 weeks mortality	14	0.05	26
Ventricular fibrillation	38	0.01	61
Congestive heart failure during convalescence	37	0.05	53
Recurrent infarction	12	—	9
Pericarditis	19	0.001	46
Cardiogenic shock	13	—	24
Dopamine/dobutamine therapy	26	0.03	42

TABLE III.

	Mean Life Expectancy		Costs		Costs per Year of
	C*	T**	C	T	Life Gained
Inferior infarction	16.3 yrs	17.0 yrs	$ 9,532	$12,869	$4,766
Anterior infarction (all patients)	14.1 yrs	16.5 yrs	$ 9,056	$13,346	$1,811
Anterior infarction (admission ≤2 hours and Σ ST ≥ 1.2 mV)	12.7 yrs	16.3 yrs	$ 8,102	$11,439	$ 905
Anterior infarction (admission 2–4 hours or Σ ST < 1.2 mV)	15.1 yrs	16.6 yrs	$10,009	$14,775	$3,193

*C = standard therapy (controls).
**T = a strategy of thrombolysis.

prevention trial, over 40,000 individuals had to be screened to find 4,020 patients with abnormal serum lipids, of whom 2,607 ultimately completed a 5-year follow-up. The eventual reduction in coronary event rates from 41 (in controls) to 27/1000 in those treated with gemfibrozil can hardly be considered a success from a cost-benefit point of view. Surely the medical profession *will* think twice before treating one thousand asymptomatic individuals for 5 years in order to avoid 14 cardiac events!

Congestive Heart Failure

The same considerations apply to serve congestive heart failure (CHF), which is now recognized to be a major cause of death, and to the cost of cardiac care in the next decade. Many epidemiological data testify to this fact, although the results of therapy are pitiful. None of the standard pharmacological approaches have shown any major benefit once the ejection fraction has dropped below 35%, although ACE inhibitors now provide hope. Mortality in one year exceeds 50% in most series despite inotropic or vasodilation therapy. Clearly, once major cardiac tissue is lost, all is lost. Cardiac transplantation, despite the excellent results that have been obtained throughout the world, is clearly not "the way to go." For one thing, the donor problem will remain a major one; secondly experience in most European centers has shown that the selection procedure only produces a few candidates for the transplantation procedure. Finally the procedure, although highly cost-effective for that rare individual who makes it, still remains a costly form of therapy (Table I).

Recent data from Europe, such as those from the CONSENSUS trial,[4] demonstrate that death can be postponed and quality of life improved by the use of angiotensin-converting enzyme inhibitors, as was shown in the United States. We must realize, however, that we are still treating an end-stage disorder.

Recent studies[5,6] suggest that ACE inhibitors may prove to be at their most useful in congestive failure, if they are given at the first sign of cardiac dysfunction, such as diastolic filling disturbances evident on two-dimensional echocardiograms combined with Doppler flow measurements. Sharpe *et al*[5] and Pfeffer *et al.*[6] have published some exciting data demonstrating that highly detrimental changes in cardiac dimensions and function following acute ischemic episodes can be avoided with resultant preservation of left ventricular function.

Clearly such concepts, coupled with early reperfusion efforts, will constitute a radical change in the therapy of (pre)symptomatic coronary heart disease. Multicenter randomized clinical trials are urgently needed to study the long-term efficacy of ACE inhibitor use for this purpose, their cost-benefit ratio, and their impact on quality of life.

CARDIOLOGY TRIALS IN EUROPE

When we come to consider the practical aspects of clinical trials, we must bear in mind that the trial can only be as good as its procedural execution allows. Not only must the underlying concept and design of a trial be scientifically sound, but the procedure itself must also be scrutinized throughout the project to ensure quality control. For this and other reasons the organization of multicenter clinical trials is at the best of times a tricky task with numerous pitfalls. The complexities involved increase by several orders of magnitude when a trial is not only multicenter but multinational. Despite the move towards a "united" Europe, the number of languages, currencies, and, most importantly, national styles of medical practice make the execution of a coordinated, uniform clinical trial much more difficult than in the U.S. Nevertheless, the ideal of such a trial seems well worth striving for, not only because it is the only way of obtaining the necessary patient numbers, but also because by its very nature it allows generalization of its results to a much broader population.

In the recent past the lumping together of small-sized national trials into one package has failed to impress the registration authorities. We have, therefore, given considerable thought to the design of an overall control structure that would be strong enough to superimpose on the disparate national units a cohesive framework within which the study must run, and that can produce uniform scientific data despite the irregularities and inconsistencies deriving from its multiple sources.

Inasmuch as such a structure has now come into being, albeit not as yet in a fully-developed state, it may be of interest to describe its basic features. Like any such enterprise it is based on a set of foundations, which in this case can be characterized as follows:

1. Knowledge of clinical trial science
2. Knowledge of European cardiology, its available techniques and leading practitioners and clinical centers.
3. Knowledge of the requirements of the pharmaceutical and medical technology industry.
4. Acceptance by the regulatory agencies.

Let us examine how we used these four foundation stones to build up our own structure, the Société pour la Recherche Cardiologique (SOCAR) SA in Switzerland.

CLINICAL TRIAL SCIENCE: SOCAR

For many years, clinical trials in cardiology have been performed to standards that were sometimes almost adequate but more often dreadful. It has now become apparent that excellence in clinical trial planning and execution requires the breadth of knowledge and attention to detail appropriate to an academic discipline *sui generis*. The early well-intentioned fumblings of clinicians were succeeded by the mechanistic strictures of the biostatisticians, each trained to view one part of the problem but unable to strike a sensible balance between academic formalism and the practicalities of dealing with human patients. What is more, the dust raised by this particular conflict has tended to obscure very fundamental questions relating to the performance of the necessary technical maneuvres by the trialist, and the reliability of methods for documenting that these maneuvres have in fact been carried out, and carried out correctly.

We therefore decided to develop a clinical trial design that would strike the required balance, and to minimize problems in the actual execution of the study by designing a case-record form (CRF) containing all the instructions necessary to conduct the trial, so that the doctor attending the patient could execute the trial perfectly without ever having to read the protocol itself. Obviously we make sure that he has done so. Moreover the whole protocol/CRF complex is subject to revision, both from within the trial structure, by the investigators themselves, or by their steering committee, on which a senior representative of the sponsoring organization has a place. It is also under scrutiny from outside, by a committee of senior cardiologists not involved with the study but constituting the Scientific Council of SOCAR, and charged with safeguarding the scientific merit of all the work which SOCAR undertakes. The end result is a study design that is not only acceptable on scientific grounds but is also eminently "doable" in a busy hospital or outpatient clinic.

We also pay considerable attention to the proper execution of the trial. We are here concerned not so much with deliberate fraud, which we do not believe to be widespread among the reputable centers with which we deal, but rather with ensuring that the prescribed procedures are carried out diligently and accurately, and that irregular occurrences such as premature termination of experimental therapy and adverse events are carefully monitored and controlled.

The tools that we have found to be of the greatest help in this context include:

1. Investigator training sessions
2. The "dummy-run"
3. Telephone allocation service
4. Clinic monitoring visits
5. Automated edit-query tracking

We make it a policy to ensure at the outset that the trialist is familiar with the necessary procedures, by holding workshops and training sessions, and by insisting that each center put two or three patients through the trial protocol (not necessarily using the trial drug) in order to check on the technical quality of the data they produce, before allowing them to join the trial proper. This is of particular importance for gauging the technical quality of coronary angio-grams, echocardiograms, exercise test procedures, Holters, and the like, most of which require core laboratories for quality control and unbiased interpretation.

The use of a telephone allocation service is an important safeguard, not so much as a means of ensuring that the allocation is totally blinded (some trialists have shown themselves remarkably adept at divining the contents of "sealed" envelopes), but rather because the act of obtaining the telephone allocation irrevocably commits the patient concerned to entering the trial, since the patient is registered then and there and can never "disappear."

Clinic visits will not be discussed here. These have been well described in the various publications relating to "Good Clinical Practice" emanating from the FDA and elsewhere. Except we should say that we regard them as the only effective method of certifying the actual existence of patients in the trial, and for that reason alone they are indispensable.

The last item on our list relates to data management. With the best will in the world, the CRF, when filled in by the trialist will contain gaps, obscurities and errors. After much work by our computing staff, we have now developed a system that detects these problems continuously as the data are being entered, generates a letter to the trialist with the appropriate queries, and checks that the letter has been answered within a suitable period of time. It is clearly much easier to find a missing piece of data in the patient's notes while he is still on the ward than to ask him to seek it out months or years later.

EUROPEAN CARDIOLOGY IN THE CONTEXT OF THE MULTICENTER CLINICAL RESEARCH TRIAL

There was a time when European cardiologists suffered from a sense of inferiority with respect to their American colleagues. This was particularly pronounced in two main areas, both of which are germane to the present discussion, namely "high-tech" cardiology and major clinical trials. The work of Andreas Gruentzig on the one hand, and the publication of the Norwegian Timolol trial on the other, may perhaps be identified as marking the respective turning-points. Although many others can be quoted, the climate nowadays is one in which European cardiology is flexing its muscles, and the enormous increase in original work on this side of the Atlantic is in no small way a reflection of the achievements of the European Society of Cardiology and its Working Groups in recent years.

Nevertheless, the geographical separation of the leading European centers, and the differing national philosophies within which they are embedded, has made it difficult to develop a uniform "brand" of cardiology that could be readily characterized as European. To be realistic, one must also recognize the particularly large difference between "British" and "Continental" cardiology, in some areas almost as marked as that between European and American, which prompted a poetic colleague to remark, after observing a three-cornered discussion:

"With each of the three perched on his little fence
The place has tricuspid (in)competence."

When it comes to talking to even one of these large groups and obtaining a consensus among its various members on the precise details of a clinical protocol, the situation can at first sight seem impossible. It is of course desirable that all the cardiologists participating in a particular project should have some say in what is to be done, but in practice we find that the best solution is to design the protocol with the help of a small committee of experts and to submit this for review by the group as a whole. The initial Investigators' Meeting should be an open forum where the participants are encouraged to express their views without being made to feel that a preordained "cut-and-dried" protocol is being imposed upon them.

All this presupposes that the group assembled is composed of the best persons for the job, and it is here, in the selection of potential trialists, that critical mistakes can be made if the coordinator of the trial — be it a pharmaceutical sponsor or a contract research organization — is not thoroughly familiar with the attributes of those chosen. When the decision is made to invite a particular trialist, the following questions must be answered:

1. Is he experienced in the therapeutic area under study (e.g., thrombolytics, ACE inhibitors)?
2. Is he expert in the technical procedures required (e.g., angiography, echocardiography)?
3. Does he have a track record as a "good trialist" (quality of CRF completion, punctuality, etc.)?
4. Does he work well as part of a team? (Or is he a loner who will "do his own thing"?)
5. Does he have an adequate patient load (and can he keep his patients for follow-up?)

All this is difficult enough, but even with an optimal team there are likely to be problems arising from differences in the everyday practice of cardiology in various countries, which can surface as technical differences (How many ways are there of doing an exercise test?), or as procedural differences (for example, in the accepted methods for obtaining patient consent). For this reason we have found it helpful to invite a senior cardiologist, one not otherwise involved with the trial, to act as chairman of the steering committee. His extra authority can be exercised where necessary, without his being accused of having his own personal axe to grind, as might have been the case if he himself were a trialist in that particular study.

This is the place perhaps to mention publication policy. Debate over the thorny question of authorship of the final report has consumed vast amounts of time at Investigators' Meetings and has occasioned the end of many promising friendships. In fact, our view is that, for any trial involving more than a handful of centers, there is only one satisfactory solution. The report should appear as the work of "The XYZ Study Group," and all those involved in the study — trialists, coordinators, and other hangers-on — should be listed at the end of the paper (or on the front page of the final publication). People should begin to realize that the status of someone appearing as 17th author at the head of the article is neither better nor worse than if he were to be included in a list of everybody at the end or the beginning of the report.

THE PHARMACEUTICAL INDUSTRY

It is understandable that most clinicians have the following order of priorities: (1) patients, (2) science, and (3) the pharmaceutical industry. This sometimes makes it difficult for them to understand or sympathize with the special requirements of the trial from the sponsor's point of view. They may bridle at being asked to perform large quantities of apparently trivial laboratory tests, or at filling in inordinately detailed CRFs. This is one reason why we are careful to undertake only those studies that we feel have genuine scientific merit, independent of any value they may have for the sponsor. Provided that the project is scientifically exciting, the slight extra load on the trialist occasioned by the sponsor's special requirements will largely go unnoticed and, in fact, is usually carried out willingly.

Difficulties may also occur if we turn the sponsor-trialist relationship around and view it from the other side. The technical aspects of cardiology have advanced so rapidly over the last few years that it is not surprising that sponsors may not be completely *au-fait* with the techniques and measurements currently available, let alone their interpretation, or still more importantly the identities of those practitioners who can be regarded as most expert in the use of the technique involved.

Under these circumstances, sponsors often fall back on inviting "friends" of the company, with whom they have enjoyed good relations and productive endeavors in the past. These may not, however, be the best people for the job at hand. We feel that the best procedure is for us, being the ones closest to the actual day-to-day work of cardiologists in Europe, to select those we think best qualified to undertake the work at hand, unless the sponsor has some particular objection. This has the added advantage that, if at some stage it is necessary to bring pressure to bear on a trialist (perhaps because of slow recruitment rate or shoddy work), this is best done by the independent organization that will not impair future harmony between the trialist and the sponsor. This takes on particular importance if one considers the payment for the services required of the trial participants.

It will be apparent from the foregoing, that an organization such as SOCAR regards itself primarily as an academic unit rather than a commercial enterprise; and although it bridges the gap between the commercial world of the pharmaceutical industry and the scientific world of the clinic, its own priorities always remain scientific. Its goal must be to harness the financial resources of the industry and to apply them in a manner that is optimally productive in scientific terms, and best assists the development of European cardiology.

LARGE TRIALS WITH SIMPLE PROTOCOLS: INDICATIONS AND CONTRAINDICATIONS

We now turn to the scientific principles underlying the design of the Multicenter Clinical Research Trial (MCRT), as it has become the most reliable way of assessing efficacy in medicine. The evidence provided by MCRTs is often the "missing link" in clarifying (aspects of) pathophysiology or mechanism(s) of action and forms the basis for the registration of new drugs. MCRTs are also done to assess the efficacy of technical procedures such as surgery or PTCA. Thus, they have become an integral part of scientific clinical medicine and an important basis for its practice.[7-20]

MCRTs are done in the setting of normal medical care but affect that care almost without exception in a major way. Care is usually highly variable, individualistic, and oriented toward the specific problems of individual patients. MCRTs impose on this care for all involved (doctors, nurses, and patients) a whole range of additional features. Among these are unusual "informed consent" procedures, randomization, frequently the use of placebo medication, protocol rather than problem directed (and often additional) tests, and rigid procedural quality assurance. The multicenteredness of these trials adds another level of complexity: central assessment of observations and measurements, a whole bureaucracy of committees, coordinating and data audit centers, and so on.

As a consequence, MCRTs have become very complicated and costly, a fact that, quite rightly, has concerned many. Some have simply become disenchanted. More seriously, others have questioned the need to do trials in the first place. In any case, it has become more difficult for trialists to find the money. Not surprisingly therefore, forceful arguments have been made in favor of mounting large but simple trials. In the following section we discuss the arguments for such trials as they have been presented and unravel their implications, indications, and contraindications.

THE ARGUMENTS *FOR* SIMPLICITY AND LARGE SIZE:

Among the protagonists of large and simple trials, Yusuf, Collins and Peto have been particularly outspoken. Their arguments, to "suggest both the possibility and the desirability of *large, simple randomized* trials of the effects on *mortality* of various *widely practicable* treatments for *common* conditions," (italics as in the quoted publication) are six-fold and are quoted below verbatim from their 1984 publication:[7]

Firstly, the identification of effective treatments is likely to be more "important" if the disease to be studied is *common* than if it is rare, and studies of common conditions *can* be large.

Secondly, the identification of effective treatments for common diseases is likely to be more "important" if the treatment is widely practicable than if it is so complex that it can be performed only in specialized centers, and treatment protocols for widely practical treatments *can* be simple.

Thirdly, study of the effects of treatments on major endpoints (e.g. death) is likely to be more "important" than study of the effects on minor endpoints, and follow-up protocols for the assessment only of major endpoints *can* often be simple.

Fourthly, no matter what prognostic features are recorded at entry, the duration of survival, etc., among apparently similar patients is likely still to be rather unpredictable, so no great increase in statistical sensitivity is likely to be conferred by stratification and/or adjustment for such features. In other words, the reliability of the main treatment comparison is improved surprisingly little by adjustment for any initial imbalances in prognostic features, which suggests that entry protocols too *can* be simple.

Fifthly, the direction (though not necessarily the magnitude) of the net effects of treatment on particular modes of death is likely to be similar for many different subcategories of randomized patients. Again, therefore, if there is no need to subcategorize patients to decide who needs which treatment, the entry protocol *can* be simple.

Sixthly, if a widely practicable treatment had a large effect on an important endpoint (e.g. mortality) in a common disease this would probably already be known, so the true effect is likely to be either null, or at most, moderate.

From the sixth argument, Yusuf *et al.* argue that trials must be large to provide reliable answers and conclude that "a number of important medical questions will be answered reliably in the next few years only if some ultra-simple, ultra-large, strictly randomized trials can be mounted."

Do the Arguments Translate to Design Options?

In a critique of the above arguments in favor of simple and large trials, it is essential to distinguish between arguments that do translate to design options open to the investigator and those that do not.

Any trial's design derives from its objective, which is in turn dictated by the biology of the disease and the nature of the treatment of interest. As far as these go, the investigator has little to choose. Thus, a *common* condition (first argument) is an **opportunity** rather than a design **option.** A simple experimental treatment (second argument) simplifies a protocol but oversimplification in the context of a trial may render a treatment that is effective when properly applied apparently ineffective. Here, the investigator has few real options to choose from (and we note in passing that MCRTs of treatments that can be performed only in specialized centers are of particular importance to a society burdened by ever-rising health care costs).

As regards the first half of the third argument, few would take issue with the notion that major endpoints that signify clinical benefit are more "important." Similarly, there is no question that trials should be large enough to yield sufficiently precise effect estimates (e.g., have sufficient statistical power) given the endpoint(s) to be studied and the magnitude of the effect to be expected (sixth argument). These principles cannot be overemphasized since they are overlooked so often. They translate, however, to responsibilities the investigator must face rather than to design choices.

The arguments that do translate to design options are the second half of the third, the fourth, and the fifth one. Here we do not necessarily agree with Yusuf *et al.*[7] In particular, we take issue below with their argument that, since the direction of the net treatment effect can be expected to be similar across patient subgroups, entry protocols can be simple (fifth argument). We also take issue with their argument that, since only major endpoints are important, follow-up protocols can be simple (second half of the third argument).

SIMILARITY OF NET TREATMENT EFFECT ACROSS SUBGROUPS

The argument that the direction of the net treatment effect can be expected to be similar across patient subgroups is perhaps the most central one in the whole debate.[13] If the argument is **credible,** trial design can indeed be simplified enormously and it will suffice to collect only the fourfold items in a table that relates the occurrence of endpoints to randomized treatment. But is it credible?

In our view, this particular argument may be attractive from a statistical point of view but has no *a priori* biological foundation, let alone credibility. A treatment may reduce the occurrence of a particular mode of death but may induce another one (truly harmless treatments do not exist). Yusuf *et al.*[7] correctly imply that trials measure net effects. A net effect is the resultant of positive and negative influences on an outcome such as total mortality. Thus, it is to be expected that subgroups that are at high risk of a particular mode of death, which is positively influenced, benefit because the positive influences outweigh the negative ones. By contrast in those subgroups at low risk of a mode of death that is not influenced positively, the net effect of treatment may be harmful due to the negative influences outweighing the positive ones. As a consequence, the net effect of treatment may change direction of risk between subgroups (Figure 1).

The reality of this statement can be seen from the following examples:

Example 1. (Sub)groups from hypertension trials[8-12] have generally shown a positive effect on total mortality if the control group has a comparatively high death rate.

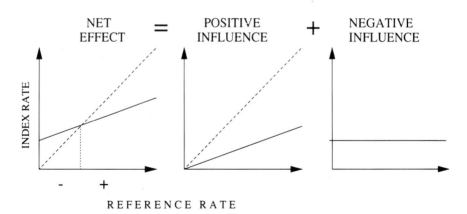

FIG. 1. Direction of net effects. If a treatment does not affect the course of disease in any way, the index and reference rates of an outcome in an MCRT will, when plotted on an X–Y graph across subgroups of patients at different levels of risk, fall (on the average) on the identity line (---). If there is a positive influence that reduces the reference rate with a constant proportion (middle panel), and a negative influence that induces a risk that is uniform over subgroups (right panel), their net effect will sum up as shown in the left panel.

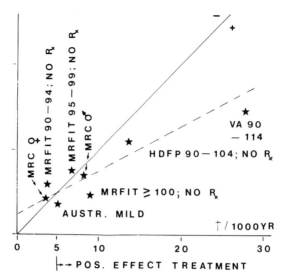

FIG. 2. Index and reference total mortality rates per 1000 observation years for subgroups of patients with "mild" hypertension from major hypertension trials. Plotted on the Y-axis are the index rates for respective intervention groups and on the X-axis those for control groups. Shown are the females from the Medical Research Council (MRC) trial,[8] the not-previously-treated (no Rx) group with an entry diastolic blood pressure of 90–94 mm Hg from the Multiple Risk Factor Intervention Trial (MRFIT),[9] the Australian Mild Hypertension trial,[10] the not-previously-treated group with an entry diastolic blood pressure of 95–99 mm Hg from MRFIT,[9] the males from MRC,[8] the not-previously-treated group with an entry diastolic blood pressure of 100 mm Hg or above from MRFIT,[9] the not-previously-treated group with an entry diastolic blood pressure of 90–104 mm Hg from the Hypertension Detection and Follow-up Programme (HDFP),[11] and the 90–114 mm Hg entry diastolic blood pressure group from the Veterans Administration (VA) trial.[12] If a cumulative proportion (CP) of death was reported rather than an incidence rate (IR), the latter was estimated from the formula (12)$CP = 1 - exp(-IR.t)$, where t represents the time period of follow-up over which a particular cumulative proportion was reported.

On the other hand, the effect has come out zero or even negative if the death rate in the control group is comparatively low (Figure 2).

Example 2. In the Italian study of thrombolysis in acute myocardial infarction (AMI) with intravenous streptokinase (GISSI),[14] the effect on total mortality was positive in patients treated early after onset of symptoms but negative in patients treated late (Figure 3).

These examples show that there may be a reversal of the direction of net treatment effects both within and between studies. As will be discussed below, this has profound consequences as regards how simple trials can be. In passing, it is worthy to note that the potential differences in the direction of net treatment effects also puts a question mark behind some of the metanalyses that have been presented by, among others, Yusuf et al.[15]

CONSEQUENCES OF SIMPLE ENTRY PROTOCOLS

"Simple" means, in this context, that very few descriptive data on patient characteristics at entry are collected. Data that have not been collected by design will never emerge, and the consequences of not collecting must be faced. There are at least three such consequences:

First, in the absence of data on entry characteristics, it will be impossible to stratify patients according to clinical characteristics that potentially modify the direction of the treatment effect or its magnitude. It follows that a simple entry protocol deliberately removes the possibility of studying effect modification in the analysis and of determining, for instance, whether effect modification is perhaps the reason why a large trial has produced an overall "no effect" result.

Second, the chance is lost to properly characterize, in the interest of scientific generalization (external validity), the patient group that was actually studied. The view that patients entered into a MCRT are a "random sample"

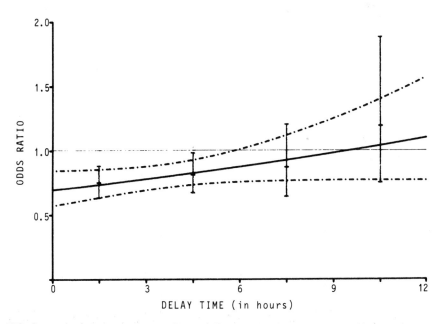

FIG. 3. Relationship between the effect on 21-day total mortality of intravenous streptokinase and the delay between onset of symptoms and entry in patients from the GISSI trial. Plotted on the Y-axis are the odds ratios of death, which compare mortality among the intervention subgroups with that of the control subgroups defined by the delay times plotted on the X-axis. Also shown is a regression line, which describes the relationship between the odds ratio and delay time with its 95% confidence boundaries. Based on data from the Gruppo Italiano per lo Studio della Streptochinasi Nell' Infarto Myocardiale (GISSI) trial.[14]

of patients to be treated in the future and that, if the trial is positive, all similar patients will have to receive the treatment is again overly simplistic. Diagnoses and certainly indications for treatment are notoriously unreliable and arbitrary in practice. Thus, it does not suffice from the point of view of scientific generalization to know that a clinician has diagnosed a condition to be present or has judged an indication for treatment to exist according to his or her own current criteria. MCRTs need to assess treatment effects in sharply defined conditions, and clinicians need explicit indications for treatment. It follows that eligibility criteria must reflect a specific nosology that represents the disease entity to be studied and that descriptive entry characteristics are required to determine what is represented by the patient group actually studied, and this in such a fashion that the practitioner of today and tomorrow can still 'recognize' his patient.

Example 3. It is now generally conceded that the diagnosis of AMI cannot be made reliably at hospital admission. At present, no data collection scheme can be proposed for an MCRT in AMI that solves the diagnostic dilemma. But AMI as an indication for treatment is very real and must be described explicitly in terms of the nature of symptoms and delay since onset, signs at physical examination, and electrocardiographic abnormalities. To paraphrase Gertrude Stein: "An infarct is *not* an infarct is *not* an infarct."

Third, the opportunity is thrown away of describing the direction and magnitude of the treatment effect observed as a function of relevant entry characteristics. Thus, not only is scientific generalization hampered, but there is limited opportunity to learn more about mechanisms of action and to describe to clinicians the indications and contraindications.

Example 4. For AMI, many clinically relevant effect modifiers can be observed at hospital admission. These include clinical signs of heart failure, extent of electrocardiographic abnormalities, previous drug treatment, type of symptoms and time since onset, heart rate, blood pressure, etc., etc. Each of these could represent a contraindication or an effect modifier of potential clinical relevance.

Data that are collected have a tendency to be used beyond the original intent. The collection of data on entry characteristics for the reasons and purposes mentioned above will inevitably imply the use of subgroup analyses and/or multivariate modeling. To avoid any misunderstanding, our argument should not be taken as a plea for *post hoc* "data dredging." We share the statistical concern in this context. It does not follow, however, that data on entry characteristics need not be collected. Trials are not done in isolation from the rest of medical science. In many situations there will be general agreement, at least in qualitative terms, on what the most important prognostic indicators are. These can, and should, be taken into account in analyzing trial data. We object in this context to "biological data-dredging" (i.e., equating statistical significance with biological relevance), but not to the incorporation in the analysis of sound arguments derived from what is known about the biology of the disease entity in question. As we have argued elsewhere,[16] rather than be overly bothered by what is right or wrong in inferential statistics, investigators should present their evidence as completely and as meaningfully as possible, but should leave inference to the consumer. In this context, we plea for the use of appropriate, descriptive, multivariate methods of the type so well-known from nonexperimental epidemiology[13] in the derivation of effect estimates and the study of effect modification. That these methods can be helpful both in effect estimation and in understanding clinically relevant prognostic indicators has been shown in a trial on unstable angina recently completed in the Netherlands.[18]

THE ROLE OF INTERMEDIARY TREATMENT EFFECTS AND SIMPLE FOLLOW-UP PROTOCOLS

In understanding mechanisms of action and in the practice of medicine, what may be called intermediary treatment effects are extremely important. To illustrate what is meant by an intermediary treatment effect, consider for instance hypertension. Patients with mild hypertension are generally free of any symptoms and signs other than a blood pressure that is elevated. Antihypertensives are given to lower blood pressure, not because this is by itself beneficial but because it is generally assumed to be a causal intermediary treatment effect in achieving what really matters, i.e., a reduction of the risk of future cerebrovascular or coronary disease events. The notion that this is so is based on the fact that blood pressure is an independent risk factor for these disease events and on the observation from MCRTs and other follow-up studies that there is a relationship between the drop in blood pressure observed and the risk of subsequent disease events (in the sense that a large drop is associated with reduced risk). Apart from its theoretical significance, blood pressure as an intermediary treatment effect is also of great practical importance, since physicians who treat patients with hypertension will use blood pressure as a basis for judging whether treatment is adequate or not.

Another example of an intermediary treatment effect is the removal of a coronary thrombus in the context of thrombolytic therapy for AMI. Here, all available evidence from animal experiments, clinical studies, and MCRTs point to the notion that the earlier the thrombus is dissolved, the smaller the eventual infarct will be and the better the patient will do subsequently.

A corollary of Yusuf et al.'s plea for choosing major endpoints[7] is that their assessment calls only for simple follow-up protocols (third argument). Presumably this means that follow-up measurements of intermediary effects can be omitted. As is shown in the following example, this advice can severely hamper the interpretation of MCRT results.

Example 5. The Multiple Risk Factor Intervention Trial (MRFIT)[9] was designed to determine whether reduction of the levels of the three major risk factors for cardiovascular disease (i.e., blood pressure, cholesterol and smoking) would reduce total mortality. The results of this enormously expensive program were disappointing because no appreciable effect on total mortality was observed. This was a large, but by no means a simple, trial. Reliable information on the levels of risk factors during follow-up was available for both groups. There were appreciable changes in a favorable direction in the intervention group. There were, however, also much bigger changes than anticipated in the same direction in the control group. The differences as regards these *intermediary treatment effects* between the two compared groups were so small that the absence of an appreciable effect on total mortality was entirely explicable on these grounds. This had enormous consequences as far as the scientific conclusions that could reasonably be drawn are concerned. Given its findings as regards intermediary treatment effects, MRFIT did not falsify in any way its underlying assumptions. Had there been no data collection on risk factor levels during follow-up, no meaningful explanation would have been possible at all.

Our contention is that Yusuf et al.'s[7] plea for major endpoints, although having definite merits, cannot and should not lead to the notion that follow-up protocols can thus be simplified to assessment of major endpoints only. To be sure, our argument holds only if there are generally accepted intermediary treatment effects in the above sense that are clinically measurable in the first place. This is not always the case. For instance, there seems to be at present no generally accepted platelet function test that can be used for intermediary treatment effect assessment in a MCRT of aspirin. If there are established intermediary treatment effects, however, omitting their assessment hampers the possibility to learn from a trial, as is exemplified by the MRFIT experience.

Apart from the need to collect reliable data on intermediary treatment effects (if such effects are present), there is also a need to collect data on rare but important side effects and to take into account the effect of extraneous influences such as co-medication. In this context, double-blinding and the use of placebo is based on sound theoretical argument, and these design features should not be omitted in the interest of keeping follow-up protocols simple. We would most likely not have known about the ophthalmologic effects of practolol[19] and the gastrointestinal effects of clofibrate[20] had the respective trials been "large and simple."

CONCLUSIONS

Indications and Contraindications for Large and Simple Trials

To the extent that the arguments in favor of large and simple trials represent design options, it follows from the above that entry protocols can be simple (1) if the disease entity at issue can be sharply defined by inclusion and exclusion criteria alone, (2) if there are no established indicators of prognosis, and (3) if there is no reason to suspect clinically relevant and detectable effect modification. However, those who simplify place the burden of proof upon themselves. If any of these three conditions cannot be agreed, appropriate data will have to be collected.

Follow-up protocols can be simple if there are no established intermediary effects that can be measured clinically inherent in the mechanism of action to be studied. Otherwise, reliable data on intermediary effects have to be collected for interpretability of the data. Furthermore, follow-up protocols can only be simple if the side-effect profile of the therapeutic principle at issue is well-established, and double-blinding can only be omitted if there is no need to safeguard the symmetry of information and of extraneous influences, such as co-medication.

REFERENCES

1. Hugenholtz PG. The significance of European integration in 1992 for the European cardiological community in the completion of a single market. Consequences and perspectives for the medical community and industry. *IAPM* 1988; 58–66.
2. Simoons ML, Serruys PW, vanden Brand M, Res J, Verheugt FWA, Krauss H, Remme WJ, Bär F, de Zwaan C, vander Laarse A, Vermeer F, Lubsen J. Early thrombolysis in acute myocardial infarction: limitation of infarct size and improved survival—for the Working Group on Thrombolytic Therapy in Acute Myocardial Infarction of the Netherlands Interuniversity Cardiology Institute. *J Am Coll Cardiol* 1986; 7:717–728.
3. Frick MH, Elo O, Haapa K, Heinonen OP, Heinsalmi P, Helo P, Huttunen JK, Kaiteneimi P, Koskinen P, Manninen V, Mäenpää H, Mälkönen M, Mänttäri M, Norola S, Pasternack A, Pikkareinen J, Romo M, Sjöblom T, Nikkilä EA. Helsinki Heart Study: Primary prevention trial with gemfibrozil in middle-aged men with dyslipidemia. *N Engl J Med* 1987; 317:1237–1245.
4. The CONSENSUS Trial Study Group. Effect of enalapril on mortality in severe congestive heart failure. *N Engl J Med* 1987; 316:1429–1435.
5. Sharpe DN, Murphy J, Smith H, Hannan S. Treatment of patients with symptomless left ventricular dysfunction after myocardial infarction. *Lancet* 1988; 1:255–259.
6. Pfeffer MA, Lamas GA, Vaughan DE, Parisi AF, Bruanwald E. Effect of captopril on progressive ventricular dilation after anterior myocardial infarction. *N Engl J Med* 1988; 319:80–86.
7. Yusuf S, Collins R, Peto R. Why do we need some large, simple randomized trials? *Statistics in Medicine* 1984; 3:409–420.
8. Medical Research Council Working Party. MRC trial of treatment of mild hypertension: principal results. *Br Med J* 1985; 291:97–104.
9. Multiple Risk Factor Intervention Trial Research Group. Multiple risk factor intervention trial: risk factor changes and mortality results. *JAMA* 1982; 248:1465–1477.
10. Management Committee: The Australian therapeutic trial in mild hypertension. *Lancet* 1980; 1:1261–1267.
11. Hypertension Detection and Follow-up Program Co-operative Group. Five-year findings of the hypertension detection and follow-up program. I. Reduction of mortality of persons with high blood pressure, including mild hypertension. *JAMA* 1979; 242:2562–2571.
12. Veterans Administration Cooperative Study Group on Antihypertensive Agents. Effects of treatment on morbidity in hypertension. II. Results in patients with diastolic blood pressure averaging 90 through 114 mm Hg. *JAMA* 1970; 213:1143–1152.
13. Miettinen OS. Theoretical Epidemiology: Principles of Occurrence Research in Medicine. New York, John Wiley & Sons, 1985.
14. Gruppo Italiano per lo Studio della Streptochinasi nell' Infarto Myocardiale (GISSI). Effectiveness of intravenous thrombolytic treatment in acute myocardial infarction. *Lancet* 1986; 1:397–401.

15. Yusuf S, Peto R, Lewis, Collins R, Sleight P. Beta-blockade during and after myocardial infarction. An overview of the randomized trials. *Prog Cardiovasc Dis* 1985; **27**:335–371.
16. Lubsen J. Problems of objectives, evidence and inference in the MIAMI and Belfast trials. *Eur Heart J* 1985; **6**:216–224.
17. Kannel WB, McGee D, Gordon T. A general cardiovascular risk profile, the Framingham study. *Am J Cardiol* 1976; **38**:46–51.
18. Tijssen JGP, Lubsen J, for the HINT Research Group: 5 data analysis. *Eur Heart J* 1987; **8 (suppl H)**:49–69.
19. Wright P. Untoward effect associated with practolol administration. Oculomucocutaneous syndrome. *Br Med J* 1975; **1**:595–598.
20. Report of a WHO Working Party: A cooperative trial in the primary prevention of ischemic heart disease using clofibrate. *Br Heart J* 1978; **40**:1069–1075.

SUMMARY

Multicentre randomized clinical trials in Europe over the past decade have made a major contribution to the practice of cardiology and will do so increasingly in the immediate future now that the Single Europe Act will become a fact of life in 1992.

Arguments for a major role for independent scientifically-based research organizations in the area of coronary artery disease include cost-benefit considerations, scientific aspects of clinical trials, data acquisition techniques, and data management requirements. The roles of the pharmaceutical industry versus the investigator-trial participant is discussed.

Finally, a critique is provided on the current fashion of "big is beautiful," with arguments why "simplicity" and "large size" notions must be opposed by the need for "credibility," applicability, and economic usefulness, as well as validity in terms of sound pathophysiological hypotheses.

RÉSUMÉ

Des études cliniques randomisées multicentriques en Europe, au cours de ces dix dernières années, ont largement contribué aux progrès effectués dans le domaine de la cardiologie et ces contributions continueront à s'accroître à l'avenir avec l'avénement de l'Europe des 12 en 1992.

Les arguments en faveur du rôle important des centres de recherche scientifique indépendants dans le domaine des maladies coronariennes artérielles comprend des considérations d'ordre économique, des aspects scientifiques d'essais cliniques, des techniques d'acquisition des données, et des exigences d'organisation des données. On discute du rôle de l'industrie pharmaceutique vis-à-vis des investigateurs cliniques.

Finalement, on passe à la critique des tendances actuelles à accepter que «tout ce qui est grand est beau». On oppose les notions de «simplicité» et de «grande taille» au besoin de «crédibilité», d'application, d'utilité économique, aussi bien que de validité en termes d'hypothèses pathophysiologiques bien fondées.

ZUSAMMENFASSUNG

In den letzten zehn Jahren haben klinische Versuche in willkürlich ausge-
wählten Zentren in Europa einen wichtigen Beitrag zur kardiologischen
Praxis geliefert; und diese Tendenz wird sich in der nahen Zukunft fortsetzen,
da der Akt Zur Vereinheitlichung Europas im Jahr 1992 in Kraft tritt.
Argumente für eine Hauptrolle der unabhängigen wissenschaftlich orien-
tierten Forschungorganisationen auf dem Gebiet der Koronararterie beziehen
sich auf Kosten-Nutzen-Betrachtungen, wissenschaftliche Aspekte der klinischen Versuche, Techniken der Datensammlung und Forderungen der Da-
tenverarbeitung. Diskutiert wird auch die Rolle der pharmazeutischen Industrie im Gegensatz zu Forschungsinstitutionen.
Schliesslich wird die gegenwätige Tendenz zu "Big is beautiful" kritisiert,
mit der Frage, warum Einfachheit und Grösse notwendig mit dem Bedürfnis
nach Glaubwürdigkeit gekoppelt sein müssen oder mit der Anwendbarkeit,
ökonomischen Verwendbarkeit oder Validität solider pathophysiologischer
Hypothesen verbunden sind.

RIASSUNTO

Saggi clinici randomizzati multicentrici in Europa nel corso dell'ultimo de-
cennio sono stati un importante contributo alla cardiologia e lo saranno
sempre maggiormente nell'immediato futuro ora che l'Europa Unita diven-
terà un fatto compiuto nel 1992. Gli argomenti a favore di un ruolo di grande
importanza per le organizzazioni indipendenti di ricerca a base scientifica nel
campo del morbo dell'arteria coronaria includono considerazioni econo-
miche, aspetti di scienza sperimentale clinica, tecniche di acquisizione dati e
requisiti di gestione dati. Vengono discussi i rispettivi ruoli dell'industria
farmaceutica e dei ricercatori/sperimentatori.
Viene infine avanzata una critica dell'attuale moda del "Grande è bello"
con argomenti su perché le nozioni di "semplicità" e "grandezza" devono
essere contrastate col bisogno di "credibilità", applicabilità ed utilità econo-
mica, nonché validità in termini di ipotesi patofisiologiche ben fondate.

SUMÁRIO

Estudos clínicos multicêntricos randomizados efetuados na Europa durante a
última década têm contribuído notavelmente á prática de cardiologia, e num
futuro imediato contribuirão cada vez mais, dado que a Lei de Uma Europa
Só torna-se uma realidade a partir de 1992. Os argumentos a favor de um
papel importante para as organizações independentes de pesquisa de base
científica na área da arteriopatia coronária incluem considerações custo/ben-

efício, aspectos científicos dos estudos clínicos, técnicas de aquisição de dados
e requisitos para o manejo de dados. Discute-se o papel da indústria farmacêutica *versus* aquele do pesquisador. Finalmente, faz-se uma crítica à moda
atual de "O grande é melhor", argumentando-se que as ideias de "simplici-
dade" e "grande tamanho" devem ser opostas pela necessidade de "credibili-
dade", aplicabilidade e utilidade econômica, assim como validez em termos
de hipóteses patofisiológicas sólidas.

RESUMEN

Estudios clínicos multicéntricos aleatorios efectuados en Europa durante la
última década han contribuido notablemente a la práctica de la cardiología, y
en el futuro inmediato esta contribución incluso aumentará ya que la Europa
Unida constituirá un hecho a partir de 1992. Los argumentos a favor de un
mayor papel para las organizaciones independientes de investigación de base
científica en el área de la arteriopatía coronaria incluyen consideraciones
costo/beneficio, aspectos científicos de los estudios clínicos, técnicas de ad-
quisición de datos y requisitos para el manejo de datos. Se discute el papel de
la industria farmacéutica versus el del investigador. Finalmente, se hace una
crítica a la moda actual de "Lo grande es mejor", argumentándose que las
ideas de "simplicidad" y "gran tamaño" deben ser opuestas por la necesidad
de "credibilidad", aplicabilidad y utilidad económica, así como validez en
términos de hipótesis patofisiológicas bien cimentadas.

要約

　ヨーロッパで過去10年間にわたって行われた多施設無作為臨床試験は，心臓病
学の実践において多大な貢献をした。そしてもうまもなく，1992年にEC統合が
実現すれば，同様に多大な貢献がなされよう。
　ここでは，冠動脈疾患の分野において，科学的基盤に基づく独立した研究組織
の主要な役割について論ずる。これには，費用と利益とのバランスの考慮，臨床
試験の科学性，データ収集技法，およびデータ管理の必要条件などの問題が含ま
れる。また，製薬業界と研究者-治験実施者との役割の問題についても考察する。
　最後に，「大きいことはいいことだ」という最近の風潮について批評し，なぜ「簡
潔さ」と「大きさ」の観念が「信頼性」の要求に反してしまうのか，適応可能性，
経済的有用性，また，確かな病態生理学的仮説という意味での妥当性，などにつ
いても論じる。

Cardiac and Renal Failure: An Expanding Role for ACE Inhibitors, edited by C. T. Dollery and L. M. Sherwood, Hanley & Belfus, Inc., Philadelphia.

Discussion

LANGMAN: It is important to recruit investigators who have genuine doubt; otherwise they will not include certain patients or will include the wrong sort. The strength of the study is strongly influenced by your ability to measure what you intended to measure. If investigators cannot be consistent, the calculations may be meaningless.

HUGENHOLTZ: This is why we use a computer-supported system which has demonstrated a much reduced inter-observer variability.

LANGMAN: Without the power of the computer, it did seem a very small difference that you could measure.

HUGENHOLTZ: That is how you see it as you are interpreting the slide. I assure you that these differences have been documented both with models and with previous studies, and the inter-observer variability as a factor has virtually been eliminated. But you are right, the differences are small but they are measurable. After all, coronary arteries begin at the ostium with a diameter of 5 mm, and end up being immeasurable after 1–2 mm.

LANGMAN: I am not against "data dredging," but you should look for a simple effect in the trial. If you wish to subdivide later you can do so.

HUGENHOLTZ: I agree.

DOLLERY: If you randomize, however good or bad the trend may be, you will find interesting data. I worry a little about your program, because you rely largely on pharmaceutical industry sponsorship. The pharmaceutical industry is a marvelous machine for developing drugs through the pharmacology/taxicology phase 1, 2 and 3 studies, though I am not sure that it is the appropriate mechanism for doing outcome trials. The industry is remarkably astute if you are doing comparative trials whereby you show their product in a slightly better light than the opponent's. Big development budgets are attached to new products as the profits of old products are no longer there. It is relatively easy to get money to study new calcium antagonists or ACE inhibitors, but if you want to study the effects of cessation of cigarette smoking or low-dose aspirin, you would have great difficulty in attracting sponsorship. If you rely largely on pharmaceutical company sponsorship, some of the most interesting questions will never get addressed.

HUGENHOLTZ: Your points are very valid, but we do have a number of plans which are not sponsored by pharmaceutical companies. One is a WHO project comparing coronary artery bypass grafting (CABG) with percutaneous transluminal coronary angioplasty (PTCA) in a certain category of patients. These are public health type issues. By 1992 in Europe we will have to change. As yet, there is nobody willing to support this type of work in a collective area. Perhaps it exists in England with the MRC or DHSS. In the smaller countries there is no such interest. We need to show there can be a degree of cooperation. WHO has shown that confidence by giving us the contract for comparing PTCA with CABG, and with their support we can approach the national government. As yet, Europe has no "federally" funded structure as there is in America.

BAYLISS: In the studies examining the effects of HMG-CoA reductase inhibitors on atheroma regression, am I correct in thinking that you intend to do angios [angiography studies] before you start the treatment group and then post-treatment angios later?

HUGENHOLTZ: Yes and no. We will need quantitative angios both before and after treatment, but the first one we obtained because there were clinical indications for it.

BAYLISS: Yes, I realize that. Therefore you have to wait for people who need an angio to enter this trial; then they will need a follow-up angio. With whom are you going to compare this group?

HUGENHOLTZ: It will be a placebo controlled trial. Half will be untreated, and we will study the natural history of the coronary artery disease.

BAYLISS: Have you worked out what proportion of every 100 people taken into the trial will never have a second angio?

HUGENHOLTZ: Previous intake data show a return rate in the high 70s, though some feel so well that they refuse to come back. The majority of the people in the various countries we are dealing with, through loyalty to their doctors, will come back for the repeat study. The physician must be interested in motivating his patient that this is really an issue to be studied. I believe that is an important factor in the success rate. I have not met a single physician who is not interested in finding out whether these compounds can arrest or even lead to regression of coronary artery disease.

BAYLISS: How long will you treat these patients?

HUGENHOLTZ: The study is designed to last for 2 years, but we have plans for carrying on longer.

BAYLISS: I'm filled with admiration.

JOHNSTON: I don't think there really is a conflict between simple and complex trials. If you are asking if a calcium antagonist benefits everyone, you can do a simple trial and the answer is no. If you are asking whether a calcium antagonist benefits a certain subset, you do a complex trial and the answer becomes yes.

HUGENHOLTZ: I agree with you, and I wish everyone would put his case in those words before starting his trial.

JOHNSTON: The most important thing in a trial is to define exactly what question you are asking. I don't think that is done in enough trials.

HUGENHOLTZ: Yes, in fact the large sample trial with simple entry criteria and exit points can only give a very partial answer and is only relevant for certain things. Also it shouldn't be done to the exclusion of more complex trials where, as you said, significant questions can and must be properly asked.

Cardiac and Renal Failure: An Expanding Role for ACE Inhibitors, edited by C. T. Dollery and L. M. Sherwood, Hanley & Belfus, Inc., Philadelphia.

Roundtable 4: *Further Research and Therapeutic Opportunities for ACE Inhibitors*

Chairman: Thomas W. Smith
Panelists: Detlev Ganten, Philip Poole-Wilson, John D. Irvin, Edmond Sonnenblick, and Klaus Thurau

ACE INHIBITORS, ANGIOTENSIN AND THE BRAIN

Whether ACE inhibitors affect the functioning of the brain is related to whether or not they penetrate the blood-brain barrier. Dose appears to be crucial, and different drugs may also act differently. Various studies, the majority of which have been performed in experimental animals, have shown that angiotensin affects central functions such as memory, performance, fertility and thirst.

Dose Dependence

A single large dose of captopril will inhibit converting-enzyme activity in the brain, whereas no clear effect can be demonstrated after chronic administration of low doses. This does not necessarily mean, however, that there are no effects. Certain parts of the brain, such as the area postrema and the subfornical organ, have no blood-brain barrier and also have high concentrations of angiotensin receptors that are affected by circulating angiotensin. Dr. Smith agreed with Dr. Ganten's summary of the properties of the area postrema, which, he explained, together with the nearby nucleus tractus solitarius, is very much involved in the control of the circulation. It must be assumed that "by inhibition of plasma angiotensin you will have central effects on the brain," said Dr. Ganten.

383

Effects on Memory

Dr. Ganten said "Dr. De Weid showed that ACTH and ADH improve memory. Because angiotensin releases ACTH and ADH, we thought that angiotensin would improve memory—but this has not been shown to be the case."[1] He went on to say that angiotensin introduced into the brain of experimental animals reduced retention performance. This effect could be inhibited by ACE inhibitors given centrally, but there is a question mark over whether penetration of the brain occurs when ACE inhibitors are given orally.

Dr. Irvin referred to recent studies that have shown that captopril modifies habituation tasks in laboratory animals.

The Central Effect on Thirst

"In some clinical conditions with high angiotensin levels there is a marked effect on thirst," said Dr. Dollery. He went on to explain that autoradiographic studies have shown that the subfornical organ and the area postrema are the major binding sites for atrial natriuretic peptide. "If the subfornical area is accessible to ACE inhibitors, why do we not notice an effect on thirst from the existing drugs?" he asked.

This point was taken up by Dr. Ganten. Studies have been performed in Cambridge by Fitzsimons et al.[2], which show that low doses of ACE inhibitor act peripherally to cause enzyme inhibition and also lead to the accumulation of angiotensin I. This may then penetrate the brain, where ACE inhibitor is not present, and increase thirst and drinking behavior in experimental animals. This is preliminary experimental work that deserves further study. It points to possible additional effects of ACE inhibition: the balance of low circulating levels of angiotensin II and high penetration of angiotensin I into the brain—and their possible local conversion.

However, Dr. Ledingham pointed out that the question of thirst as one aspect of drinking behavior is a difficult one. In the rat it can be measured by quantifying fluid intake in defined circumstances. In man it is much more difficult because of satiation, cultural habits and oropharyngeal sensations, and much else (Rolls and Rolls).[3]

Angiotensin and the Sense of Well-Being

Dr. Sonnenblick brought up the question of angiotensin and the sense of "well-being." He pointed out that patients in warm shock can continue for a long time with little anxiety. However, if their angiotensin system becomes activated they become cold and clammy and suffer a great deal of anxiety. He asked whether high levels of angiotensin may cause a "negative sense of well-being." This idea of well-being was expanded upon by Dr. Poole-Wilson. He postulated that a sense of well-being may affect, for example, exercise capacity. In this case, he said, ". . . you are essentially giving a 'happy pill,'" rather than affecting the heart failure itself. Alternatively the drug might interfere with the brain's perception of the consequences of heart failure, which he described as "a very different and unusual treatment of heart failure." Dr. Smith compared this to the beneficial CNS effects of morphine in patients with pulmonary edema, which occur independent of the preload reducing effects.

ACE RECEPTORS, ANGIOTENSIN AND THE HEART

Dr. Poole-Wilson felt that, although the role of the renin-angiotensin system in myocardial ischemia had recently been reviewed, the subject was still not entirely clarified. It has been suggested that beta-blockers and calcium antagonists cause alterations in myocardial electrolytes, and Dr. Poole-Wilson attributed their action to "altering the distribution of the blood flow at the time of myocardial reperfusion." The distribution of blood flow at this time may contribute to development of arrhythmias, reperfusion damage, and "no reflow" phenomena, he said.

Although ACE inhibitors were originally thought to be scavengers of free radicals, the role of free radicals in ischemia is under debate. In addition, contradictory results are now being published, and there appear to be big differences between animal models and human disease. Dr. Ganten commented further on the effects of ACE inhibitors on the heart, saying that "circulating angiotensin is converted in the endothelium, and there are coronary vascular effects." He also suggested that there are direct and metabolic effects on cardiomyocytes. This view was supported by Dr. Smith, who felt that the presence of angiotensin receptors on the cardiomyocytes is a fact that may be turned to an advantage.

The Pathophysiology of Ischemic Heart Disease

Dr. Langman queried the extent to which knowledge of pathophysiology helps in finding a treatment for a disease. He cited peptic ulcer as an example in which pathophysiology has not been of use. The general response of the panel was that pathophysiology should not be ignored, and Dr. Smith described the pathophysiology of ischemic cell death as "a remarkably refractory area" in which many theories have come and gone.

Dr. Sonnenblick introduced the topic of "saving the myocardium." This approach initially failed because of a lack of good animal models and the temptation to try multiple drugs rather than study pathophysiology. He went on to suggest, however, that polypharmacy may have a role to play in salvaging cells that have been damaged by different mechanisms. A brief discussion centered on whether infarct size can be reduced by depleting the body of certain components such as complement or white cells. Dr. Poole-Wilson felt that although there may be many factors that contribute to the original damage, and to its repair, the key problem in myocardial infarction is blood flow. "This has to be maximized," he said, "particularly at the moment of reperfusion." This was supported by Dr. Sonnenblick: "Now we have come back to the idea that unless you preserve flow you cannot preserve tissue," he said.

ANGIOTENSIN AS A GROWTH FACTOR

After an infarction, the condition of the heart may not worsen further for a time, but the peripheral vasculature undergoes hypertrophy or hyperplasia. This prevents the normal dilation of the vessels and affects the delivery of blood. The patient finally develops terminal heart failure. This is where agents that can prevent cell growth may be of use.

Many of the panel members reported experiments in which ACE inhibitors reduced the size of tissues or organs. Kidneys and vasculature from hypertensive rats, which would normally show hypertrophy, were maintained at the same size as those from normotensive animals by treatment with ACE inhibitors, said Dr. Ganten. Dr. Keane agreed with this: in his rat model "ACE inhibitor therapy reduces the size of the kidney," although the mechanism is not clear.

In the discussion of other factors that affect cell growth, Dr. Smith mentioned that non-anticoagulant fragments of heparin can prevent the hyperplasia of vascular smooth muscle that is associated with atherosclerotic lesions. The importance of gastrin receptors on colonic polyps was also briefly raised.

The question of allowing differential cell growth was raised by Dr. Sonnenblick, who felt that "when considering coronary collaterals, it would be good to have hyperplasia going on in the heart, but not in the kidney." He suggested the need for a tissue-specific growth factor, and Dr. Keane pointed out that the environment of the cell may also be an important determinant in cell growth.

SUMMARY

All of the panel agreed that angiotensin has important effects on both the brain and the heart. The development of ACE inhibitors has provided agents that can, in effect, block the activation of angiotensin receptors, altering the functioning of both of these organs. The need for further research into this class of compounds was emphasized by Dr. Irvin, in his summing up, when he said "If we could focus on antagonists of the angiotensin II receptor or some other area of the renin-angiotensin system perhaps we could improve on the safety profile of the ACE inhibitors."

REFERENCES

1. Köller M, Krause HP, Hoffmeister F, Ganten D. Endogenous brain angiotensin II disrupts passive avoidance behavior in rats. *Neurosci Lett* 1979; **14**:71–75.
2. Fitzsimons JT. Angiotensin stimulation of the central nervous system. *Rev Physiol Biochem Pharmacol* 1980; **87**:117–167.
3. Rolls BJ, Rolls ET. Thirst. In *Problems in Behavioural Sciences* (Series). New York, Cambridge University Press, 1982.

INDEX

Page numbers in **boldface** indicate complete chapters.